SCIENTIFIC REVIEW OF THE PROPOSED RISK ASSESSMENT BULLETIN FROM THE OFFICE OF MANAGEMENT AND BUDGET

Committee to Review the OMB Risk Assessment Bulletin

Board on Environmental Studies and Toxicology

Division on Earth and Life Studies

NATIONAL RESEARCH COUNCIL
OF THE NATIONAL ACADEMIES

THE NATIONAL ACADEMIES PRESS
Washington, D.C.
www.nap.edu

THE NATIONAL ACADEMIES PRESS   500 Fifth Street, NW   Washington, DC 20001

NOTICE: The project that is the subject of this report was approved by the Governing Board of the National Research Council, whose members are drawn from the councils of the National Academy of Sciences, the National Academy of Engineering, and the Institute of Medicine. The members of the committee responsible for the report were chosen for their special competences and with regard for appropriate balance.

This project was supported by Contract No. 68-C-03-081 between the National Academy of Sciences and the U.S. Environmental Protection Agency, the U.S. Department of Agriculture, the U.S. Department of Defense, the U.S. Department of Energy, the U.S. Department of Health and Human Services, the U.S. Department of Labor, and the National Aeronautics and Space Administration. Any opinions, findings, conclusions, or recommendations expressed in this publication are those of the authors and do not necessarily reflect the views of the organizations or agencies that provided support for this project.

International Standard Book Number-13: 978-0-309-10477-7
International Standard Book Number-10: 0-309-10477-7

Additional copies of this report are available from

The National Academies Press
500 Fifth Street, NW
Box 285
Washington, DC 20055

800-624-6242
202-334-3313 (in the Washington metropolitan area)
http://www.nap.edu

Printed in the United States of America

THE NATIONAL ACADEMIES
Advisers to the Nation on Science, Engineering, and Medicine

The **National Academy of Sciences** is a private, nonprofit, self-perpetuating society of distinguished scholars engaged in scientific and engineering research, dedicated to the furtherance of science and technology and to their use for the general welfare. Upon the authority of the charter granted to it by the Congress in 1863, the Academy has a mandate that requires it to advise the federal government on scientific and technical matters. Dr. Ralph J. Cicerone is president of the National Academy of Sciences.

The **National Academy of Engineering** was established in 1964, under the charter of the National Academy of Sciences, as a parallel organization of outstanding engineers. It is autonomous in its administration and in the selection of its members, sharing with the National Academy of Sciences the responsibility for advising the federal government. The National Academy of Engineering also sponsors engineering programs aimed at meeting national needs, encourages education and research, and recognizes the superior achievements of engineers. Dr. Wm. A. Wulf is president of the National Academy of Engineering.

The **Institute of Medicine** was established in 1970 by the National Academy of Sciences to secure the services of eminent members of appropriate professions in the examination of policy matters pertaining to the health of the public. The Institute acts under the responsibility given to the National Academy of Sciences by its congressional charter to be an adviser to the federal government and, upon its own initiative, to identify issues of medical care, research, and education. Dr. Harvey V. Fineberg is president of the Institute of Medicine.

The **National Research Council** was organized by the National Academy of Sciences in 1916 to associate the broad community of science and technology with the Academy's purposes of furthering knowledge and advising the federal government. Functioning in accordance with general policies determined by the Academy, the Council has become the principal operating agency of both the National Academy of Sciences and the National Academy of Engineering in providing services to the government, the public, and the scientific and engineering communities. The Council is administered jointly by both Academies and the Institute of Medicine. Dr. Ralph J. Cicerone and Dr. Wm. A. Wulf are chair and vice chair, respectively, of the National Research Council.

www.national-academies.org

OTHER REPORTS OF THE
BOARD ON ENVIRONMENTAL STUDIES AND TOXICOLOGY

Copies of these reports may be ordered from the National Academies Press
(800) 624-6242 or (202) 334-3313
www.nap.edu

Preface

In an effort to improve the overall practice of risk assessment in the federal government, the Office of Management and Budget (OMB) released its Proposed Risk Assessment Bulletin on January 9, 2006, with a stated objective to "enhance the technical quality and objectivity of risk assessments prepared by federal agencies." The bulletin presents specific standards for risk assessments disseminated by federal agencies. OMB and the sponsoring agencies (Environmental Protection Agency, U.S. Department of Agriculture, Department of Defense, Department of Energy, Department of Health and Human Services, Department of Labor, and National Aeronautics and Space Administration) requested that the National Research Council (NRC) conduct a scientific review of the bulletin.

In this report, the NRC's Committee to Review the OMB Risk Assessment Bulletin provides its assessment of the OMB bulletin. The committee evaluates the standards presented in the bulletin, comments on the impact of the bulletin on the practice of risk assessment in the federal government, identifies critical elements missing from the bulletin, evaluates the consistency of the bulletin with previous reports of NRC and other organizations, and determines whether the draft bulletin has met OMB's stated objective.

This report has been reviewed in draft form by persons chosen for their diverse perspectives and technical expertise in accordance with procedures approved by NRC's Report Review Committee. The purpose of this independent review is to provide candid and critical comments that will assist the institution in making its published report as sound as possible and to ensure that the report meets institutional standards of objectivity, evidence, and responsiveness to the study charge. The review comments and draft manuscript remain confidential to protect the integrity of the deliberative process. We wish to thank the following for their review of this report: Lawrence Barnthouse, LWB Environmental Services, Inc.; Robert J. Budnitz, Lawrence Livermore National Laboratory; David Gaylor, Gaylor and Associates; J. Paul Gilman, Oak Ridge Center for Advanced Studies; Daniel Krewski, University of Ottawa; Jonathan Levy, Harvard School of Public Health; Roger O. McClellan, Albuquerque, New Mexico; Ali Mosleh,

University of Maryland; Gilbert Omenn, University of Michigan Medical School; and Paul Slovic, Decision Research.

Although the reviewers listed above have provided many constructive comments and suggestions, they were not asked to endorse the conclusions or recommendations, nor did they see the final draft of the report before its release. The review of this report was overseen by B. John Garrick, Laguna Beach, California, and John C. Bailar, III, University of Chicago. Appointed by NRC, they were responsible for making certain that an independent examination of this report was carried out in accordance with institutional procedures and that all review comments were carefully considered. Responsibility for the final content of this report rests entirely with the committee and the institution.

The committee gratefully acknowledges the following for making presentations to the committee: Linda Abbott, U.S. Department of Agriculture; Nancy Beck, Office of Management and Budget; Al Cobb, U.S. Department of Energy; Shannon Cunniff, U.S. Department of Defense; Homayoon Dezfuli, National Aeronautics and Space Administration; Steve Galson, Christopher Portier, and Christine Sofge, U.S. Department of Health and Human Services; John Graham, RAND Graduate School; Judith Graham, American Chemistry Council; George Gray, U.S. Environmental Protection Agency; Stephen Heinig, Association of American Medical Colleges; Alan Krupnick, Resources for the Future; Gilbert Omenn, University of Michigan Medical School; William Perry, U.S. Department of Labor; Lorenz Rhomberg, Gradient Corporation; Jennifer Sass, Natural Resources Defense Council; and Robert Shull, OMB Watch.

The committee is also grateful for the assistance of the NRC staff in preparing this report. Staff members who contributed to this effort are Jennifer Saunders, associate program officer; Norman Grossblatt, senior editor; John Brown, program associate; Radiah Rose, senior editorial assistant; and James J. Reisa, director of the Board on Environmental Studies and Toxicology. Primary among the staff was Ellen K. Mantus, project director, whose knowledge, careful working with the committee, and extreme diligence brought this report to completion.

I would especially like to thank the members of the committee for their efforts throughout the development of this report.

John F. Ahearne, *Chair*
Committee to Review the OMB Risk
Assessment Bulletin

Contents

BOXES

TABLES

SCIENTIFIC REVIEW OF THE PROPOSED RISK ASSESSMENT BULLETIN FROM THE OFFICE OF MANAGEMENT AND BUDGET

Summary

In January 2006, the Office of Management and Budget (OMB) released a draft bulletin that proposes technical guidance for risk assessments produced by the federal government. The bulletin defines *risk assessment* broadly, states several goals for risk assessment, and proposes general risk assessment and reporting standards and special standards for influential risk assessments. The stated intent of the bulletin is "to enhance the technical quality and objectivity of risk assessments prepared by federal agencies by establishing uniform, minimum standards," and it follows several other influential documents issued by OMB, including the Information Quality Guidelines, the Information Quality Bulletin on Peer Review, and Circular A-4, which pertains primarily to benefit-cost analysis and cost-effectiveness analysis. Recognizing the potential impact on federal agencies, OMB—with the Environmental Protection Agency (EPA), the U.S. Department of Agriculture (USDA), the Department of Defense (DOD), the Department of Energy (DOE), the Department of Health and Human Services (DHHS), the Department of Labor (DOL), and the National Aeronautics and Space Administration (NASA)—asked the National Research Council (NRC) to conduct an independent review of the bulletin. In response to that request, NRC convened the Committee to Review the OMB Risk Assessment Bulletin, which prepared this report.

COMMITTEE'S CHARGE AND APPROACH TO ITS CHARGE

The committee was asked to conduct a scientific and technical review of the proposed bulletin and to determine whether it meets OMB's objective to "enhance the technical quality and objectivity of risk assessments prepared by federal agencies." In performing its task, the committee was asked to comment, in general terms, on how the guidance will affect the practice of risk assessment in the federal government, to identify critical elements that might be missing from the guidance, and to assess whether there are scientific or technical circumstances that might limit applicability of the guidance. In addition, the committee was asked whether OMB appropriately incorporated recommendations from previous reports of the NRC and other organizations into the proposed risk assessment guidance.

To accomplish its task, the committee held a large public meeting during which it heard presentations from the study sponsors and other invited speakers from private industry, universities, trade associations, and environmental groups. The committee reviewed numerous documents cited in the bulletin and reviewed public comments submitted to OMB on the bulletin. The committee also requested information from the federal agencies on their risk assessment practices and their view of the potential impact of the bulletin on current practices. The committee reviewed both the bulletin and the accompanying supplementary information, and reference to "the bulletin" in this summary includes both the bulletin and the supplementary information.

Although this report touches on some statutory, policy, and budgetary issues, it is not a comprehensive review of all potential impacts of the bulletin. Rather, it is primarily a review of the science involved and the technical applications of the bulletin. Furthermore, much of the language used (and the examples provided) in the bulletin is related to human health risk assessment and not engineering, ecologic, or behavioral risk assessment. The committee recognizes that each of these fields has generated risk assessment methods that address specific interests. However, the committee was tasked with reviewing the bulletin and not providing a comprehensive treatment of risk assessment, so its comments focus mainly on human health risk assessment, as did the OMB bulletin.

COMMITTEE'S REVIEW

Consistency with NRC and Other Reports

The general thrust of the bulletin appears to be consistent with many of the themes and recommendations in reports by previous NRC committees and other expert organizations. The bulletin emphasizes the need to define objectives clearly and to ensure that assessments yield results that are both faithful to underlying scientific knowledge and useful for decision-making. The committee, however, is concerned that the bulletin is inconsistent with previous recommendations in a number of ways, including its presentation of a new definition of risk assessment, its omission of discussion of the important role of default assumptions and clear criteria to modify or depart from defaults, its proposal of risk *assessment* standards related to activities traditionally regarded as risk *management* activities, and its requirement for formal analyses of uncertainty and presentation of "central" or "expected" risk estimates. In several respects, the bulletin attempts to move standards for risk assessment into territory that is beyond what previous reports have recommended and beyond the current state of the science. Such departures from expert studies are of serious concern, because any attempt to advance the practice of risk assessment that does not reflect the state of the science is likely to produce the opposite effect.

Definition of Risk Assessment and the Bulletin's Goals

The bulletin defines risk assessment as "a scientific and/or technical document that assembles and synthesizes scientific information to determine whether a potential hazard exists and/or the extent of possible risk to human health, safety or the environment." That definition conflicts with long-established concepts and practices that have defined risk assessment as a *process* that involves hazard identification, hazard characterization or dose-response assessment, exposure assessment, and risk characterization. The definition in the bulletin is too broad and encompasses not only traditional risk assessments but the *components* of risk assessment. Such a definition, which captures a variety of analyses under the same name, could cause great confusion. Moreover, several standards proposed in the bulletin are not applicable to individual components of risk assessment or other types of documents that might be classified as risk assessment under the proposed definition.

The bulletin defines five goals of risk assessment that are related to problem formulation, completeness, character of risk assessment, resources expended, and peer review and public participation. Taken as a whole, the five goals indicate that a risk assessment should be tailored to the specific need for which it is undertaken; balanced in scope, time, and cost with the importance of the issue; and peer-reviewed and released for public comment. The goals mostly emphasize efficiency, rather than quality, in the conduct of risk assessment. Thus, the goals do not all support the primary purpose of the bulletin—"to enhance the technical quality and objectivity of risk assessments."

Proposed Standards for Risk Assessment

The bulletin proposes seven standards for general risk assessment—one of which refers to risk assessments for regulatory analysis—and nine special standards for influential risk assessments. The committee found this structure problematic, because one may not know at the outset whether an analysis will constitute an "influential" risk assessment. Furthermore, arbitrarily separating risk assessment into two broad categories (general and influential) ignores the continuum of risk assessment efforts. The committee reviewed each standard and provides comments on them in this report. In general, the committee found many of the standards to be unclear or flawed. Standards on presentation of specific information, uncertainty, and adversity of health effects exemplify the problems.

Several standards require the presentation of "a range of plausible risk estimates" that includes "central or expected estimates." The discussion regarding this requirement is incomplete and confusing. Those numerical quantities are meaningful only in the context of some distribution that arises when variability and uncertainty are taken into consideration. A central estimate and a risk range might be misleading in situations when sensitive populations are of primary concern. Thus, the choice of summary statistics cannot be a blanket prescription but must reflect the specific context.

Standards for influential risk assessments require a formal characterization of uncertainty. However, the description of uncertainty and variability in the bulletin is oversimplified and does not recognize the complexities of different types of risk assessments or the need to tailor uncertainty analysis to a given agency's particular needs. Furthermore, there is no scientific consensus to support the bulletin's universal prescriptions for how uncertainty should be evaluated. In the absence of clear guidance regarding the conduct of uncertainty analysis, there is a serious danger that agencies will produce ranges of meaningless and confusing risk estimates, which could result in risk assessments of reduced rather than enhanced quality and objectivity.

Finally, for influential risk assessments, the bulletin states that "where human health effects are a concern, determinations of which effects are adverse shall be specifically identified and justified." The bulletin's definition of *adverse effect* implies a *clinically* apparent effect, which ignores a fundamental public-health goal to control exposures well before the occurrence of any possible functional impairment of an organism. Dividing effects into "adverse" and "nonadverse" ignores the scientific reality that adverse effects may be manifest along a continuum. The committee concludes that the bulletin's treatment of adverse effects is too simplistic and restrictive and ignores important factors in determining appropriate effects to evaluate, the scientific information available, and an understanding of the underlying biochemical mechanisms for an effect of interest.

Omissions from the Bulletin

Omission of several relevant topics limits the utility of the bulletin as balanced and comprehensive risk assessment guidance. Specifically, OMB has proposed a bulletin addressing risk assessment in the federal government; however, the bulletin focuses mainly on biologic systems, with an emphasis on human health risk assessment. The vast majority of examples it presents (and the authorities cited) apply to toxicologic and other human health end points. By reducing risks to human health risks, as important as they may be, OMB commits a serious error in neglecting risk assessment of technology and engineered structures. Those are of vital importance to such agencies as DOE, DOD, and NASA and therefore to the general public and the economic vitality of the United States. The bulletin's incomplete and unbalanced approach to engineering risk assessment (as well as ecologic and other types of risk assessment) contradicts its stated objective of improving the quality of risk assessment throughout the federal government. Unless all risk assessment disciplines are considered, any government-wide guidance on risk assessment would be unacceptable.

Furthermore, the bulletin gives little attention to sensitive populations, the often pivotal role of risk assessment policy in choices regarding default options, the integral role of risk communication, and standards for risk assessments submitted by outside parties for use in the rule-making process. With reference to risk communication, the committee agrees with previous NRC reports that view risk communication as a dialogue with users of risk assessment throughout the process that helps to ensure its relevance and credibility and does not see it as a one-way, end-of-the process activity. The bulletin also fails to explain the basis for exempting risk assessments associated with licensing and approval processes.

Perhaps the most glaring omission is the absence of criteria and information for gauging the benefits to be achieved by implementing the bulletin (that is, a benefit-cost analysis). Although OMB has implied that the agencies currently do not meet the standards that it seeks to establish, it has not established a baseline of each agency's risk assessment proficiency, including the extent to which generally satisfactory and high-quality risk assessments are produced or how some agencies fall short of the specified standards. Specifically, OMB has not established which agencies do not appear to know what good practices are and which agencies do not have the ability, resources, or incentives to meet the standards. Similarly, OMB has not identified the costs that could be encountered in implementing the bulletin. Thus, OMB has not determined the impact of the bulletin on federal agencies.

Impact on Risk Assessment Practices in the Federal Government

Although OMB did not construct a baseline reflecting current agency risk assessment practices, the committee concludes on the basis of agency comments and its own knowledge of risk assessment practices that some aspects of the bulletin could be beneficial but that the costs—in terms of staff resources, timeliness of completing risk assessments, and other factors—are likely to be substantial. Overall, the committee concludes that the potential for negative impacts on the practice of risk assessment in the federal government, although varied and uncertain to some extent, would be very high if the currently proposed bulletin were implemented.

COMMITTEE'S CONCLUSIONS AND RECOMMENDATIONS

On the basis of its review, the committee concludes that the OMB bulletin is fundamentally flawed and recommends that it be withdrawn. Although the committee fully supports the goal of increasing the quality and objectivity of risk assessment in the federal government, it agrees unanimously that the OMB bulletin would not facilitate reaching this goal. The committee also agrees that OMB should encourage the federal agencies to describe, develop, and coordinate their own technical risk assessment guidance. Therefore, the committee recommends that, after additional study of current agency practices and needs, a different type of risk assessment bulletin be issued by OMB. That bulletin should outline goals and general principles of risk assessment designed to enhance the quality, efficiency, and consistency of risk assessment in the federal government. It should direct the agencies to develop technical guidance that would implement the general principles, be consistent with the individual agencies' legislative mandates and missions, and draw on the expertise that exists in federal agencies and other organizations. The technical guidance developed or identified by the agencies should be peer-reviewed and contain procedures for ensuring compliance with the guidance within the agencies. Although OMB should determine whether the technical guidance developed by the agencies fully addresses the general principles, the committee recommends that development and peer review of agency technical guidance be left to the agencies. The committee strongly recommends that federal agencies addressing similar hazards or risks work together to develop common technical guidance for risk assessment; that would help to achieve the appropriate consistency among agencies in risk assessment practices.

The committee arrived at its position after deliberate consideration of many factors. The committee began with the working assumption that its role would be to recommend modifications, if necessary. After digging deeply into the bulletin and after extensive discussion, the committee reluctantly came to its conclusion that the bulletin could not be rescued.

Risk assessment is not a monolithic process or a single method. Different technical issues arise in assessing the probability of exposure to a given dose of a chemical, of a malfunction of a nuclear power plant or air-traffic control system, or of the collapse of an ecosystem or a dam. Thus, one size does not fit all, nor can one set of technical guidance make sense for the heterogeneous risk assessments undertaken by federal agencies. Although the bulletin generally acknowledges that diversity and attempts to meet it with frequent references to "where appropriate" or "where feasible," the bulletin does not reflect an adequate understanding of the many risk assessment disciplines, particularly those devoted to analyzing the risks of engineered structures and natural systems. Its narrow focus on human health risk assessment makes it inappropriate as across-the-board guidance for all risk assessments conducted throughout the federal government. Furthermore, as stated above, the committee strongly recommends that technical guidance be produced by the individual agencies and that agencies dealing with the same or similar hazards work together to produce common guidance to ensure an appropriately consistent approach.

The committee agrees that there is room for improvement in risk assessment practices in the federal government and that additional guidance would help "to enhance the technical quality and objectivity of risk assessments prepared by federal agencies." However, the committee concludes that OMB should limit its efforts to stating goals and general principles of risk assessment. The details should be left to the agencies or expert committees appointed by the agencies, wherein lies the depth of expertise to address the issues relevant to their specific types of risk assessments.

1

Introduction

In 1983, the National Research Council (NRC) issued the seminal report *Risk Assessment in the Federal Government: Managing the Process*, which provided a framework for the conduct of risk assessment. It defined risk assessment as "the qualitative or quantitative characterization of the potential health effects of particular substances on individuals or populations" (NRC 1983, p. 38) and indicated four components of risk assessment: hazard identification, dose-response assessment, exposure assessment, and risk characterization. Over the last 2 decades, the practice of risk assessment has evolved in the federal government. Some agencies, such as the Environmental Protection Agency (EPA) and the National Aeronautics and Space Administration (NASA), have formalized guidelines for various types of risk assessment (EPA 1996, 1998, 2005; NASA 2002); others have no formal process. Thus, the practice of risk assessment in the federal government varies considerably. To improve the overall practice of risk assessment, the Office of Management and Budget (OMB) issued the Proposed Risk Assessment Bulletin, which sets forth specific standards for risk assessments used and disseminated by federal agencies, and asked NRC to review it. In response to OMB's request, NRC convened the Committee to Review the OMB Risk Assessment Bulletin, which prepared this report.

THE OFFICE OF MANAGEMENT AND BUDGET

OMB is responsible for ensuring that information, analyses, and regulatory actions issued by federal agencies meet high quality standards.

Executive Order 12866 (58 Fed. Reg. 51735 [1993]) directs OMB to provide guidance to federal agencies on regulatory development and emphasizes the need for each agency to "base its decisions on the best reasonably obtainable scientific, technical, economic, and other information." The Paperwork Reduction Act (44 U.S.C. § 3504 [1995]) requires OMB to "develop and oversee the implementation of policies, principles, standards, and guidelines to...apply to Federal agency dissemination of public information." The Information Quality Act (Public Law 106-554 § 515(a) [2000]), a supplement to the Paperwork Reduction Act, directs OMB to develop guidelines that "provide policy and procedural guidance to Federal agencies for ensuring and maximizing the quality, objectivity, utility and integrity of information" released by federal agencies.

In 2002, in response to the many directives, OMB finalized *Guidelines for Ensuring and Maximizing the Quality, Objectivity, Utility, and Integrity of Information Disseminated by Federal Agencies*, which defines *quality*, *objectivity*, *utility*, and *integrity* and requires federal agencies to issue their own information-quality guidelines (67 Fed. Reg. 8452 [2002]). In 2003, OMB issued *Circular A-4, Regulatory Analysis*, which defines the key elements of a regulatory analysis and provides specific guidance on conducting cost-benefit and cost-effectiveness analyses (OMB 2003). In 2005, OMB published *Final Information Quality Bulletin for Peer Review*, which requires peer review of important scientific information by qualified experts before release by federal agencies (70 Fed. Reg. 2664 [2005]). In its continuing effort to improve the quality of information and analyses disseminated by federal agencies, OMB issued the draft bulletin (OMB 2006) providing guidance for the conduct of risk assessment.

THE BULLETIN AND SUPPLEMENTARY INFORMATION

OMB's draft bulletin consists of a preamble (22 pages) containing primarily "supplementary information" followed by the actual bulletin (3½ pages) (see Appendix B). The bulletin provides key definitions, goals for risk assessment, general risk assessment and reporting standards, and special standards for influential risk assessment. The bulletin also presents information on applicability, updates, certification, deferrals and waivers, responsibilities of executive offices, effective date, and judicial review. The supplementary information includes background on risk assessment, OMB's legal authority to issue the bulletin, and details on the requirements listed in the bulletin.

It is important to understand the relationship between the preamble and the bulletin. When a federal agency publishes a rule, it also provides a statement of the reason and basis for the rule. Those who are subject to the regulation are bound by the words in the regulation itself. If the regulation is challenged and the dispute reaches the courts, the courts look first at the text of the regulation; if the text is unclear, the courts will generally refer to the preamble to determine what the promulgating agency meant in the regulation. As indicated in the draft OMB bulletin, judicial review and hence judicial interpretation are explicitly precluded, and challenges to agency action under the bulletin would go to OMB, which would invariably be guided by the statements in the preamble as to scope and content. The committee therefore reviewed both the bulletin and the supplementary information and discusses both in its report. Generic references to the bulletin here typically refer to both the bulletin and the supplementary information.

COMMITTEE'S TASK AND APPROACH

The committee members were selected for their expertise in risk assessment, clinical medicine, toxicology, industrial hygiene, statistics, engineering, epidemiology, ecology, decision and uncertainty analysis, and cost-benefit analysis. Specifically, the committee was asked to conduct a scientific review of OMB's draft risk assessment bulletin and to complete the following tasks: (1) determine whether the application of the draft bulletin will meet OMB's stated objective to "enhance the technical quality and objectivity of risk assessments prepared by federal agencies"; (2) comment, in general terms, on how the bulletin will affect the practice of risk assessment in the federal government; (3) identify critical elements that might be missing from the bulletin; (4) determine whether OMB appropriately incorporated recommendations from previous reports of NRC and other organizations into the draft bulletin; and (5) assess whether there are scientific or technical circumstances that might limit applicability of the bulletin (see Appendix C for a verbatim statement of task). The study sponsors were EPA, NASA, the U.S. Department of Agriculture, the Department of Defense, the Department of Energy, the Department of Health and Human Services, and the Department of Labor.

To accomplish its task, the committee held three meetings from May to August 2006. The first included a public meeting during which the committee heard presentations from the sponsors; invited speakers from private industry, universities, trade associations, and environmental groups also provided a diverse perspective on risk assessment and the draft bulletin (see Appendix D for an agenda of the public meeting). At that meeting, OMB asked the committee to comment in its report on specific aspects of the proposed bulletin, including the definition of risk assessment, the goals, the proposed standards, possible omissions or errors, and examples to serve as models for risk assessment. The committee reviewed numerous documents cited in the supplementary information and reviewed public comment submitted to OMB on the bulletin. The committee also requested information from the federal agencies on their risk assessment practices and their view of the impact of the bulletin on current practices. Appendix E presents the questions submitted to the agencies and their responses.

Much of the language used and the examples provided in the bulletin and the supplementary information are related to human health risk assessment and not engineering, ecologic, or behavioral risk assessments. Specifically, little is said about the failure of engineered systems, the degradation of ecosystems, and the risk of malicious human behavior. The committee recognizes that each class of risks has generated risk assessment methods to address its unique set of issues (see Box 1-1). However, the committee was tasked with reviewing the bulletin and not providing a comprehensive treatment of risk assessment; therefore, the committee comments focus primarily on human health risk assessment.

ORGANIZATION OF THE REPORT

The committee's report is organized into seven chapters. Chapter 2 evaluates the consistency of the bulletin with previous NRC and other expert reports. Chapter 3 addresses issues surrounding the definition of risk assessment provided in the bulletin and the goals listed in it. The risk assessment standards articulated in the bulletin are reviewed in Chapter 4. Chapter 5 highlights key omissions from the bulletin. Chapter 6 discusses the impact of the bulletin on risk assessment practices in the federal government. The committee's conclusions and recommendations are summarized in Chapter 7.

BOX 1-1 Types of Risk Assessment

Historically, risk assessment has been dominated by two parallel methodologic developments: (1) *public-health risk assessment*, with a major focus on the health effects of chronic exposures to chemicals, contaminants, and pollutants in the water we drink, the air we breathe, and the food we eat, and (2) *engineered-systems risk assessment*, with a primary focus on immediate and delayed effects due to the failure of systems, such as aerospace vehicles, chemical process plants, and nuclear power plants. More recently, there has been heightened interest in other risks, including ecologic risks, such as the degradation of ecologic systems due to nonnative invasive species, global warming, and genetically modified organisms; risks related to severe natural phenomena, such as hurricanes, earthquakes, fires, and floods; and risks associated with malicious human acts, such as terrorism. Each domain raises its own intellectual challenges, sometimes involving extension of public-health and engineered-systems methods, at other times requiring dedicated methods. Differences and similarities of risk assessment for public health and engineered systems provide insight into the issues faced in the development of scientifically sound methods.

Risk assessment, in both cases, involves a search for "causal links" or "causal chains" verified by "objective" analytic and experimental techniques, such as quantifying the behavior of various elements (for example, pumps, valves, operators, maintenance supervisors, and physicians) in terms of failure-rate data or exposure and dose-response data. Risk assessments for engineered systems focus on the questions, What can go wrong? How likely is it to happen? (Kaplan and Garrick 1981). The analysis is typically organized around fault and event trees, delineating the impacts of initiating events and failure rates. Public-health risk assessment focuses on the question, What are the consequences in terms of exposure assessment and dose-response assessment, using quantitative estimates of behaviors like ingestion and metabolism. Each field has generated its own analytic methods and experimental protocols, with the common goal of quantifying overall system performance in terms of valued consequences.

REFERENCES

EPA (U.S. Environmental Protection Agency). 1996. Guidelines for Reproductive Toxicity Risk Assessment. EPA/630/R-96/009. Risk Assessment Forum, U.S. Environmental Protection Agency, Washington, DC [online]. Available: http://www.epa.gov/ncea/raf/pdfs/repro51.pdf [accessed July 27, 2006].

EPA (U.S. Environmental Protection Agency). 1998. Guidelines for Ecological Risk Assessment. EPA/630/R-95/002F. Risk Assessment Forum, U.S. Environmental Protection Agency, Washington, DC [online]. Available: http://cfpub.epa.gov/ncea/cfm/recordisplay.cfm?deid=12460 [accessed July 27, 2006].

EPA (U.S. Environmental Protection Agency). 2005. Guidelines for Carcinogen Risk Assessment. EPA/630/P-03/001B. Risk Assessment Forum, U.S. Environmental Protection Agency, Washington, DC [online]. Available: http://www.epa.gov/iris/cancer032505.pdf [accessed July 27, 2006].

Kaplan, S., and B.J. Garrick. 1981. On the quantitative definition of risk. Risk Anal. 1(1):11-27.

NASA (National Aeronautics and Space Administration). 2002. Probabilistic Risk Assessment Procedures Guide for NASA Managers and Practitioners, Version 1.1. Prepared for Office of Safety and Mission Assurance NASA Headquarters, Washington, DC [online]. Available: http://www.hq.nasa.gov/office/codeq/doctree/praguide.pdf [accessed Oct. 11, 2006].

NRC (National Research Council). 1983. Risk Assessment in the Federal Government: Managing the Process. Washington, DC: National Academy Press.

OMB (U.S. Office of Management and Budget). 2003. Regulatory Analysis. Circular A-4 to the Heads of Executive Agencies and Establishments, September 17, 2003 [online]. Available: http://www.whitehouse.gov/omb/circulars/a004/a-4.pdf [accessed Oct. 12, 2006].

OMB (U.S. Office of Management and Budget). 2006. Proposed Risk Assessment Bulletin. Released January 9, 2006. Washington, DC: Office of Management and Budget, Executive Office of the President [online]. Available: http://www.whitehouse.gov/omb/inforeg/proposed_risk_ assessment_bulletin_010906.pdf [accessed Oct. 11, 2006].

2

Consistency with National Research Council and Other Reports

The committee was asked to evaluate the consistency of the proposed risk assessment bulletin issued by the Office of Management and Budget (OMB) with the recommendations of previous committees of the National Research Council (NRC) and those of other expert organizations. Some recommendations arose in general studies of risk assessment and its relationship to other activities, whereas others came from studies directed at specific substances or classes of substances. Some studies are cited by OMB as the source of guidance on general principles, and others are cited to document specific statements. The committee has focused on the studies concerning broader principles, although other studies were also useful. The reports reviewed by the committee are primarily those cited by the bulletin in footnotes 4 and 5. In this report, the committee refers to the entire collection as "the cited studies."

In this chapter, the committee identifies a set of common themes and recommendations that emerge from the cited studies and bear most directly on the bulletin. The content of the bulletin, most especially that pertaining to standards for risk assessment, is discussed in relation to the cited studies, and areas lacking consistency are identified.

Consistency with the cited studies is important for ensuring the quality and continuing advance of risk assessment. Those studies have drawn on the collective skills and experience of the leading practitioners of risk assessment, and the committee believes that any departures should be fully explained and be based on a consensus of scientific experts.

THEMES AND RECOMMENDATIONS
FROM CITED STUDIES

The major recommendations that have emerged from nearly 25 years of study of risk assessment have much in common. The seminal NRC study on risk assessment, cited several times by OMB, yielded the 1983 report *Risk Assessment in the Federal Government: Managing the Process* (the *Red Book*).

The recommendations set forth in the 1983 *Red Book* appear to have been widely accepted in the regulatory and public health communities; indeed, all the cited studies on risk assessment that have followed the 1983 report appear to have adopted the principles first presented in it. Those later reports have done much to clarify and solidify thinking about risk assessment and related activities, but all seem to adopt or accept the following:

• The process of risk assessment is carried out within a framework within which diverse sets of scientific information are organized and evaluated for specific uses. The first step, generally called hazard identification, involves assembling and evaluating information on the harmful properties of the substance or activity under review. The second step, called dose-response assessment, describes the relationship between exposure to the substance or activity and the nature and extent of resulting harm. The third step, usually termed human exposure assessment, describes the nature and extent of human exposure to the substance or activity. The fourth step, called risk characterization, integrates the information assembled in the first three steps to assess the likelihood that the hazardous properties of the substance or activity will be expressed in humans. Risk characterization generally has both qualitative and quantitative components, and it also includes a description of the uncertainties in the assessment (NRC 1983). The results of risk characterization have many uses that lie outside the bounds of risk assessment.

• The same conceptual framework for risk assessment and the four-step analytic process were adopted and promoted in NRC's *Science and Judgment in Risk Assessment* (1994), in *Understanding Risk: Informing Decisions in a Democratic Society* (1996), and in all the other reports cited in footnote 5 in the OMB bulletin.

• The *Red Book* clarified the distinction between risk assessment and risk management, and the same distinction is maintained in the other cited studies. The first recommendation of the *Red Book* is the following:

We recommend that regulatory agencies take steps to establish and maintain a clear conceptual distinction between assessment of risks and consideration of risk management alternatives; that is, the scientific findings and policy judgments embodied in risk assessments should be explicitly distinguished from the political, economic, and technical considerations that influence the design and choice of regulatory strategies (NRC 1983, p. 7).

• Ideally, relevant scientific data and other information are available for any particular risk assessment. Scientific principles and risk assessment practices establish unequivocally that such data are always preferred to the use of the defaults and inference options discussed here and elsewhere in this report. However, virtually all risk assessments are undertaken in the absence of complete knowledge and information. Risk characterization is thus necessarily uncertain. Moreover, in most cases the results of risk assessments are not scientifically testable in the traditional sense. In the absence of relevant knowledge and information, risk assessments often can be completed only if models and assumptions of uncertain scientific standing are adopted. For that reason, the *Red Book* committee and others pointed to the need for agencies engaged in risk assessments to specify and make explicit the models and assumptions they would use in advance of the conduct of specific risk assessments.

• The *Red Book* used the term *inference options* to describe alternative models and assumptions that are needed to complete risk assessments in the absence of complete scientific information or knowledge. *Inference guideline* was defined as "an explicit statement of a predetermined choice among alternative...options" (NRC 1983, p.4). The predetermined choices of models and assumptions have come to be called defaults. Such standardized defaults are critical if one is to avoid case-by-case manipulations of individual risk assessments to achieve predetermined risk management outcomes. The NRC report *Science and Judgment in Risk Assessment* (1994) urged the Environmental Protection Agency (EPA)[1] to pursue the issue of justifying and specifying the defaults more aggressively in its guidelines for risk assessment. The committee noted that "EPA does not fully explain in its guidelines the basis for each default option" (NRC 1994, p. 7). Selection of defaults has both

---

[1] To be consistent with its congressional mandate, the report focused entirely on the risk assessment practices of EPA, particularly EPA's air program, and not those of other agencies.

scientific and policy components, although risk assessment policies are different in kind and distinguishable from those involved in risk management decisions, as indicated in the first recommendation of the *Red Book*, which clarified the distinction between risk assessment and risk management.

• Although recognizing the need for defaults to achieve consistency and to avoid case-by-case manipulations of risk assessments, the *Red Book* committee and other committees have urged that the agencies incorporate procedures that allow departures from the defaults in specific cases in which a scientific basis for alternative assumptions or models can be found. Flexibility to incorporate new scientific knowledge, when it becomes available, is urged in most expert studies of risk assessment. The *Science and Judgment* committee examined the question of whether EPA had "clear and consistent principles for...departing from default options" and found the agency wanting on this point (NRC 1994, p. 79).

• The cited studies all emphasize the important issue of uncertainty in risk assessment. Some focus on issues related to its evaluation and expression for purposes of informing risk managers and the public. Others focus on the need to describe uncertainties so that the research community is informed about what is needed to improve risk assessments. Most of the studies discuss both qualitative (descriptive) and quantitative aspects of uncertainty in risk assessment, but none seems to offer highly explicit guidance to agencies. Several caution that the level of uncertainty analyses and description should be influenced by the needs of decision-makers in specific cases. The difficult problem of uncertainty analysis is well-described in *Understanding Risk* (1996):

> Much attention has been given to quantitative, analytic procedures for describing uncertainty in risk characterizations. Participants in decisions need to consider both the magnitude of uncertainty and its sources and character: whether it is due to inherent randomness or to lack of knowledge; and whether it is recognized and quantifiable, recognized and indeterminate; or perhaps unrecognized. Unfortunately, the unrecognized sources of uncertainty—surprise and fundamental ignorance about the basic processes that drive risk—are often important sources of uncertainty, and formal analysis may not help if they are too large. Thus, uncertainty analysis should be conducted with care and in conjunction with deliberation and in full awareness of its limitations, especially in the face of unrecognized sources of uncertainty. It is best to focus on uncertainties that mat-

ter most to ongoing processes of deliberation and decision. The users of uncertainty analysis should remember that both the analysis and people's interpretations of it can be strongly affected by the social, cultural, and institutional context of the decision (NRC 1996, p. 5).

These cautionary notes regarding the descriptions of uncertainties in risk assessments are echoed in other cited studies, but none offers explicit guidance on the analytic methods best suited to evaluate and express uncertainties in specific contexts.

• Although the cited studies generally do not offer explicit guidance on the conduct of uncertainty analysis, much work has been done in probabilistic risk assessment (PRA) to develop standards that explicitly incorporate such analysis. Perhaps the leading efforts are the PRA standards for nuclear power plants that have been developed by various professional societies. For example, the American National Standards Institute, in conjunction with the American Nuclear Society and the American Society of Mechanical Engineers, has developed risk assessment standards for internal and external initiating events at nuclear power plants (ASME 2002; ANS 2003). OMB does not cite those and other such studies. Whether and to what extent the technical details of those standards apply to other types of risk assessments—those for chemical toxicity, for example—is not clear, but it is possible that some of the methods used in them are applicable.

• A consistent theme in the cited studies concerns the value of well-described purposes for risk assessments, balanced and clear presentations of all relevant data, and the bases of inferences drawn from the data. Most reports offer general guidance on these matters but do not offer highly explicit instructions. An important theme regarding the risk assessment process is given explicit treatment in *Understanding Risk*:

The analytic-deliberative process leading to a risk characterization should include early and explicit attention to *problem formulation*; representation of the spectrum of interested and affected parties at this early stage is imperative. The analytic-deliberative process should be *mutual and recursive*. Analysis and deliberation are complementary and must be integrated throughout the process leading to risk characterization: deliberation frames analysis, analysis informs deliberation, and the process benefits from feedback between the two (NRC 1996, p. 6).

• Some NRC reports on specific substances (perchlorate, methylmercury, and arsenic) were reviewed. Those reports appear to adhere to the general principles set forth above although they vary in their presentations of risk results and uncertainties. All discuss uncertainties, but two provide only "point" estimates of risk, and the third (on arsenic) provides a relatively limited range of risk estimates based on application of a single dose-response model. Thus, uncertainties are not expressed quantitatively but are to various degrees discussed qualitatively.

Other themes and recommendations can be found in the many cited studies, but those described in the foregoing are judged to be critical to an understanding and evaluation of the standards proposed in the OMB bulletin.

INFLUENCE OF THE CITED STUDIES

It is difficult to judge the influence of all the many studies on the practices of federal agencies other than EPA. It appears that only EPA has explicitly adopted the general recommendations that have emerged from the reports, and the agency has put much effort into developing guidelines for risk assessment that, at least in principle, are consistent with the themes and recommendations that are described here. (Whether EPA consistently adheres to the guidelines is a different matter and is beyond the scope of the committee's review.) The need for greater consistency among federal agencies in risk assessment approaches might be satisfied by the development of government-wide guidelines as they have been developed in EPA. Whether the bulletin accomplishes that objective is discussed below.

Although the issue is not explicitly discussed in any of the cited studies, there is no obvious reason why the principles and themes elucidated in them should apply only to risk assessments conducted by federal agencies. Most are directed more broadly at the risk assessment community, and that includes operators of facilities who are seeking licenses and manufacturers submitting risk-related data and assessments to agencies to gain product approvals, licenses, or registrations.

THE OFFICE OF MANAGEMENT AND BUDGET BULLETIN: CONSISTENCY WITH MAJOR THEMES AND RECOMMENDATIONS

The bulletin emphases the need for a clear declaration of objectives, for discussion between risk assessors and the users of risk information, and for ensuring that assessments yield results that are faithful to underlying scientific knowledge and are useful for decision-making. In its call for balanced presentations of all relevant data and the inferences drawn from them, the bulletin is consistent with the many expert recommendations that have shaped current risk assessment practice. And as a general matter, the bulletin's requirements for a thorough characterization of risk and its associated uncertainties and for a level of effort "commensurate with the importance of the risk assessment" (OMB 2006, p. 23) reflect what most expert studies have recommended. In those many general respects, the bulletin is consistent with the themes and recommendations outlined above.

However, the proposed bulletin is inconsistent with the recommendations that have been discussed on a number of important issues. Concerning its call for formal uncertainty analyses, it attempts to move the standards for risk assessment beyond what the many cited studies have provided. Furthermore, the bulletin does not seem to be a guideline, but rather a highly prescriptive mandate. Therefore, there is a danger that in its present form the bulletin may reduce rather than enhance the quality and objectivity of agency risk assessments. The committee's principal concerns are the following:

- The bulletin does not recognize the importance of what several NRC committees have called policy judgments in risk assessment. As described above, there is a continuing need for defaults to complete risk assessments; without a consistent and justified set of defaults (based on both scientific and policy considerations), there is a danger that risk assessments will be manipulated case by case through the arbitrary selection of models and assumptions that guarantee a predetermined outcome. NRC committees have strongly recommended that agencies throughout the government develop guidelines that justify and specify general defaults. The bulletin's inattention to this issue might open the door to less well-standardized risk assessment practices.
- As described above, most expert studies have recognized that agencies should evaluate new scientific information and knowledge that

suggest that particular defaults may no longer be justified and need to be changed. That may happen in the general case (as, for example, in EPA's recent proposal to change the model for "scaling" animal doses to equivalent human doses) or in the case of specific substances or activities (as, for example, in EPA's adoption of a nonlinear model for low-dose extrapolation of carcinogenicity data for chloroform [EPA 2001]). The move away from defaults, either general or substance-specific, has been plagued with difficulties in that there are always questions regarding the scientific rigor with which an alternative model or assumption has been established. One interpretation of the bulletin is that it implicitly recognizes that proposals to depart from defaults often result in protracted and contentious scientific debates and that requiring agencies always to report risk results on the basis of alternative models and assumptions might both circumvent the debate and also provide more balanced views of risk. If that is what OMB is calling for, it might be presented better in the context of the use of defaults, as is described here, and a requirement to consider alternatives to the defaults in specific cases when new data become available. Such a presentation by OMB would be consistent with the body of expert recommendations described.

• Alternative models and assumptions based on new scientific data will, like the defaults they may replace, always have some degree of scientific uncertainty. In considering such alternatives, agency risk assessors should not be placed in the position of having to decide "how much evidence is sufficient" to adopt the alternative. Rather, they should attempt to describe the scientific bases of a proposed alternative and describe how certain it is. Deciding whether it is "sufficiently certain" to replace a default or is to be given more weight, equal weight, or less weight than the default may be seen as requiring a combination of scientific and policy considerations that go beyond risk assessment. With this approach, risk assessors do not discard alternative models and assumptions unless they clearly lack substantial scientific merit; rather, they attempt to judge and describe the relative scientific merits. If the bulletin were recast to suggest such consideration of alternatives, it would be more consistent with past expert recommendations.

• The bulletin proposes "standards" for the evaluation and description of uncertainties in risk characterization that lack clarity and may foster a reduction in the quality and consistency of risk assessments. Its discussion of "risk ranges" and "central or expected risks" is superficial (see Chapter 4) and mandates analyses that could, if not done with care, yield misleading estimates. The scientific literature on uncertainty analysis has not been translated into explicit and peer-reviewed guidelines except for the standards that have been developed for PRA (see Chapter 4). In an apparent leap beyond what is offered in the previous reports, OMB is proposing approaches that might be reduced to inappropriate statistical analyses (see the next paragraph). Explicit guidelines are needed to support scientifically sound and useful characterization of uncertainties. Some "demonstration projects" on this topic might be called for, and much might be learned from the PRA standards discussed above and more fully in Chapter 4. In many fields of risk assessment, there is much to be learned about this topic; although the many cited studies clearly point to the need for well-conceived uncertainty analyses, none offers agencies much more than general guidance. Indeed, the NRC reports on perchlorate, arsenic, and methyl mercury do not contain the type of uncertainty analyses with an emphasis on central estimates and risk ranges that the bulletin appears to mandate. The committee notes that the data available to conduct the proposed analyses are often not available.

• Several NRC committees have clearly warned that descriptions of "central estimates" of risk, when they are applied to models for high-dose to low-dose extrapolation, have little meaning—the model that best describes the "fit" of the observed dose-response relationship cannot be claimed to describe accurately the dose-response relationship at low doses. If this type of low-dose extrapolation is intended by OMB to yield "central estimates," the requirement will produce misleading results. If "central estimate" is used only in connection with observed data, it can be highly valuable if properly calculated. The bulletin lacks clarity on this point.

• The bulletin says little about the biologic bases of the various models and assumptions that might be used in risk assessments and about how judgments regarding their relative scientific merits are to be encompassed in the expressions of risk and of uncertainty. Perhaps the bulletin intends that such efforts be inherent in the analyses called for, but it could also be read as simply calling for the use of alternative statistical models that have unknown biologic bases. The OMB ambition with regard to uncertainty analyses seems appropriate; but because there are no well-examined and widely accepted guidelines for such analyses outside of some narrow applications of PRA, there is a risk that the bulletin's requirements will be followed in a rote way and compromise the quality of risk assessments. That outcome also runs the risk of creating even more confusion among the users of risk assessments, and the public they serve, than is now the case. Before steps are taken to mandate the vague proposals set forth by OMB, the committee urges the development of rigorous scientific methods for uncertainty analysis that meet the information needs of decision-makers.

• With respect to chemical toxicity, much of the effort of risk assessors is devoted to substances that are thought to act through threshold mechanisms. EPA reference doses for toxicity, for example, are the products of such efforts. A variety of approaches to uncertainty analysis for such measures could be suggested, but which of these would be preferred is unclear. Further study would be needed before an approach could be selected.

• The committee is not suggesting that risk characterizations ignore uncertainties or omit reasonable depictions of the ranges of risk that might be suggested by the data. Indeed, as stated above, the committee urges the use of defaults and, when possible, alternatives to them. But the bulletin seems to go well beyond these modest approaches and can be read as calling for more fully quantitative expressions of the uncertainties in risk than have been offered in most applications of risk assessment. In the absence of clear guidance regarding the conduct of uncertainty analysis, there is a danger that agencies will produce meaningless and confusing ranges of risk estimates and that the development of risk assessments will be delayed to no clear benefit. The possibility of large inconsistencies in risk assessments between and even within agencies is also increased in the absence of explicit and peer-reviewed guidance on this issue.

• The bulletin's inclusion, in its definition of risk assessment, of agency efforts that are directed only to specific steps of the risk assessment process is inconsistent with the definition preferred by the cited studies. Furthermore, OMB redefines risk assessment to include some activities associated with risk management decision-making. See Chapter 3 for a further discussion of OMB's definition of risk assessment.

• The cited NRC studies have focused primarily on general principles for risk assessment and have left development of specific guidelines to the agencies, whereas the proposed bulletin has attempted to prescribe specific approaches. In this respect, the bulletin is inconsistent with the cited studies.

Given the points elaborated above, the committee finds that the bulletin is inconsistent with the cited studies in important ways. It adopts a new definition of risk assessment and ignores without explanation the important role that policy judgments play in risk assessment. Its call for formal analyses of uncertainties and for undefined "central estimates" may, in the absence of peer-reviewed technical guidance on the evaluation and expression of uncertainties, result in risk characterizations of reduced rather than enhanced quality and consistency. These are serious concerns because any attempt to advance the practice of risk assessment that does not lean heavily on nearly 25 years of expert study of the topic and reflect scientific consensus is likely to produce the opposite effect. The chapters that follow in this report provide further discussion of those concerns.

REFERENCES

ASME (American Society of Mechanical Engineers). 2002. Standard for Probabilistic Risk Assessment for Nuclear Power Plant Applications. ASME RA-S-2002. American Society of Mechanical Engineers. December 20, 2002.

ANS (American Nuclear Society). 2003. External-Events PRA Methodology: ANSI/ANS-58.21-2003. American National Standard. American Nuclear Society. December 2003.

EPA (U.S. Environmental Protection Agency). 2001. Toxicological Review of Chloroform (CAS No. 67-66-3): In Support of Summary Information on the Integrated Risk Information System (IRIS). EPA/635/R-01/001. U.S. Environmental Protection Agency, Washington, DC [online]. Available: http://www.epa.gov/iris/toxreviews/ 0025-tr.pdf [accessed Oct. 2, 2006].

NRC (National Research Council). 1983. Risk Assessment in the Federal Government: Managing the Process. Washington, DC: National Academy Press.

NRC (National Research Council). 1994. Science and Judgment in Risk Assessment. Washington, DC: National Academy Press.

NRC (National Research Council). 1996. Understanding Risk: Informing Decisions in a Democratic Society. Washington, DC: National Academy Press.

OMB (U.S. Office of Management and Budget). 2006. Proposed Risk Assessment Bulletin. Released January 9, 2006. Washington, DC: Office of Management and Budget, Executive Office of the President [online]. Available: http://www.whitehouse.gov/omb/inforeg/ proposed_risk_ assessment_bulletin_010906.pdf [accessed Oct. 11, 2006].

PCCRARM (Presidential/Congressional Commission on Risk Assessment and Risk Management). 1997. Risk Assessment and Risk Management in Regulatory Decision-Making, Vol. 2. Washington, DC: U.S. Government Printing Office [online]. Available: http://www.riskworld.com/Nreports/ 1997/riskrpt/volume2/pdf/v2epa. PDF [accessed Oct. 3, 2006].

3

Risk Assessment Definition and Goals

This chapter addresses the definition of risk assessment proposed by the Office of Management and Budget (OMB). The definition is important because it determines which agency analyses are subject to the standards set forth in the bulletin. As discussed here, the committee finds that some departures from long-standing concepts could create confusion and controversy. The chapter also reviews the goals set forth in the bulletin. The goals are generally constructive but raise questions about the emphasis on efficiency rather than scientific quality.

The committee notes that the bulletin does not define *risk*, which lies at the core of "risk assessment." *Risk* can be defined as a hazard, a probability, a consequence, or a combination of probability and severity of consequences. Although the bulletin hints at taking both probability and severity into account, it appears to treat risk primarily as the probability of adverse effect, which is an incomplete conceptualization of risk.

DEFINITION OF RISK ASSESSMENT

Section I of the bulletin defines risk assessment as "a scientific and/or technical document that assembles and synthesizes scientific information to determine whether a potential hazard exists and/or the extent of possible risk to human health, safety or the environment" (OMB 2006a, p. 23). The supplementary information explains that "for the purposes of this Bulletin, this definition applies to documents that could be used for risk assessment purposes, such as an exposure or hazard assessment that might not constitute a complete risk assessment as defined by the National Research Council [NRC 1983]. This definition includes documents that evaluate baseline risk as well as risk mitigation activities" (OMB 2006a, p. 8).

It is important to note that the bulletin's definition of risk assessment is closely tied to which documents need to comply with the standards of the bulletin. That is, the applicability of the bulletin is intrinsically related to the definition of risk assessment because anything defined as a risk assessment will need to comply with the standards as indicated in Section II of the bulletin ("Applicability"), which states that "to the extent appropriate, all agency risk assessments available to the public shall comply with the standards of this Bulletin" (OMB 2006a, p. 23).

A recurring theme in comments received by OMB on the bulletin from organizations, associations, and individuals concerned the definition of risk assessment. Of the 78 public comments submitted to OMB (OMB 2006b), 50 (64%) discussed the definition of risk assessment. Most of those comments mentioned that the proposed definition is too broad and may create confusion and other problems. Several agencies responding to the committee's questions also pointed to potential confusion and the need for further clarification.[1]

The definition of risk assessment in the bulletin is extremely broad. Specifically, OMB defines risk assessment as a document. That characterization conflicts with standard risk assessment definitions. Risk assessment is a process from which documents can result. To define risk assessment as a document is problematic. It can capture many "documents" that are not risk assessment. More important, OMB defines risk assessment in such a way that its individual components, such as hazard assessment and exposure assessment, are inappropriately classified as "risk assessment." Expanding the definition of risk assessment in such a way has a number of disadvantages:

• Hazard and exposure assessments are components of a risk assessment but do not in themselves constitute a risk assessment. A hazard assessment—which describes and assesses the nature of a hazard—and an exposure assessment—which estimates the expected intensity, frequency, and duration of an exposure—clearly are different from a risk

---

[1]See Appendix E, pp. CPSC-2 to -3, DOE-8, HHS-A, HHS-7 to -12, DOL-4 to -5, DOT-6, and NASA-7.

assessment, which incorporates these components with hazard characterization or dose-response assessment to determine the likelihood and severity of an adverse effect or event given specified conditions. Equating risk assessment with components of risk assessment creates confusion by referring to different types of analyses with the same name. In addition, including hazard and exposure assessments would require application of the requirements of the bulletin to an extremely large number of documents, adding substantial time and resource burdens to the agencies (see "Costs" in Chapter 6 for further discussion of this issue). The committee emphasizes that although the technical requirements indicated in the proposed bulletin should not necessarily be applied to each component, the goals of higher quality and transparency should be met by all components of risk assessment.

- Previous NRC documents and other relevant documents (NRC 1983, 1989, 1993, 1994, 1996) use definitions of risk assessment that clearly differentiate risk assessment from its components. Similarly, the glossary of the 1997 Presidential/Congressional Commission on Risk Assessment and Risk Management (PCCRARM 1997) and the glossary of the Society for Risk Analysis (SRA 2003) include definitions of risk assessment that differentiate risk assessment from its components or "steps."

- Uniform general guidelines may not be able to be issued for exposure assessment. Authors of the 1983 NRC report *Risk Assessment in the Federal Government: Managing the Process* concluded that "exposure guidelines, in contrast with guidelines for other risk assessment steps, are not now readily amenable to uniform application in various agencies," and "the agencies have rather narrowly defined interests regarding exposure" (NRC 1983, p. 81).

- Several requirements of Sections IV and V of the bulletin are aimed at risk assessments and cannot be applied to exposure or hazard assessment or other components of risk assessment (for example, evaluation of risk reduction alternatives). Because it is not clear how those standards of the bulletin could be applied to hazard or exposure assessments, it also is not clear how the agencies could issue certificates of compliance for those documents.

- Some of the documents listed as examples of influential risk assessments in the supplementary information collect and summarize information from a variety of sources and studies and provide it in a format that is useful to both health professionals and the public. Many of the documents contain hazard identification, dose-response assessments, or both but do not include exposure assessments or risk characterizations. Subjecting those documents to the requirements for risk assessment detailed in the bulletin could greatly delay release of important health information to the public.

• It is unclear whether the broad definition pertains to many safety guidelines that are now issued without going through a detailed risk assessment process. That could lead to delays in putting out important guidelines, warnings, and alerts. Examples include guidelines for healthcare workers on the handling of hazardous biologic materials, such as body fluids from HIV patients; guidelines for respirator fit testing; National Institutes of Health guidelines for research practices, particularly in relation to new therapies and technologies (for example, those on the use of recombinant-DNA products); and health information alerts or warnings, which may result from reports of adverse effects of a therapy or medication. At the public meeting for this committee, the Food and Drug Administration (FDA) representative warned that OMB's definition would include most FDA safety alerts and that the risk assessment standards could delay the issuance of safety alerts regarding the adverse effects of drugs, medical devices, or foods.

• It also is not clear whether epidemiologic or toxicologic research used in risk assessments to identify factors that affect human health would now be classified as risk assessment and thus be subject to the standards in the bulletin.

OMB appears to redefine risk assessment to include some aspects of risk mitigation, such as analysis of risk reduction measures to inform risk management decision-making. The bulletin and the supplementary information approach this point in different ways, creating the potential for inconsistent interpretation and implementation of the standards. Specifically, the bulletin refers to risk mitigation only in relation to regulatory analyses (see Section IV[7]), where this reference is appropriate, and not in the definition of risk assessment (see Section I), where such a reference would be a sharp departure from the long-established conceptual distinction between risk assessment and risk management. However, the supplementary information specifies that the definition of risk assessment "includes documents that evaluate baseline risk as well as risk mitigation activities" (OMB 2006a, p. 8)—an auxiliary definition that highlights the departure from the conceptual distinction. If the definition from the supplementary information is incorporated into the risk assessment definition, the bulletin would conflict with the 1983 NRC recommendation, reinforced in numerous reports, to "take steps to establish and maintain a clear conceptual distinction between assessment of risk and consideration of risk management alternatives" (NRC 1983, p. 7). In making that recommendation, the 1983 NRC committee noted that experience shows that difficulties can arise from not having a clear distinction between those closely related, but different, aspects of setting regulatory standards. For example, if nonrisk factors, such as the expected economic or political consequences of proposed regulatory action, were seen to affect either the interpretation of scientific information or the choice of default options, the credibility of the assessment inside and outside an agency could be compromised, and this might reduce the legitimacy of the risk management decision itself.

Since the publication of the 1983 NRC report, there has been some debate as to how much one can separate risk management from risk assessment. Nevertheless, the 1994 NRC report *Science and Judgment in Risk Assessment* stated that "protecting the integrity of the risk assessment, while building more productive linkages to make risk assessment more accurate and relevant to risk management, will be essential as the agency [EPA] proceeds to regulate the residual risks of hazardous air pollutants" (NRC 1994, p. 260). Furthermore, the 1996 NRC report *Understanding Risk* stated that "what is needed for successful characterization of risk must be considered at the very beginning of the process and must to a great extent drive risk analysis. If a risk characterization is to fulfill its purpose, it must (1) be decision driven, (2) recognize all significant concerns, (3) reflect both analysis and deliberation, with appropriate input from the interested and affected parties, and (4) be appropriate to the decision" (NRC 1996, p. 16). Thus, the committee believes that risk assessors and risk managers should talk with each other; that is, a "conceptual distinction" does not mean establishing a wall between risk assessors and risk managers. Indeed, they should have constant interaction. However, the dialogue should not bias or otherwise color the risk assessment conducted, and the activities should remain distinct; that is, risk assessors should not be performing risk management activities.

GOALS

The bulletin and the supplementary information lay out five goals, also called "aspirational goals" (see Table 3-1). The goals can be seen as having to do with both the efficiency and the quality of a risk assessment.

TABLE 3-1 Goals for Risk Assessment as Stated in Bulletin and Clarified in Supplementary Information

Goal	Bulletin Description	Supplementary Description
1	"The objectives of an assessment shall be a product of an iterative dialogue between the assessor(s) and the agency decision maker(s)" (OMB 2006a, p. 23)	Goal related to problem formulation: "there will be many choices regarding the objectives, scope and content of the assessment, and an iterative dialogue will help ensure that the risk assessment serves its intended purpose and is developed in a cost-effective manner" (OMB 2006a, p. 10)
2	"The scope and content of the risk assessment shall be determined based on the objectives of the assessment and best professional judgment, considering the benefits and costs of acquiring additional information before undertaking the assessment" (OMB 2006a, p. 23).	Goal related to completeness: "there is often a tension between…completeness in the scientific sense and…a well-defined scope that limits the inquiry to a set of practical, tractable and relevant questions." "The scope…should reflect a balance between the desire for scientific completeness and the need to provide relevant information to decision makers" (OMB 2006a, p. 10).
3	"The type of risk assessment prepared shall be responsive to the nature of the potential hazard, the available data and the decision needs" (OMB 2006a, p. 23).	Goal related to effort expended: "level of effort should be commensurate with the importance of the risk assessment… nature of the potential hazard, the available data, and the decision needs" (OMB 2006a, p. 11).
4	"The level of effort put into the risk assessment shall be commensurate with the importance of the risk assessment" (OMB 2006a, p. 23).	Goal related to resources expended: "take into account the importance of the risk assessment in gauging the resources, including time and money, required to meet the requirements of this Bulletin" (OMB 2006a, p. 11).
5	"The agency shall follow appropriate procedures for peer review and public participation in the process of preparing the risk assessment" (OMB 2006a, p. 23).	Goal related to peer review and public participation: "when a draft assessment is made publicly available for comment or peer review, the agency is required to clarify that the report does not represent the official view of the federal government." "Public comments play an important role in helping to inform agency deliberations…when people are engaged early in the process, the public typically has an easier time concurring with government documents and decisions which may affect them" (OMB 2006a, p. 11).

All federal-agency risk assessments are subject to OMB's Information Quality Guidelines (67 Fed. Reg. 8452 [2002]), which require utility, objectivity, and integrity. As a first approximation, goals 1, 3, and 5 focus on quality, and goals 2 and 4 on efficiency. Objectivity and integrity are addressed by the five goals to the extent that peer review and public participation contribute to these attributes.

Goal related to problem formulation (1). This is principally the goal of good communication between the risk assessor and the agency decision-maker or client. Although the emphasis is on an iterative discussion in the bulletin, the supplementary information adds a cost-effectiveness component.

Goal related to completeness (2). This is principally the goal of balancing the completeness of a risk assessment in providing relevant information to the agency decision-maker with the decision-maker's immediate needs. The goal calls for a cost-benefit balancing of scientific completeness with practical usefulness in making decisions in keeping with OMB's Information Quality Guidelines (67 Fed. Reg. 8452 [2002]). Having the scope and content linked to the assessment seems logical, and one would hope that this recommendation is already implicit in most risk assessments. The supplementary information raises a number issues about satisfying the goal. For example, the supplementary information refers to a well-defined scope as one that "limits the inquiry to a set of practical, tractable and relevant questions" (OMB 2006a, p. 10). However, how should the properties of practical, tractable, and relevant be established? In addition, the supplementary information indicates that "the scope of an assessment should reflect a balance between the desire for scientific completeness and the need to provide relevant information to decision makers" (OMB 2006a, p. 10). One might expect that decision-makers would want nothing less than scientifically relevant information. What constitutes scientifically complete information might be a contentious issue. A risk assessment might be conducted on a new class of hazards or a new engineered system before extensive data are available. Then, the question would be, How does the magnitude of the uncertainty affect the policy decision?

Goal related to effort expended (3). In what may be only an oversight, this goal differs somewhat between the bulletin and the supplementary information. The goal according to the bulletin addresses the type of risk assessment performed, whereas the goal according to the supplementary information addresses effort and resources. These are not contradictory, but different. The former seems to be what was intended. But the meaning of "the type of risk assessment prepared" is not self-evident and is not clarified in the bulletin or the supplementary information.

Goals related to resources expended (4). This goal is a corollary of the aforementioned goal related to completeness. This goal says that the time and money invested in the risk assessment should be commensurate with the use to which the results are to be put, that is, the "importance of the risk assessment." That is redundant in light of goal 3 in the supplementary information; goal 3 might be better represented by its description in the bulletin than by that in the supplementary information.

Goal related to peer review and public participation (5). This goal involves principally adequate review of the product of the risk assessment. Although the bulletin suggests peer review and public participation in the "process of preparing the risk assessment," the supplementary information emphasizes the product.

Taken as a whole, the five goals say, in essence, that a risk assessment should be tailored to the narrow need for which it is undertaken; balanced in scope, time, and cost with the importance of the issue; and peer-reviewed and subject to public participation. To the extent that current practice is inadequate in coordinating the focus and scope of a risk assessment with the objectives of the agency decision-maker, and to the extent that the outcomes of a risk assessment are inadequately reviewed and not subject to public comment, goals 1 and 5 are beneficial in promoting higher-quality risk assessments. Whether those conditions exist is a separate question.

A risk assessment usually involves incomplete data, scientific uncertainty, and the need for expert judgment. The pressure to narrow the scope becomes a pressure to give inadequate attention to those complications. Thus, the goals may lead to less expensive and quicker risk assessments, but they do not necessarily lead to higher-quality risk assessments.

The dominating theme of the bulletin and the supplementary information is improving the quality of risk assessments undertaken by federal agencies, but the stated goals do not all support this theme. The goals stated in the bulletin and the supplementary information emphasize *efficiency* in the conduct of risk assessment activities more than *quality*.

REFERENCES

NRC (National Research Council). 1983. Risk Assessment in the Federal Government: Managing the Process. Washington DC: National Academy Press.

NRC (National Research Council). 1989. Improving Risk Communication. Washington DC: National Academy Press.

NRC (National Research Council). 1993. Issues in Risk Assessment, Volumes I, II and III. Washington DC: National Academy Press.

NRC (National Research Council). 1994. Science and Judgment in Risk Assessment. Washington DC: National Academy Press.

NRC (National Research Council). 1996. Understanding Risk: Informing Decisions in a Democratic Society. Washington DC: National Academy Press.

OMB (U.S. Office of Management and Budget). 2006a. Proposed Risk Assessment Bulletin. Released January 9, 2006. Washington, DC: Office of Management and Budget, Executive Office of the President [online]. Available: http://www.whitehouse.gov/omb/ inforeg/proposed_risk_assessment_bulletin_010906.pdf [accessed Oct. 11, 2006].

OMB (Office of Management and Budget). 2006b. Comments on Proposed Risk Assessment Bulletin. Office of Management and Budget, Washington, DC [online]. Available: http://www.whitehouse.gov/omb/inforeg/comments_rab/list_rab2006.html [accessed Oct. 13, 2006].

PCCRARM (Presidential/Congressional Commission on Risk Assessment and Risk Management). 1997. Glossary. Pp. 153-157 in Risk Assessment and Risk Management in Regulatory Decision-Making, Vol. 2. Washington, DC: U.S. Government Printing Office [online]. Available: http://www.riskworld.com/Nreports/1997/risk-rpt/volume2/pdf/v2epa.PDF [accessed Oct. 3, 2006].

SRA (Society for Risk Analysis). 2003. Risk Analysis Glossary [online]. Available: http://www.sra.org/resources_glossary_p-r.php [accessed Oct. 13, 2006].

4

Standards for Risk Assessment

This chapter evaluates the standards that are proposed in the Office of Management and Budget (OMB) bulletin. The standards are defined for general and influential risk assessment, and the committee first comments on that structure. It then discusses major themes, such as uncertainty. The chapter concludes with a summary of comments on each of the individual standards that are proposed in the bulletin.

DIFFERENT LEVELS OF STANDARDS

The bulletin articulates standards for general risk assessments and special standards for influential risk assessments (see Appendix B). One standard listed for general risk assessments is specifically directed at risk assessments used for regulatory analysis. The bulletin defines an influential risk assessment as one that the responsible "agency reasonably can determine will have or does have a clear and substantial impact on important public policies or private sector decisions" (OMB 2006, p. 23). Thus, the categories of risk assessments, and thus the standards, are not based on inherent properties of risk assessments but on aspects of risk management.

In defining special standards for influential risk assessments, OMB appropriately recognizes that risk assessments that have potentially greater impact should be more detailed, be better supported by data and analyses, and receive a greater degree of scrutiny and critical review than risk assessments likely to have smaller impacts. However, proposing different standards for general and influential risk assessments is problematic for at least three reasons. First, the determination of what constitutes an influential risk assessment may be unclear at the outset. Although some agencies may be able to identify an influential risk assessment at the onset of the analysis,[1] others may not be able to.[2] The impact of an agency activity that led to the development of the risk assessment may not be known a priori. Some degree of iteration is necessary and appropriate, but the application of additional standards when some arbitrary impact threshold is crossed may lead to needless and inappropriate delays in implementation of the action.

Second, the effort to separate risk assessments arbitrarily into two broad categories does not appropriately recognize the continuum of risk assessment efforts in terms of potential impact on economic, environmental, cultural, and social values. Any attempt to divide that continuum into two categories is unlikely to succeed and will not substantially improve the quality of risk assessments. The use of two categories will tend to lead to costly and slow iterative processes in which a risk assessment may not be judged influential initially but on completion may be found to cross an arbitrary threshold that triggers the additional standards. It may be that additional evaluation and analysis may be appropriate as the impacts of the risk assessment are better identified, but an arbitrary triggering of a new set of standards is not appropriate.

Third, the specific standards to be required of all influential risk assessments appear to be targeted at types of risk assessments and supporting information that may not be appropriate for the broad array of risk assessments that are conducted by federal agencies. Several standards proposed for influential risk assessments appear to be related specifically to human health risk assessments; these standards might not be appropriate for engineering risk assessments that evaluate the safety of structures or systems. Other issues associated with the standards are discussed in the remainder of this chapter.

RANGE OF RISK ESTIMATES AND CENTRAL ESTIMATES

One focus in the bulletin is the presentation of a range of risk estimates and a central estimate; statements on this topic in the bulletin and

---

[1]See Appendix E, pp. DOE-4 and DOL-5.
[2]See Appendix E, pp. HHS-13, DOD-9, and CPSC-4.

supplementary information are summarized in Table 4-1. Previous National Research Council (NRC) reports have made relevant comments on this and related topics; selected comments from those reports are provided in Table 4-2. The committee agrees with OMB that in some cases "presentation of single estimates of risk is misleading" and that ranges of "plausible risk" should be presented; however, the challenge is in the operational definitions of such words as *central*, *expected*, and *plausible*. The committee's concerns regarding the use of those words in the bulletin are presented in this section.

Central Estimates of What?

In the supplementary information, a central estimate is defined as a mean of a distribution, the most representative value of a distribution, or a weighted estimate of risk. However, a central estimate is defined in context, and those definitions raise the question of what is being considered.

Distributions arise in considerations of uncertainty and variability. Variability is an inherent property of a system. Ventilation rates, water-consumption amounts, and body-mass indexes all differ in a population of individuals. Obtaining more data will not reduce variability but will provide a better description of the distribution of a variable trait. In contrast, uncertainty reflects ignorance. The mean body-mass index of a population of individuals is typically an unknown value. Similarly, the true statistical model for a dose-response relationship is unknown. Unlike variability, uncertainty might be reduced by obtaining more data. Potential confusion arises because distributions might be used to represent both variability and uncertainty. For variability, the distribution corresponds to the different values of a trait or characteristic in a population. For the uncertainty of a parameter value, a distribution might correspond to the sampling distribution of the parameter in repeated samples (a frequentist perspective) or to the actual distribution of the parameter (a Bayesian perspective).

Variability and uncertainty can lead to a distribution of risk. Consider the use of a single dose-response model (without the additional complexity of model uncertainty) to predict the risk of adverse response as a function of dose, and assume that the coefficients of the model must be estimated (that is, uncertainty) and that there is a distribution of exposures in the population (that is, variability). The point estimates of the

TABLE 4-1 Summary of Bulletin and Supplementary Information on Range of Risk Estimates and Central Estimates

Type of Risk Assessment	Bulletin	Supplementary Information
General risk assessment	A risk assessment should "provide a characterization of risk, qualitatively and, whenever possible, quantitatively. When a quantitative characterization of risk is provided, a range of plausible risk estimates shall be provided" (OMB 2006, p. 24).	The reporting of "multiple estimates of risk (and the limitations associated with these estimates)" is recommended to "convey the precision associated with these estimates" (OMB 2006, p. 13). A discussion of the Safe Drinking Water Act (SDWA) noted the need to describe the population addressed by each risk estimate, the expected risk or central estimate for affected populations, and the upper-bound or lower-bound risk estimates, with uncertainty issues, supporting studies, and methods used in the calculations. The SDWA reporting standards "should be met, where feasible, in all risk assessments which address adverse health effects" (OMB 2006, p. 14).
Risk assessment for regulatory analysis	A risk assessment should include "whenever possible, a range of plausible risk estimates, including central or expected estimates, when a quantitative characterization of risk is made available" (OMB 2006, p. 24).	The supplementary information expands on issues related to risk assessments used for regulatory analysis. A "range of plausible risk estimates, including central estimates," are required with any quantitative characterization of risk. A "central estimate" is defined to be "(i) mean or average of the distribution; (ii) number which contains multiple estimates of risk based on different assumptions, weighted by their relative plausibility; or (iii) any estimate judged to be most representative of the distribution." This quantity should "neither understate nor overstate the risk, but rather, should provide the risk manager and the public with the expected risk" (OMB 2006, p. 16).
Influential risk assessment	All influential risk assessment shall "highlight central estimates as well as high-end and low-end estimates of risk when such estimates are uncertain" (OMB 2006, p. 25).	The supplementary information expands on issues related to standards for influential risk assessment. An influential risk assessment should meet the standards for regulatory-analysis risk assessment and additional standards. In particular, the standard for

the presentation of numerical estimates directly addresses issues related to central estimates of risk and ranges of risk estimates. Reporting a range avoids a "false sense of precision" when there is uncertainty. Reporting the range and central estimate "conveys a more objective characterization of the magnitude of the risks." The highlighting of only high-end or low-end risk estimates is discouraged (OMB 2006, p. 17). The supplementary information further notes that "central" and "expected" are used synonymously. If model uncertainty is present, this central model could reflect a weighted average of risk estimates from alternative models or some synthesis of "probability assessments supplied by qualified experts" (OMB 2006, p. 17).

TABLE 4-2 Previous NRC Reports Addressing Issues of Uncertainty and Central Risk Estimates

Topic	Comment	Reference
Uncertainty and risk assessment	NRC (1989), a report on risk communication, discusses uncertainty in the risk assessment process: "*Any scientific risk estimate is likely to be based on incomplete knowledge combined with assumptions, each of which is a source of uncertainty that limits the accuracy that should be ascribed to the estimate.* Does the existence of multiple sources of uncertainty mean that the final estimate is that much more uncertain, or can the different uncertainties be expected to cancel each other out? The problem of how best to interpret multiple uncertainties is one more source of uncertainty and disagreement about risk estimates" (p. 44).	NRC 1989
Central estimates (point estimates) and range of risk estimates	"When a risk estimate is uncertain, it can be described by a point or 'maximum likelihood' estimate or by a range of possibilities around the point estimate. But estimates that include a wide range of uncertainties can imply that a disastrous consequence is 'possible,' even when expert opinion is unanimous that the likelihood of disaster is extremely small. The amount of uncertainty to present is a judgment that can potentially influence a recipient's judgment" (p. 83).	NRC 1989
Averaging predictions	"Simply put, although classical decision theory does encourage the use of expected values that NRC take account of all sources of uncertainty, it is not in the decision-maker's or society's best interest to treat *fundamentally different predictions as quantities that can be 'averaged' without considering the effects of each prediction on the decision that it leads to*" (p. 173). "To create a single risk estimate or PDF [probability density function] out of various different models not only could undermine the entire notion of having default models that can be set aside for sufficient reason, but could lead to misleading and perhaps meaningless hybrid risk estimates" (p. 174).	NRC 1994
Range of plausible values	"One important issue related to uncertainty is the extent to which a risk assessment that generates a point estimate, rather than a range of plausible values, is likely to be too 'conservative' (that is, to excessively exaggerate the plausible magnitude of harm that might result from specified environmental exposures)" (p. 180).	NRC 1994

model coefficients are obtained (for example, central estimates of a sampling distribution or of some posterior distribution). The mean of the exposure distribution (a central estimate) could be substituted into the dose-response model by using the point estimates of the coefficients to yield a central risk estimate. If the exposure distribution is unimodal and symmetric, the estimate seems like a reasonable central risk estimate. If the exposure distribution is skewed or multimodal, the central estimate may be unreasonable. At this point, uncertainty might enter into the calculation, and confidence or credible intervals for the model coefficients might be used to reflect parameter uncertainty. The bulletin requires the reporting of a plausible range of risk when a quantitative risk assessment is conducted. How should *plausible* be defined in this context? For example, would substituting the 2.5th percentile and 97.5th percentile from the exposure distribution in the dose-response model yield a plausible range? Without more guidance and operational definitions of terms, the bulletin's guidance on central estimates and plausible risk ranges is unclear.

More on "Central" Estimates

Expected value has a technical statistical meaning that corresponds to the mean of some random variable. Many central estimates can be constructed, including arithmetic means, geometric means, harmonic means, medians, and trimmed means; however, it is misleading to say that "central" and "expected" estimates are synonymous, as is suggested in the bulletin (see Table 4-1). As noted in NRC (1994, p. 173), "it is not in the decision-maker's or society's best interest *to treat fundamentally different predictions as quantities that can be 'averaged' without considering the effects of each prediction on the decision that it leads to.*" In fact, a simple "expected" value may not convey an appropriate message.

It may be reasonable to provide a calculation of the central risk estimate along with the lower and upper bounds of the 95% confidence or credible intervals and thus provide a sense of the degree of uncertainty in a particular risk assessment. Usually, some number will need to be selected for a risk management decision, such as to set an "action level" to control a toxicant under consideration or to offer guidance about how much exposure is acceptable or "safe," as in the determination of a reference dose or an allowable limit in the workplace. Variability is an important consideration because people might respond differently to a given exposure because of personal vulnerability to exposure or behavior that alters the actual exposure. Often in public-health practice and prevention, the goal is to protect the *most vulnerable* in the population—children, the elderly, people with illnesses (such as respiratory or cardiac disease), the developing fetus, and workers. Using the mean or central estimate would not accomplish that goal unless it reflected the mean response of the distribution of vulnerable or susceptible individuals.

Risk communication is hampered by the use of vague or meaningless terms. For example, there is no such thing as the "average person." Is the average person male or female? Does this person weigh 70 kg? Instead, we have average values of measurable attributes of people. Similarly, terms like *central, expected,* and *plausible* should be replaced with precise language.

Reporting Plausible Ranges and Central Estimates

The purpose and context of risk assessments frequently influence the need for, and indeed the advisability of, reporting a range and a central estimate. For example, consider a risk assessment that evaluates risks associated with operations conducted in an extreme environment. The setting of National Aeronautics and Space Administration (NASA) spacecraft exposure guidelines (SEGs) illustrates how decisions made in advance can determine the kinds of data that need to be presented and how risks should be reported.

NASA guidelines for chemical exposure on spacecraft, which include SEGs and their predecessors, spacecraft maximum acceptable concentrations (SMACs) and spacecraft water exposure guidelines (NRC 1994, 1996a, 1996b, 2000b, 2004), are set to protect astronauts whose health and job fitness are closely monitored. However, they are engaged in an inherently dangerous activity and are in an environment that presents unique stressors, such as exposure to high levels of solar radiation (associated risks include cancer and hematopoietic toxicity) and microgravity (associated risks include loss of muscle mass and lowered hematocrit). In addition to protecting the health of astronauts, great emphasis is placed on avoiding exposure that would prevent astronauts from performing mission-critical tasks. The guidelines for chemical exposures are derived with those risks in mind.

Because of NASA's emphasis on safety and the devastating consequences of accidents, relatively conservative assumptions are used in setting exposure guidelines. In addition, the chemical exposure guidelines are used as design points for the environmental control systems for the spacecraft. In early discussions concerning SMACs, NASA engineers working on those systems indicated their preference for a single guideline to use as a design target. Thus, although SEG documentation discusses uncertainties and limitations and transparently describes the derivation of all SEG values, SEG values are set at levels thought to be protective, and central estimates or ranges are not reported.

UNCERTAINTY

This section assesses the extent to which the proposed bulletin achieves its goal of enhancing technical quality and objectivity with respect to the treatment of uncertainty. Understanding the current state of best practice is a precondition for improving that practice. Therefore, this section first provides a historical perspective on uncertainty in risk assessment. That discussion provides the best examples of approaches to uncertainty analysis in the federal agencies. This section then briefly reviews methods used to address uncertainty in risk assessment and next notes relevant statements from previous NRC reports. The section concludes with the committee's comments on the bulletin's standards related to uncertainty analysis. This section differs from other sections of the report in that it provides more in-depth discussion of this topic; the level of detail was considered appropriate, given the focus on uncertainty in the bulletin.

Historical Perspective

The desire to do risk assessment properly led to the development of many of the methods for uncertainty analysis, particularly probabilistic risk assessment (PRA, also referred to as probabilistic safety analysis [PSA] in Europe). Although the aerospace industry led the development of reliability engineering, the basic methods for the use of PRA in engineering were developed in the nuclear industry. The concepts of formal and structured development of accident risk scenarios using event trees, extension of the causal models using fault trees, probabilistic treatment of physical dependencies, separation of external and internal sources of risk, and quantification and propagation of parameteric uncertainties first appeared in the Reactor Safety Study. This historical perspective on the development of PRA is discussed below.

The Aerospace Sector

A systematic concern with PRA began in the aerospace sector after the fire in Apollo flight test AS-204 on January 27, 1967, in which three astronauts were killed. Before the Apollo accident, NASA relied on its contractors to apply "good engineering practices" to provide quality assurance and quality control. NASA's Office of Manned Space Flight initiated the development of quantitative safety goals in 1969. Quantitative safety goals were not adopted; the reason given at the time was that managers would not appreciate the uncertainty in risk calculations: "the problem with quantifying risk assessment is that when managers are given numbers, the numbers are treated as absolute judgments, regardless of warnings against doing so" (Wiggins 1985). After the inquiry into the Challenger accident of January 28, 1986, it came to light that distrust of reassuring risk numbers was not the only reason for abandoning quantitative risk assessment. Rather, initial estimates of catastrophic failure probabilities were so high that their publication would have threatened the political future of the entire space program (Bedford and Cooke 2001).

Since the shuttle accident, NASA has instituted programs of quantitative risk analysis to support safety during the design and operation phases of space travel. On the basis of an earlier U.S. Nuclear Regulatory Commission document, a PRA procedures guide was published in 2002; it included a chapter on uncertainty analysis (NASA 2002). The current NASA Procedural Requirements NPR-8705.5, effective as of July 2004, mandates PRA procedures for NASA programs and projects and stipulates that "any PRA insights reported to decision makers shall include an appreciation of the overall degree of uncertainty about the results and an understanding of which sources of uncertainty are critical. Presentation of PRA results without uncertainties significantly detracts from the quality and credibility of the PRA study" (NASA 2004, p. 12).

The Nuclear Sector

Throughout the 1950s, in accordance with President Eisenhower's

Atoms for Peace program, the Atomic Energy Commission pursued an approach to risk management that emphasized using high-quality components and construction; conservatism in the engineering codes and standards for design, construction, and operation of plants; and conservative analysis of accident scenarios using the "maximum credible accident." Because "credible accidents" were covered by plant design, residual risk was estimated by studying the hypothetical consequences of "incredible accidents." A study released in 1957 focused on three scenarios of radioactive releases from a 200-megawatt (200-MW) nuclear-power plant operating 30 miles from a large population center. Regarding the probability of such releases, the study concluded that "no one knows now or will ever know the exact magnitude of this low probability" (AEC 1957).

Successive design improvements were intended to reduce the probability of a catastrophic release of the radioactive material from the reactor. However, because of the limitations of the analytic methods, such improvements were not able to have a significant effect on the accident estimates. Moreover, as larger reactors were planned, such as 1,000-MW reactors, the increase in radioactive material in the cores led to larger consequences in the "incredible accident" scenarios.

The desire to quantify and evaluate the effects of those improvements led to the introduction of *probabilistic* risk assessment. Whereas the earlier studies had dealt with uncertainty by making conservative assumptions, the goal now was to provide a *realistic*, as opposed to conservative, assessment of risk. A realistic risk assessment necessarily involved an assessment of the uncertainty in the risk calculation. The basic methods of PRA developed in the aerospace program in the 1960s found their first full-scale application, including accident-consequence analysis and uncertainty analysis, in the Reactor Safety Study of 1975 (U.S. NRC 1975), which is rightly considered to be the first modern PRA.

The Reactor Safety Study caused considerable concern within the scientific community. In response to letters from Representative Udall, chairman of the House Committee on Interior and Insular Affairs, the U.S. Nuclear Regulatory Commission created an independent group of experts to review its "achievements and limitations." The report of that review group (Lewis et al. 1978) led to a policy statement by the commission (U.S. NRC 1979). The policy statement (1) endorsed the review group's strong criticism of the executive summary, stating that it was misleading and was not a summary of the report, (2) acknowledged that the peer-review process followed in publishing the Reactor Safety Study was inadequate, and (3) stated that the commission "does not regard as reliable the Reactor Safety Study's numerical estimates of the overall risk of reactor accident." However, the commission also noted that the review group cited major achievements of the Reactor Safety Study and stated that "WASH 1400 [the Reactor Safety Study] was a substantial advance over previous attempts to estimate the risks of the nuclear option. WASH -1400 was largely successful in at least three ways: in making the study of reactor safety more rational, in establishing the topology of many accident sequences, and in delineating procedures through which quantitative estimates of the risk can be derived for those sequences for which a data base exits."

After the Three Mile Island accident, two influential independent studies (Kemeny 1979; Rogovin and Frampton 1980) recommended greater use of probabilistic analyses in assessing nuclear-plant risks. A new generation of PRAs appeared in which some of the methodologic defects of the Reactor Safety Study were avoided. The Nuclear Regulatory Commission released the *Fault Tree Handbook* in 1981 (Vesely et al. 1981) and the *PRA Procedures Guide* in 1983 (U.S. NRC 1983), which shored up and standardized much of the risk assessment methodology. An extensive chapter was devoted to uncertainty and sensitivity analysis. An authoritative review of PRAs conducted after the Three Mile Island accident noted the necessity of modeling uncertainties properly in using PRA as a management tool (Garrick 1984).

In 1990, a suite of studies known as NUREG 1150 (U.S. NRC 1990) appeared; these used structured expert judgment to quantify uncertainty and set new standards for uncertainty analysis. They were followed by a joint U.S.-European program in 1994-1998 (Harper et al. 1995; Goossens et al. 1996; Brown et al. 1997; Goossens et al. 1997; Haskin et al. 1997; Little et al. 1997) for quantifying uncertainty in accident-consequences models. Expert-judgment methods were further elaborated, as were screening and sensitivity analysis. European studies, spun off that work, have applied uncertainty analysis to European consequences models and provided extensive methodologic guidance (Brown et al. 2001; Goossens et al. 2001; Jones et al. 2001a,b,c,d,e). In particular, they address methods for identifying important variables; selecting, interviewing, and combining experts; propagating uncertainty; inferring distributions of model parameter values; and communicating results. The guidance is summarized in a special 2000 issue of *Radiation Protection*

Dosimetry.[3] All the documents in those reports have undergone peer review.

In August 2006, the Nuclear Regulatory Commission Office of Nuclear Regulatory Research issued *Draft Regulatory Guide: An Approach for Determining the Technical Adequacy of Probabilistic Risk Assessment Results for Risk-Informed Activities* (U.S. NRC 2006). The document cites related activities of the American Nuclear Society (ANS 2003), the American Society of Mechanical Engineers (ASME 2005), and the Nuclear Energy Institute (NEI 2000); the committee notes guidelines by the Department of Energy (DOE 1996). The *Draft Regulatory Guide* lists principles and objectives for a standard for PRA and clarifies what a standard should be and do (see Box 4-1). In particular, a standard should identify current good practice, thoroughly define what is technically required, and require a peer-review process that identifies where the technical requirements of the standard are not met.

The committee notes that PRA is often performed without a full-scale uncertainty analysis. Examples include PRAs of individual power plants and of individual chemical plants. In such cases, it is customary to take uncertainty ranges from generic PRAs or other generic sources. Such sources include *Federal Guidance Report 13* for cancer risk coefficients for radionuclides (Eckerman et al. 1999) and the Integrated Risk Information System (IRIS) database (IRIS 2006).

Current Good Practice in the Evaluation of Uncertainty in Risk Analysis

Risk analysis typically involves substantial uncertainties, and the quantification of uncertainty has become an integral part of PRA. Standards for PRA therefore require standards for uncertainty analysis that are based on current good practice. Three levels of good practice are distinguished here.

Level 1—uncertainty methods that are accepted and standardized. These are methods and techniques about which there is near unanimity in the scientific community. The subjective, or Bayesian, interpretation of probability for representing uncertainty would be in this category, as

---

[3]Volume 90 (Issue 3).

BOX 4-1 Principles and Objectives of a PRA Standard
(U.S. NRC 2006, p. 22)

1. The PRA standard provides well-defined criteria against which the strengths and weaknesses of the PRA may be judged so that decision makers can determine the degree of reliance that can be placed on the PRA results of interest.

2. The standard is based on current good practices (see Note below) as reflected in publicly available documents. The need for the documentation to be publicly available follows from the fact that the standard may be used to support safety decisions.

3. To facilitate the use of the standard for a wide range of applications, categories can be defined to aid in determining the applicability of the PRA for various types of applications.

4. The standard thoroughly and completely defines what is technically required and should, where appropriate, identify one or more acceptable methods.

5. The standard requires a peer review process that identifies and assesses where the technical requirements of the standard are not met. The standard needs to ensure that the peer review process:

— determines whether methods identified in the standard have been used appropriately;

— determines that, when acceptable methods are not specified in the standard, or when alternative methods are used in lieu of those identified in the standard, the methods used are adequate to meet the requirements of the standard;

— assesses the significance of the results and insights gained from the PRA of not meeting the technical requirements in the standard;

— highlights key [emphasis added] assumptions that may significantly [emphasis removed] impact the results and provides an assessment of the reasonableness of the assumptions;

— is flexible and accommodates alternative peer review approaches; and

— includes a peer review team that is composed of members who are knowledgeable in the technical elements of a PRA, are familiar with the plant design and operation, and are independent with no conflicts of interest that may influence the outcome of the peer review [this clause was not in the ASME definition].

6. The standard addresses the maintenance and update of the PRA to incorporate changes that can substantially impact the risk profile so that the PRA adequately represents the current as-built and as operated plant.

7. The standard is a living document. Consequently, it should not impede research. It is structured so that, when improvements in the state of knowledge occur, the standard can be easily updated.

Note: Current good practices are those practices that are generally accepted throughout the industry and have shown to be technically acceptable in documented analyses or engineering assessments.

---

would Monte Carlo methods of propagation, including Latin hypercube sampling, stratified sampling, and pseudo-random-number sampling. Standard statistical techniques for quantifying the uncertainty associated with estimates of model parameters also belong here.

Level 2—uncertainty methods that are used but not standardized. Many techniques are being applied and have passed muster in peer review but cannot claim universal assent. One example is expert-judgment methods. NUREG 1150 (U.S. NRC 1990) developed techniques to capture experts' modeling assumptions and used equal weighting to combine their distributions. The U.S. Nuclear Regulatory Commission and EU studies applied performance-based weighting in addition to equal weighting, leaving the choice to the discretion of the problem-owner (Harper et al. 1995). They also developed a different method for dealing with model uncertainty by using expert judgment to derive a distribution over models with probabilistic inversion. Guidelines for probabilistic inversion (Jones et al. 2001a) and structured expert judgment (Cooke and Goossens 1999) were published in that project. The Senior Seismic Hazard committee has developed a third approach (Budnitz et al. 1997). Model uncertainty is another subject for which several techniques populate the field of applications. Examples include Bayesian model averaging (Raftery 1995; Hoeting et al. 1999; Kang et al. 2000; Morales et al. 2006; NRC 2000a; Bailer et al. 2005), expert model elicitation (U.S. NRC 1990), and probabilistic inversion (Jones et al. 2001a). Where the scientific community has not yet resolved which techniques are most suitable in which situations, the only prudent course for technical guidance is to delineate the relevant techniques and their current status.

Level 3—uncertainty methods in the research mode. These are methods and techniques that address recognized problems but that the research community is still developing. Techniques do not have full procedures, applicable computer codes are of "research grade" (to be used only by the developer), and other, possibly better, techniques are on the drawing board. Perhaps the most important category still in the research mode is dependence modeling. Mathematical methods for representing dependence in high-dimensional distributions are still in development. One can consider graphical models (Markov trees, Bayesian belief nets, and Vines) as probes. Other aspects are the efficient sampling of high-dimensional dependent distributions and the elicitation or learning of dependence structures. The common distinction of uncertainty vs variability is clear enough in many applications, but it can glide easily into thorny issues of dependence modeling. The final point in the principles and objectives of a PRA standard cited earlier is worth recalling: "The standard is a living document. Consequently, it should not impede research. It is structured so that, when improvements in the state of knowledge occur, the standard can easily be updated" (U.S. NRC 2006, p. 22).

The committee finds that where practice is not standardized it is not judicious to mandate methods. Research methods and techniques need research support to evolve into practical tools that can be evaluated in the field. Any "ongoing effort to improve the quality, objectivity, utility, and integrity of information disseminated by the federal government to the public" must be cognizant of the state of the art (OMB 2006, p. 1).

Uncertainty Addressed in Previous National
Research Council Reports

The standards and related discussion in the proposed OMB bulletin and supplementary information on uncertainty echo previous NRC reports. For example, NRC (1989, p. 12) noted that "risk messages and supporting materials should not minimize the existence of uncertainty." That report also noted the importance of considering the distribution of exposure and sensitivity in a population as components of an evaluation of total population risk. Uncertainties about risks and benefits are described, including those in assumptions and models that serve as the basis of risk estimates.

The issue of uncertainty was clearly of concern in the NRC report on human exposure assessment for airborne pollutants (NRC 1991):

> Limited information is available regarding the accuracy of most contaminant concentration models and less is known about exposure models because most models have not been adequately validated. Model users should understand that model outputs have uncertainties, not just those arising from the uncertainties in the input data, and that actual exposure lies somewhere in the range of that uncertainty. The results of models should be presented with their estimated uncertainties. To the extent possible, the description of the model results should distinguish between input and model uncertainty. A major objective for improving models should be to reduce uncertainty due to the model itself so that the estimated exposure

is closer to the real exposure and the uncertainties are primarily associated with the uncertainties in the input data (p. 173).

Uncertainty was also considered in detail in the NRC (1993) report in the context of ecologic risk assessment. In that report, uncertainty was classified as being related to measurements (including inadequacy of data, measurement difficulties, and variability in organismal response), to conditions of observation (including laboratory-field condition differences), and to inadequacies of models (including parameter-value uncertainty, mechanistic uncertainty, and extrapolation) (see p. 261). NRC (1993) contained some of the most expansive discussions of uncertainty and variability among all the documents prepared in the last 2 decades.

The importance of reflecting uncertainty in risk assessments was underscored by NRC (1994, p. 161), which stated that the "committee believes that uncertainty analysis is the only way to combat the 'false sense of certainty,' which is *caused* by a refusal to acknowledge and (attempt to) quantify the uncertainty in risk predictions." NRC (1994, Table 9-1) provided a taxonomy of uncertainty in risk analysis that emphasized parameter-value uncertainty and model uncertainty. That report also suggested a strategy for improving a quantitative estimate of uncertainty (Table 9-2) and suggested "that analysts present *separate* assessments of the parameter uncertainty that remains for *each* independent choice of the underlying model(s) involved" (NRC 1994, p. 173).

The NRC (2002) report *Estimating the Public Health Benefits of Proposed Air Pollution Regulations* identified three barriers to the acceptance of recent Environmental Protection Agency (EPA) health benefit analyses: large amounts of uncertainty inherent in such analyses, EPA's manner of dealing with them, and the fact that "projected health benefits are often reported as absolute numbers of avoided death or adverse health outcomes" (p. 126). A primary analysis provides a quantification of uncertainty, but "the probability models in EPA's primary analyses incorporate only one of the many sources of uncertainty in these analyses: the random sampling error in the estimated concentration-response function" (p. 128).

NRC (2002) stated that modelers often assume that their models are correct and base estimates of the models' parameter values on single studies. If a different sample of the same size has been drawn from the population, that procedure would result in different estimates. Uncertainty in the estimated concentration-response function arising in that way is termed random sampling error. Obviously, the model may not be correct or may not be complete, and uncertainties from these sources may be significant.

Ancillary uncertainty analyses list other sources of uncertainty and provide supplementary calculations based on alternative hypotheses. Those uncertainties "may be characterized only subjectively by reference to expert judgment" (NRC 2002, p. 135). EPA is encouraged to "explore alternative options for incorporating expert judgment into its probabilistic uncertainty analyses" (NRC 2002, p. 137).

The Bulletin and the Committee's Response to Proposed Uncertainty Standards

The implications of variability and uncertainty with regard to central estimates and plausible ranges of risks have been discussed. The focus here is on the bulletin sections that address uncertainty directly. The bulletin's special standards for influential risk assessments include the following requirements:

> 4. Characterize uncertainty with respect to the major findings of the assessment including: a. document and disclose the nature and quantitative implications of model uncertainty, and the relative plausibility of different models based on scientific judgment; and where feasible; b. include a sensitivity analysis; and c. provide a quantitative distribution of the uncertainty (OMB 2006, p. 25).

Requiring strict adherence to point 4.c would make the analyst's job very difficult in many circumstances. Such a quantitative distribution of uncertainty can often be produced, but the numerical values of the uncertainty distribution may not be highly accurate. The qualifying "where feasible" is too vague to serve as technical guidance. How is feasibility determined? Could studies with unwelcome results be held to higher feasibility standards? Clear guidance regarding uncertainty defaults would involve recognizing the necessity of such defaults while recognizing their provisional character. At the same time, research is needed to improve and validate default uncertainty factors.

Model uncertainty is mentioned only in the supplementary information:

A model is a mathematical representation—usually a simplified one—of reality. Where a risk can be plausibly characterized by alternative models, the difference between the results
of the alternative models is model uncertainty...When risk assessors face model uncertainty, they need to document and
disclose the nature and degree of model uncertainty. This can
be done by performing multiple assessments with different
models and reporting the extent of the differences in results. A
weighted average of results from alternative models based on
expert weightings may also be informative (OMB 2006, p.
18).

Model uncertainty has been addressed in various ways. For example, parameter uncertainty can be described by placing (joint) distributions over the parameters of a particular model (Jones et al. 2001a), and
then model uncertainty can be addressed by defining a distribution over
possible models (Bailer et al. 2005). Although there are applicable methods for evaluating model uncertainty, there is not yet a standard method
(level 2 of good practice). Methods for determining "a weighted average
of results from alternative models based on expert weightings" (OMB
2006, p. 18) would constitute a research program rather than a body of
applicable techniques. Thus, the committee emphasizes that although
methods exist for addressing model uncertainty, there are no standard
methods, and some methods are still in the initial stages of development.
Furthermore, model uncertainty may dominate parameter uncertainty in
many situations and, as indicated by the lack of standard methods, may
be more difficult, if not impossible, to quantify. That problem is a key
limitation to the bulletin's call for model uncertainty analysis. The committee notes that the selection of the models considered for any averaging process should reflect candidate models that are plausible. The averaging of output from plausible and implausible models is a useless exercise.
    The bulletin is silent on dependence modeling. OMB Circular A-4
does broach this issue briefly:

You should pay attention to correlated inputs. Often times, the
standard defaults in Monte Carlo and other similar simulation
packages assume independence across distributions. Failing to
correctly account for correlated distributions of inputs can
cause the resultant output uncertainty intervals to be too large,

although in many cases the overall effect is ambiguous. You should make a special effort to portray the probabilistic results—in graphs and/or tables—clearly and meaningfully (OMB 2003, pp. 41-42).

Neglecting dependence can lead to large errors, both conservative and nonconservative. The bulletin's silence in this regard is a serious omission. As indicated previously, techniques for inferring, eliciting, and modeling dependence are still the subjects of active research in risk assessment. Technical guidance is premature, but the issue of dependence modeling should be acknowledged and targeted for research.

The ability to quantify and propagate uncertainty is still in development. However, uncertainty analysis has developed further and faster than our ability to *use* the tools in decision-making. Questions, such as how uncertainty analysis should be used to set action levels and make regulatory decisions, deserve more attention.

ADVERSE EFFECTS

The core task of risk assessment is the analysis of risks associated with a particular activity, outcome, or event. The choice of the end point of interest is a critical step in risk assessment. The end point could be a human health effect, such as death, or other events, such as collapse of a bridge or failure of a nuclear reactor. In the discussion of adverse effects, the bulletin limits its discussion almost exclusively to adverse human health effects, with no discussion of adverse effects regarding engineering or other types of adverse effects. This section reviews the statements that are found in the bulletin regarding adverse effects and thus focuses on human health effects.

The bulletin focuses on the choice and determination of an "adverse effect" as the end point of risk assessment and states that "where human health effects are a concern, determinations of which effects are adverse shall be specifically identified and justified based on the best available scientific information generally accepted in the relevant clinical and toxicological communities" (OMB 2006, p. 25).

The supplementary information further emphasizes the choice of the adverse effect rather than a nonadverse effect as the end point and states:

It may be necessary for risk assessment reports to distinguish effects which are adverse from those which are non-adverse...In chemical risk assessment, for example, measuring the concentration of a chemical metabolite in a target tissue of the body is not a demonstration of adverse effect, though it may be a valid indicator of chemical exposure. Even the measurement of a biological event in the human body resulting from exposure to a specific chemical may not be a demonstration of an adverse effect. Adversity typically implies some functional impairment or pathologic lesion that affects the performance of the whole organism or reduces an organism's ability to withstand or respond to additional environmental challenges. In cases where qualified specialists disagree as to whether a measured effect is adverse or likely to be adverse, the extent of the differences in scientific opinion about adversity should be disclosed in the risk assessment report. In order to convey how the choice of the adverse effect influences a safety assessment, it is useful for the analyst to provide a graphical portrayal of different "safe levels" based on different effects observed in various experiments. If an unusual or mild effect is used in making the adverse-effect determination, the assessment should describe the ramifications of the effect and its degree of adversity compared to adverse effects that are better understood and commonly used in safety assessment (OMB 2006, p. 20).

The above definition of a human adverse effect as typically one in which "some functional impairment or pathologic lesion...affects the performance of the whole organism or reduces an organism's ability to withstand or respond to additional environmental challenges" (OMB 2006, p. 20) implies a *clinically* apparent effect.[4] However, a goal of public health is to control exposures before the occurrence of functional impairment of the whole organism. Recent efforts have been made to identify measurable adverse effects or biologic changes that occur at a point in which they are minor, reversible, or subclinical and that do not

---

[4]The proposed definition of *adverse effect* generally follows the approach of EPA. However, the distinction is that previous EPA guidance on this matter has been relatively flexible and could be adjusted or changed as science advanced.

result in functional impairment of the whole organism, even in the most vulnerable or susceptible individuals in the population.

Dividing effects into dichotomous categories of adverse and nonadverse is problematic. Adverse effects usually develop along a continuum, starting with uptake of a toxicant, distribution and metabolism, contact with a target organ, biologic change, physiologic response and repair, and clinical disease. Thus, with some doses and hosts, biologic changes occur, but the body has sufficient defense mechanisms for detoxification or adaptation, and there is little or no adverse cumulative effect, particularly at a low dose. In other situations, biologic changes are measurable and are precursors of an adverse clinical change, so an adverse effect, or precursor of an adverse effect, could be defined in terms of a chemical metabolite or biologic change that is an indicator of both exposure and effect. The same biologic change could have little impact at a small dose (and so be termed nonadverse using the bulletin's approach) but produce a much larger impact at a greater dose or in a more vulnerable person (and thus be termed adverse).

Two common examples are exposure to carbon monoxide (CO) and exposure to an organophosphorus pesticide. CO binds to hemoglobin about 200 times better than oxygen and thus reduces the amount of oxygen carried and released to the body's tissues. For CO, a biologic (biochemical) monitoring test is used to measure carboxyhemoglobin concentration. At very low concentrations, such as current background concentrations (1-2%), enough oxygen is usually brought to the tissues for there to be no discernible clinical or subclinical effects. However, even mild increases (to 4-6%) can cause symptoms in vulnerable populations. For example, those with underlying heart conditions can experience an increase in cardiac arrhythmias (Sheps et al. 1990) and a decrease in exercise performance (Allred et al. 1989). The developing fetus is also more susceptible to decreases in oxygen content and increases in CO. Therefore, ambient-air standards for CO are set well below the concentrations that would be expected to cause clinical effects even in more susceptible populations.

Organophosphorus and carbamate insecticides can inhibit the metabolism of a variety of enzymes called esterases. An important one is the enzyme acetylcholinesterase, which breaks down the neurotransmitter acetylcholine. If too much acetylcholine accumulates, there is excessive stimulation of cholinergic nerves, which can lead to a variety of symptoms, including blurry vision, increased salivation, diarrhea, muscle twitching, and, at higher doses, lowered heart rate, cardiac collapse, and death. Biologic monitoring relies on the measurement of blood cholinesterase activity. The percentage reduction of cholinesterase activity is a measurement of the extent of exposure and often correlates with adverse effects. Medical surveillance and regulations have been based on changes in cholinesterase activity (see, for example, Cal. Code of Regs. tit. 3 § 6728 [2003]). Actions are ordered, even if workers have no clinical symptoms, to avoid continued exposure, reduce the risk of further inhibition of acetylcholinesterase, and prevent the development of acute clinical poisoning or subclinical effects. Toxicologic risk assessment of these insecticides could be based on an end point related to the mode of action (for example, a drop in acetylcholinesterase to 70% of baseline) even if exposed people have no symptoms at that concentration. Rather than dwell on whether an effect can be technically classified as adverse or nonadverse, it seems preferable to explain the rationale for the choice of whatever end point is chosen for the risk assessment, using the best available scientific information generally accepted in the relevant clinical and toxicology communities.

The characterization of adversity as "some functional impairment or pathologic lesion that affects the performance of the whole organism" (OMB 2006, p. 20) is not appropriate for microbial risk assessment. Microbial risk assessment often focuses on the risk of infection rather than directly on the manifestation of adverse effects. Infection (replication of an organism in a host) does not always result in illness, death, or symptoms that affect the performance of the whole organism. The outcome depends on the virulence of the organism, immune responses, and other host factors, such as other underlying diseases. In many enteric infections, many people may have a relatively asymptomatic infection or mild illness but be able to spread the infection through the community. For example, young children infected with hepatitis A have a relatively mild or subclinical illness but shed the virus and are important vehicles of transmission in households and day-care settings (Wallace 1998, pp. 174-178). Similarly, the vast majority of poliovirus infections are asymptomatic, but infected people can excrete the virus in their stools for several weeks (Wallace 1998, pp. 123-127). Others infected with the same enteric organisms may experience frank illness that in some cases can have serious sequelae, including paralysis and other residual neurologic impairment (in the case of poliovirus). Thus, EPA established a goal for the treatment of surface waters of 1:10,000 per year to reduce the annual risks of infection (not illness or disease outcome) (Regli et al. 1991).

Another problem with the focus on effects on the whole organism is that it does not address toxicants that preferentially affect one organ (the target organ), such as cadmium and the kidney. The Occupational Safety and Health Administration standard for cadmium mandates both measurement of an exposure (blood and urine cadmium) and evidence of potential injury to the kidney tubule (in the form of beta-2-microglobulin). Actions are taken at various levels of exposure and increases in beta-2-microglobulin to prevent irreversible kidney damage; those actions are taken at levels well below those expected to result in clinically detectable impairment of kidney function (such as a rise in blood urea nitrogen or creatinine) (29 CFR1910.1027 [2006]).

Sometimes, a biologic effect is chosen because there are more reliable data available for it, and it is a precursor of a more serious adverse outcome. That is the rationale offered in the recent NRC report *Health Implications of Perchlorate Ingestion* (NRC 2005). The NRC committee acknowledged that perchlorate's inhibition of iodide uptake "is the key biochemical event and not an adverse effect [and] should be used as the basis of the risk assessment. Inhibition of iodide uptake is a more reliable and valid measure, it has been unequivocally demonstrated in humans exposed to perchlorate, and it is the key event that precedes all thyroid-mediated effects of perchlorate exposure" (NRC 2005, p. 14). In this situation, the NRC perchlorate committee recommended using a "nonadverse" effect rather than an "adverse" effect as the point of departure for the perchlorate risk assessment as a health-protective approach. One reason for that approach was the lack of data on the association of perchlorate exposure with thyroid dysfunction in the groups of greatest concern: low-birthweight or preterm newborns, offspring of mothers who had iodide deficiency during gestation, and offspring of hypothyroid mothers.

Among the questions to OMB, the committee asked whether the bulletin supports using a precursor of an adverse effect or other mechanistic data as the basis of a risk assessment, as was recommended in the perchlorate review. OMB responded that although the bulletin does not speak to specific use of precursor effects, it does not preclude the use of a precursor of an adverse effect or other mechanistic data as the basis of a risk assessment. The committee nevertheless concludes that the bulletin's focus on the choice of an adverse effect and the description of what is and is not an adverse effect give a strong message for what would be considered acceptable and nonacceptable end points for toxicologic risk assessment.

In summary, on the topic of risk assessment end points and adverse effects, the committee concludes that the bulletin has ventured into a technical realm of the risk assessment process that is scientifically complex and uncertain and has offered simplistic and restrictive guidance concerning adverse effects. The committee notes that this issue is one of many scientifically difficult matters that much be confronted in the conduct of risk assessment. Why OMB has chosen to emphasize this one matter as opposed to any of a number of other complex issues is unclear.

RISK COMPARISIONS

The bulletin's Standard 6 under general risk assessment standards states that a risk assessment should "provide an executive summary including.... d. information that places the risk in context/perspective with other risks familiar to the target audience" (OMB 2006, p. 24). The supplementary information adds, "Due care must be taken in making risk comparisons. Agencies might want to consult the risk communication literature when considering appropriate comparisons. Although the risk assessor has considerable latitude in making risk comparisons, the fundamental point is that risk should be placed in context that is useful and relevant to the intended audience" (OMB 2006, p. 15).

There are two conceivable legitimate purposes for risk comparisons. Readers who consult the risk communication literature will find that serving either purpose requires both formal analysis to ensure that defensible comparisons are being made and dedicated empirical research to ensure that the result is understood as intended. Readers of that literature will also find that poorly done risk comparisons can confuse, mislead, and antagonize recipients. Unless done in a scientifically sound way, risk comparisons are unlikely to be useful and relevant and hence should be avoided.

One conceivable legitimate purpose is giving recipients an intuitive feeling for just how large a risk is by comparing it with another, otherwise similar, risk that recipients understand. For example, roughly one American in a million dies from lightning in an average year (NOAA 1995). "As likely as being hit by lightning" would be a relevant and useful comparison for someone who has an accurate intuitive feeling for the probability of being hit by lightning, faces roughly that "average" risk, and considers the comparison risk to be like death by lightning in all important respects. It is not hard to imagine each of these conditions failing, rendering the comparisons irrelevant or harmful:

(a) Lightning deaths are so vivid and newsworthy that they might be overestimated relative to other, equally probable events. But "being struck by lightning" is an iconic very-low-probability risk, meaning that it might be underestimated. Where either occurs, the comparison will mislead (Lichtenstein et al. 1978; NRC 1989).

(b) Individual Americans face different risks from lightning. For example, they are, on the average, much higher for golfers than for nursing-home residents. A blanket statement would mislead readers who did not think about this variability and what their risk is relative to that of the average American (Slovic 2000; Tversky and Kahneman 1974).

(c) Death by lightning has distinctive properties. It is sometimes immediate, sometimes preceded by painful suffering. It can leave victims and their survivors unprepared. It offers some possibility of risk reduction, which people may understand to some degree. It poses an acute threat at some very limited times but typically no threat at all. Each of those properties may lead people to judge them differently—and undermine the relevance of comparisons with risks having different properties (Fischhoff et al. 1978; Lowrance 1976).

(d) It is often assumed that the risks being used for comparison are widely considered acceptable at their present levels. The risks may be accepted in the trivial sense that people are, in fact, living with them. But that does not make them acceptable in the sense that people believe that they are as low as they should or could be. It would be wrong to make comparisons with risks that responsible organizations are working diligently to reduce. For example, the National Lightning Safety Institute (NLSI) and the United States Golf Association do not consider contemporary risks of injury and death from lightning strikes to be acceptable: "A strong case can be made for reducing lightning's human and economic costs through the adoption of proactive defensive guidelines" (Kithil 1995).

The second conceivable use of risk comparisons is to facilitate making consistent decisions regarding different risks. Other things being equal, one would want similar risks from different sources to be treated the same. However, many things might need to be held equal, including the various properties of risks (discussed above) that might make people want to treat them differently despite similarity in one dimension (for example, annual fatality rate among Americans) (HM Treasury 2005; Wittenberg et al. 2003).

The same risk may be acceptable in one setting but not another if the associated benefits are different (for example, being struck by lightning while golfing or working on a road crew). Even when making voluntary decisions, people do not accept risks in isolation but in the context of the associated benefits. As a result, *acceptable risk* is a misnomer except as shorthand for a voluntarily assumed risk accompanied by acceptable benefits (Fischhoff et al. 1981).

The bulletin does not convey how difficult it is to produce useful and relevant risk comparisons. Unless such comparisons are developed in a scientifically sound and empirically evaluated way that addresses the values and circumstances of all recipients, risk comparisons should not be made.

SUMMARY OF COMMITTEE COMMENTS ON INDIVIDUAL STANDARDS

The proposed bulletin describes 16 standards for risk assessment; they are listed in Table 4-3. Many of the standards have multiple components. Section IV of the bulletin describes seven general risk assessment and reporting standards of which the seventh refers to risk assessments for regulatory analysis. Section V describes nine special standards for influential risk assessments. The standards comprise a mixture of qualitative and quantitative requirements. The committee reviewed each standard and component separately for soundness and clarity. The committee also considered the general question of developing and implementing the risk assessment guidance for all federal agencies.

The committee found many of the standards to be unclear or flawed. It also evaluated whether each proposed standard pertained to risk assessment and hence should be addressed by risk assessors or should guide risk managers or others. The committee's concerns are described below and summarized in Table 4-3. Because of the major changes required to rectify the proposed standards, the lack of a clear rationale for proposing the particular standards, and the heterogeneity of risk assessment applications in the federal government, the committee concludes that OMB should not be issuing these standards as technical guidance and that, as discussed in Chapter 7, the development of technical guidance should be left to the individual agencies.

TABLE 4-3 Technical and Scientific Circumstances That Prevent the Current Applicability of the Bulletin

General Risk Assessment Standards (from Bulletin)	Technical and Scientific Evaluation (from Committee)
1. Provide a clear statement of the informational needs of decision makers, including the objectives of the risk assessment. 2. Clearly summarize the scope of the assessment, including a description of: a. the agent, technology and/or activity that is the subject of the assessment; b. the hazard of concern; c. the affected entities (population(s), subpopulation(s), individuals, natural resources, ecosystems, or other) that are the subject of the assessment; d. the exposure/event scenarios relevant to the objectives of the assessment; and e. the type of event-consequence or dose-response relationship for the hazard of concern.	These qualitative standards (1-2. e) could improve the clarity of risk assessment in the federal government for any risk assessments that do not already implement such standards (although the existence of such problems is not established by the bulletin). They are consistent with recommendations of cited studies.
3. Provide a characterization of risk, qualitatively and, whenever possible, quantitatively. When a quantitative characterization of risk is provided, a range of plausible risk estimates shall be provided.	The standard does not provide clear guidance on how such a range is to be defined. As a result, it may produce confusion that could erode the quality of risk assessment. The term *plausible risk estimate* is undefined in the bulletin. If a distribution is substantially skewed or bimodal, identifying a single estimate considered a "plausible" estimate of the distribution is not meaningful. In that case, a "central" estimate will not reasonably represent the distribution. When distributions reflect variability, the ambiguous term *plausible* appears to be at odds with the fundamental orientation of public-health practice and prevention, especially when the applicable laws seek to protect the most

	vulnerable in the population: infants, children, the elderly, and those with illnesses or predispositions to illness. Using a mean or central estimate to identify the most "plausible" individual would undermine public-health goals.

This and related standards represent technical guidance. Although the issues of uncertainty and variability are topics of general concern in risk assessment, the detailed implementation of uncertainty and variability analyses is best addressed by individual agencies to reflect their expertise in the relevant science as applied to their mandate. |
| 4. Be scientifically objective:

a. as a matter of substance, neither minimizing nor exaggerating the nature and magnitude of risks;

b. giving weight to both positive and negative studies in light of each study's technical quality; and

c. as a matter of presentation:

i. presenting the information about risk in an accurate, clear, complete and unbiased manner; and

ii. describing the data, methods, and assumptions used in the assessment with a high degree of transparency. | Components 4.a and 4.c could improve the clarity of a risk assessment in any context where they are not already practiced (although the existence of such problems is not established by the bulletin). Component 4.a could, however, degrade risk analysis if it were interpreted so as to deprive decision-makers of important information on sensitive subpopulations on the grounds that such information may generate risk estimates considerably higher than a central tendency or general population estimates. Information on the variability of effects across potentially affected populations is essential to decision-making.

Component 4.b is problematic because it requires assigning weights, despite the lack of a standard procedure for doing so. Assigning weights is a matter of judgment and explicitly introduces another element of uncertainty. Thus, specific weights should not be assigned to studies. Rather, the most appropriate scientific information should be considered during preparation of risk assessments. |
| 5. For critical assumptions in the assessment, whenever possible, include a quantitative evaluation of reasonable alternative assumptions and their implications for the key findings of the assessment. | This standard's lack of specificity prevents any meaningful application. If the standard is referring to model assumptions, it may be ignoring more important assumptions in other aspects of the risk assessment. If it is referring to default assumptions, it may be ignoring critical science-policy concerns or statutory requirements, such as protection of sensitive people. The vagueness of the standard could open the door to endless guesswork. |

(Continued)

TABLE 4-3 Continued

General Risk Assessment Standards (from Bulletin)	Technical and Scientific Evaluation (from Committee)
6. Provide an executive summary including: a. key elements of the assessment's objectives and scope; b. key findings; c. key scientific limitations and uncertainties and, whenever possible, their quantitative implications; and d. information that places the risk in context/perspective with other risks familiar to the target audience.	These qualitative standards (6a-c) could improve the clarity of risk assessment in the federal government if risk assessments do not implement them already (although the existence of such problems is not established by the bulletin). They are consistent with recommendations of cited studies. However, there are numerous problems in the bulletin's treatment of uncertainty. Standard 6.d does not pertain to risk assessment, but to risk communication. This component is at variance with the scientific literature, and the reference to risk communication is inconsistent with current scientific understanding, as set forth by NRC and other bodies. The bulletin suggests one-way risk communication. Instead, risk communication is an essential element of all stages of risk assessment. Unless the risk communication occurs at all stages of the risk assessment and to all stakeholders, it may be misdirected and mistrusted. The wording of this standard is so vague as to be useless. It also recommends a practice (risk comparison) that has been widely criticized as potentially illogical and as potentially reducing rather than enhancing the usefulness of such an assessment.
General Risk Assessment Standards for Risk Assessments Applicable to Regulatory Analysis (from Bulletin)	Technical and Scientific Evaluation (from Committee)
7. For risk assessments that will be used for regulatory analysis, the risk assessment also shall include: a. an evaluation of alternative options, clearly establishing the baseline risk as well as the risk reduction alternatives that will be evaluated;	The standards identified as 7a-c should not be part of risk assessment guidance. The first recommendation of the *Red Book* is this: "We recommend that regulatory agencies take steps to establish and maintain a clear conceptual distinction between assessment of risks and consideration of risk management alternatives; that is, the scientific findings and policy judgments embodied in risk assessments should be explicitly distinguished from the political, economic, and technical considerations that influence the design and choice of regulatory strategies" (NRC 1983, p. 7).

b. a comparison of the baseline risk against the risk associated with the alternative mitigation measures being considered, and assess, to the extent feasible, countervailing risks caused by alternative mitigation measures;

c. information on the timing of exposure and the onset of the adverse effect(s), as well as the timing of control measures and the reduction or cessation of adverse effects;

d. estimates of population risk when estimates of individual risk are developed; and

The standards described in 7a-c ignore the essential distinction between risk assessment and risk management. Although it is important that there be communication between risk assessor and risk manager, risk management tasks and decisions should not be delegated to the risk assessment. Furthermore, although risk assessors may evaluate various risk management options (for example, mitigation options for a Superfund site), the risk assessment should remain distinct from the political, economic, and technical considerations of risk management.

The issue of resources also arises with these standards. For example, standard 7b requires that the countervailing risks caused by alternative mitigation measures be considered. That requirement would substantially broaden the content and scope of risk assessments. Resources to accomplish that task would probably not be available, and information on choices of alternative measures would probably reside with the risk manager, not the risk assessor.

The reference to population risk is unclear and undefined in the bulletin. A common practice in health risk assessment is to estimate population risk by calculating the total population impact (that is, risk times population exposure). That estimate may be referred to as "population burden" rather than "population risk." In other cases, population risk may be evaluated by considering the distribution of risks within a population or the shift of the population with regard to a risk. Thus, although the health risk assessment field usually follows the total-population-impact convention, the situation is dynamic, and as methods evolve, the applicability of one convention to all types of risk assessments and situations is not likely to be practical or possible.

Another important consideration is that estimates of individual risk are generally developed to address concerns for the most vulnerable people in a population—who, almost by definition, lie in the tails of the probability distribution. To protect the entire population, one often evaluates the risk to the most vulnerable. Thus, the risk to the entire population includes the risk to the most vulnerable. For example, if one were to evaluate the risk of

(Continued)

TABLE 4-3 Continued

General Risk Assessment Standards for Risk Assessments Applicable to Regulatory Analysis (from Bulletin)	Technical and Scientific Evaluation (from Committee)
	death for a particular ambient-air quality standard, those mostly likely to die from exposure would be the most vulnerable in the population.
e. whenever possible, a range of plausible risk estimates, including central or expected estimates, when a quantitative characterization of risk is made available.	The bulletin's discussion of central and expected estimates and uncertainty is confused and prevents useful application of the standard. It is misleading to suggest as the bulletin does that "central" and "expected" estimates are synonymous. As discussed in the section on "Range of Risk Estimates and Central Estimates," the presentation of single estimates may provide an incomplete picture, and without proper definitions and context, use of the range or "central estimate" will be misleading. The bulletin does not state the distribution to be considered in the evaluation or even whether it is to reflect uncertainty or variability. Instead, the bulletin appears to suggest "averaging" the information from a combined distribution of uncertainty and variability. It is not in decision-makers' or society's interest to treat fundamentally different predictions as quantities that can be "averaged."

Influential Risk Assessment Standards (from Bulletin)	Technical and Scientific Evaluation (from Committee)
General comments on the category	Whether an analysis constitutes an "influential risk assessment" may not be clear at the outset. Moreover, this standard's focus on economic impacts imposes risk management concerns on risk assessment. Arbitrarily separating risk assessments into two broad categories (influential and noninfluential) ignores the continuum of risk assessment efforts.
All influential agency risk assessments shall: 1. Be "capable of being substantially reproduced" as defined in the OMB Information Quality Guidelines	Appears to represent a good practice activity for any risk assessments that do not already implement such standards (although the existence of such problems is not established by the bulletin).

2. Compare the results of the assessment to other results published on the same topic from qualified scientific organizations.	It may be appropriate for some assessments to compare their results with those derived by other scientific organizations regarding such issues as the affected population, geography, time scales, and the definition of adverse effects. However, the bulletin fails to define which comparisons are required. With specialized risk assessments, substantial assumptions may be needed to make comparisons. When external risk assessments have not followed an agency's own standards, comparisons may undermine the quality of its work. Finally, requiring resources to compare results with external risk assessments that do not meet the standards may result in less time to devote to risk assessments by the agency and thus affect the quality and output of agency products.
3. Highlight central estimates as well as high-end and low-end estimates of risk when such estimates are uncertain.	The bulletin's discussion of central estimates and uncertainty is confusing and prevents useful application of the standard. The detailed requirement of a central estimate, as well as high- and low-end estimates, is clearly inapplicable and inappropriate for some types of risk assessments. Some NRC committees have warned that descriptions of "central estimates" of risk may have little meaning when applied to models for high- to low-dose extrapolation.
	Finally, the strong emphasis on central estimates in the bulletin means that the most vulnerable people in a population—who, almost by definition, lie in the tails of the probability distribution—might be underrepresented, depending on the characterization of the central estimate.
4. Characterize uncertainty with respect to the major findings of the assessment including: a. document and disclose the nature and quantitative implications of model uncertainty, and the relative plausibility of different models based on scientific judgment; and where feasible:	The aspiration level in the bulletin is at the edge of the current state of the art and exceeds what is practically feasible. The recent NRC assessments of perchlorate, arsenic, and methyl mercury discussed uncertainties qualitatively, not quantitatively. This standard will force agencies into an unsuitable role of requiring basic research before they can perform their assigned roles. These requirements are not fully articulated, either by the bulletin or by the research community. Many terms are vague, leaving the requirements

(Continued)

TABLE 4-3 Continued

Influential Risk Assessment Standards (from Bulletin)	Technical and Scientific Evaluation (from Committee)
b. include a sensitivity analysis; and c. provide a quantitative distribution of the uncertainty.	not operational. The bulletin does not constitute "technical guidance" and hence cannot "enhance the technical quality....of risk assessments" (OMB 2006, p. 3).
5. Portray results based on different effects observed and/or different studies to convey how the choice of effect and/or study influences the assessment.	The wording of this standard may undermine good scientific practice. In many cases, basing results on alternative effects can be counterproductive. For example, for methyl mercury, the assessment should be based on the most sensitive effect and not on a less sensitive or "alternate" effect. The presentation of alternative analyses may not be informative. The standard does not allow risk assessors sufficient flexibility to adapt to the nature of the available data and science.
6. Characterize, to the extent feasible, variability through a quantitative distribution, reflecting different affected population(s), time scales, geography, or other parameters relevant to the needs and objectives of the assessment.	If this standard is implemented literally, few risk assessments could be completed without significant new research and tool development.
7. Where human health effects are a concern, determinations of which effects are adverse shall be specifically identified and justified based on the best available scientific information generally accepted in the relevant clinical and toxicological communities.	The bulletin's definition of *adverse effect* implies a *clinically* apparent effect. This ignores public health's fundamental goal of controlling exposures well before the occurrence of functional impairment of the whole organism. Dividing effects into dichotomous categories of "adverse" and "nonadverse" ignores the scientific reality that adverse effects may be manifested along a continuum. Furthermore, many effects of central importance to public health (and risk assessment) are not adverse themselves but associated with healthy functioning, for example, carboxyhemoglobin formation, acetylcholinesterase inhibition, and microbial infection. The bulletin proposes simplistic and restrictive guidance concerning adverse effects, which is at odds with relevant science and legislation.

8. Provide discussion, to the extent possible, of the nature, difficulty, feasibility, cost and time associated with undertaking research to resolve a report's key scientific limitations and uncertainties.	This standard appears to address how much the uncertainty could be reduced with various investments in research. That is not risk assessment, but management of risk assessment. Because each risk assessment involves many "default" assumptions, it would be more cost-effective to undertake this activity as an overarching research activity and not as a component of each influential risk assessment.
9. Consider all significant comments received on a draft risk assessment report and: a. issue a "response-to-comment" document that summarizes the significant comments received and the agency's responses to those comments; and b. provide a rationale for why the agency has not adopted the position suggested by commenters and why the agency position is preferable.	Appears to represent a good practice for any risk assessments that do not already implement such standards (although the existence of such problems is not established by the bulletin). However, requiring a federal agency to provide a rationale for why its position is preferable to positions proposed by commenters is likely to expend excessive resources and might result in less time to devote to agency risk assessments, thus affecting the quality and output of agency products.

REFERENCES

AEC (U.S. Atomic Energy Commission). 1957. Theoretical Possibilities and Consequences of Major Accidents in Large Nuclear Power Plants. WASH-740. Washington, DC: U.S. Atomic Energy Commission.

Allred, E.N., E.R. Bleecker, B.R. Chaitman, T.E. Dahms, S.O. Gottlieb, J.D. Hackney, M. Pagano, R.H. Selvester, S.M. Walden, and J. Warren. 1989. Short term effects of carbon monoxide exposure on the exercise performance of subjects with coronary artery disease. N. Engl. J. Med. 321(21):1426-1432.

ANS (American Nuclear Society). 2003. ANSI/ANS-58.21-2003. External-Events PRA Methodology: American National Standard. American Nuclear Society. December 2003.

ASME (American Society of Mechanical Engineers). 2005. ASME RA-Sb-2005. Standard for Probabilistic Risk Assessment for Nuclear Power Plant Applications: Addendum B to ASME RA-S-2002. American Society of Mechanical Engineer. December 30, 2005.

Bailer, A.J., R.B. Noble, and M.W. Wheeler. 2005. Model uncertainty and risk estimation for experimental studies of quantal responses. Risk Anal. 25(2):291-299.

Bedford, T., and R.M. Cooke. 2001. P. 5 in Probabilistic Risk Analysis: Foundations and Methods. Cambridge: Cambridge University Press.

Brown, J., L.H.J. Goossens, F.T. Harper, B.C.P. Kraan, F.E. Haskin, M.L. Abbott, R.M. Cooke, M.L. Young, J.A. Jones S.C. Hora, A. Rood and J. Randall. 1997. Probabilistic Accident Consequence Uncertainty Study: Food Chain Uncertainty Assessment, Vols. 1 and 2. NUREG/CR-6523, EUR 16771, SAND97-0335. Prepared for Division of Systems Technology, Office of Nuclear Regulatory Research, U.S. Nuclear Regulatory Commission, Washington, DC and Commission of the European Communities, Brussels. Luxembourg: Office for Publications of the European Communities [online]. Available: http://www.osti.gov/bridge/servlets/purl/510290-keuF8T/webviewable/510290.pdf and http: //www.osti.gov/bridge/servlets/purl/510291-eUsNPE/webviewable/510291.pdf [accessed Oct. 16, 2006].

Brown, J., J. Ehrhardt, L.H.J. Goossens, R.M. Cooke, F. Fischer, I. Hasemann, J.A. Jones, B.C.P. Kraan, and J.G. Smith. 2001. Probabilistic Accident Consequence Uncertainty Assessment Using COSYMA: Uncertainty from the Food Chain Module. EUR 18823. FZKA 6309. European Communities [online]. Available: ftp://ftp.cordis.europa.eu/pub/fp5-euratom/docs/eur18823_en.pdf [accessed Oct. 17, 2006].

Budnitz, R.J., G. Apostolakis, D.M. Boore, L.S. Cluff, K.J. Coppersmith, C.A. Cornell, and P.A. Morris. 1997. Recommendations for Probabilistic Seismic Hazard Analysis: Guidance on Uncertainty and Use of Experts. NUREG/CR-6372. Prepared for Division of Engineering Technology,

Office of Nuclear Regulatory Research, U.S. Nuclear Regulatory Commission, Washington DC, Office of Defense Programs, U.S. Department of Energy, Germantown, MD, and Electric Power Research Institute, Palo Alto, CA, by Senior Seismic Hazard Analysis Committee (SSHAC) [online]. Available: http://www.osti.gov/ energycitations/servlets/purl/479072-krGkYU/webviewable/479072.pdf [accessed Oct. 18, 2006].

Cooke, R.M., and L.H.J. Goossens. 1999. Nuclear Science and Technology: Procedures Guide for Structured Expert Judgment. EUR 18820EN. Prepared for Commission of European Communities Directorate-general XI (Environment and Nuclear Safety), Luxembourg, by Delft University of Technology, Delft, The Netherlands. June 1999 [online]. Available: ftp://ftp.cordis.europa.eu/pub/fp5-euratom/docs/eur18820_en.pdf [accessed Oct. 17, 2006].

DOE (U.S. Department of Energy). 1996. Characterization of Uncertainties in Risk Assessment with Special Reference to Probabilistic Uncertainty Analysis. RCRA/CERCLA Information Brief. EH 413-068/0496. U.S. Department of Energy, Office of Environmental Policy and Assistance [online]. Available: http://www.eh.doe.gov/oepa/guidance/risk/uncert.pdf [accessed Oct. 16, 2006].

Eckerman, K.F., R.W. Leggett, C.B. Nelson, J.S. Puskin, and A.C.B. Richardson. 1999. Cancer Risk Coefficients for Environmental Exposure to Radionuclides. Federal Guidance Report No.13. EPA 402-R-99-001. Prepared for Office of Radiation and Indoor Air, U.S. Environmental Protection Agency, Washington, DC, by Oak Ridge National Laboratory, Oak Ridge, TN. September 1999 [online]. Available: http://www.epa.gov/radiation/docs/federal/402-r-99-001.pdf [accessed Oct. 16, 2006].

Fischhoff, B., P. Slovic, S. Lichtenstein, S. Read, and B. Combs. 1978. How safe is safe enough? A psychometric study of attitudes towards technological risks and benefits. Policy Sci. 9(2):127-152.

Fischhoff, B., S. Lichtenstein, P. Slovic, S.L. Derby, and R.L. Keeney. 1981. Acceptable Risk. New York: Cambridge University Press.

Garrick, B.J. 1984. Recent case studies and advancements in probabilistic risk assessments. Risk Anal. 4(4):267-279.

Goossens, L.H.J., R.M. Cooke, and B.C.P. Kraan. 1996. Evaluation of Weighting Schemes for Expert Judgement Studies. Prepared for Commission of the European Communities, Directorate-General for Science, Research and Development, XII-F-6, by Delft University of Technology, Delft, The Netherlands. 75 pp.

Goossens, L.H.J., J. Boardman, F.T. Harper, B.C.P. Kraan, R.M. Cooke, M.L. Young, J.A. Jones, and S.C. Hora. 1997. Probabilistic Accident Consequence Uncertainty Study: Uncertainty Assessment for Deposited Material and External Doses, Vols. 1 and 2. NUREG/CR-6526. EUR 16772. SAND97-2323. Prepared for Division of Systems Technology,

Office of Nuclear Regulatory Research, U.S. Nuclear Regulatory Commission, Washington, DC and Commission of the European Communities, Brussels. Luxembourg: Office for Publications of the European Communities [online]. Available: http://www.osti.gov/ bridge/servlets/purl/291006-pL3L0D/webviewable/291006.pdf http:// www.osti.gov/bridge/servlets/purl/291007-7XzROO/webviewable/291 007.pdf [accessed Oct. 16, 2006].

Goossens, L.H.J, J.A. Jones, J. Ehrhardt, B.C.P. Kraan, and R.M. Cooke. 2001. Probabilistic Accident Consequence Uncertainty Assessment: Countermeasures Uncertainty Assessment. EUR 18821. FZKA 6307. European Communities [online]. Available: ftp://ftp.cordis.europa.eu/ pub/fp5-euratom/docs/eur18821_en.pdf [accessed Oct. 17, 2006].

Harper, F.T., L.H.J. Goossens, R.M. Cooke, S.C. Hora, M.L. Young, J. Päsler-Sauer, L.A. Miller, B. Kraan, C. Lui, M.D. McKay, J.C. Helton and J.A. Jones. 1995. Probabilistic Accident Consequence Uncertainty Study: Dispersion and Deposition Uncertainty Assessment, Vol. 1 and 2. NUREG/CR-6244. EUR 15855 EN, SAND94-1453. Prepared for Division of Systems Technology, Office of Nuclear Regulatory Research, U.S. Nuclear Regulatory Commission, Washington, DC, and Commission of the European Communities, Brussels. Luxembourg: Office for Publications of the European Communities [online]. Available: http://www.osti.gov/bridge/servlets/purl/10125585-aArQNy/web viewable/10125585.pdf, http://www.osti.gov/bridge/servlets/purl/2504 1-SZccBx/webviewable/25041.pdf [accessed Oct. 17, 2006].

Haskin, F.E., F.T. Harper, L.H.J. Goossens, B.C.P. Kraan, J.B. Grupa, and J. Randall. 1997. Probabilistic Accident Consequence Uncertainty Study: Early Health Effects Uncertainty Assessment, Vols. 1 and 2. NUREG/CR-6545. EUR 16775. SAND97-2689. Prepared for Division of Systems Technology, Office of Nuclear Regulatory Research, U.S. Nuclear Regulatory Commission, Washington, DC, and Commission of the European Communities, Brussels. Luxembourg: Office for Publications of the European Communities [online]. Available: http://www. osti.gov/bridge/servlets/purl/291010-cH8Oey/webviewable/291010.pdf and http://www.osti.gov/bridge/servlets/purl/291011-8Nk nmm/web viewable/291011.pdf [accessed Oct. 17, 2006].

HM Treasury (Her Majesty's Treasury). 2005. Managing Risks to the Public: Appraisal Guidance. London: HM Treasury. June 2005 [online]. Available: http://www.hm-treasury.gov.uk/media/8AB/54/Managing_risks _to_the_public.pdf [accessed Oct. 18, 2006].

Hoeting, J.A., D. Madigan, A.E. Raftery, and C.T. Volinsky. 1999. Bayesian model averaging: A tutorial. Stat. Sci. 14(4):382-417.

Jones, J., J. Ehrhardt, L.H.J. Goossens, J. Brown, R.M. Cooke, F. Fischer, I. Hasemann, and B.C.P. Kraan. 2001a. Probabilistic Accident Consequence Uncertainty Assessment Using COSYMA: Methodology and Processing Techniques. EUR 18827. FZKA-6313. European Communities [online]. Available: ftp://ftp.cordis.europa.eu/pub/fp5-euratom/ docs/eur18827_en.pdf [accessed Oct.17, 2006].

Jones, J., J. Ehrhardt, L.H.J. Goossens, J. Brown, R.M. Cooke, F. Fischer, I. Hasemann, and B.C.P. Kraan. 2001b. Probabilistic Accident Consequence Uncertainty Assessment Using COSYMA: Overall Uncertainty Analysis. EUR 18826. FZKA 6312. European Communities [online]. Available: ftp://ftp.cordis.europa.eu/pub/fp5-euratom/docs/eur18826_ en.pdf [accessed Oct. 17, 2006].

Jones, J., J. Ehrhardt, L.H.J. Goossens, J. Brown, R.M. Cooke, F. Fischer, I. Hasemann, B.C.P. Kraan, A. Khursheed, and A. Phipps. 2001c. Probabilistic Accident Consequence Uncertainty Assessment Using COSYMA: Uncertainty from the Dose Module. EUR 18825. FZKA-6311. European Communities [online]. Available: ftp://ftp.cordis. europa.eu/pub/fp5-euratom/docs/eur18825_en.pdf [accessed Oct. 17, 2006].

Jones, J., J. Ehrhardt, L.H.J. Goossens, R.M. Cooke, F. Fischer, Hasemann, and B.C.P. Kraan. 2001d. Probabilistic Accident Consequence Uncertainty Assessment Using COSYMA: Uncertainty from the Early and Late Health Effects Module. EUR 18824. FZKA-6310. European Communities [online]. Available: ftp://ftp.cordis.europa.eu/pub/fp5-euratom/ docs/eur18824_en.pdf [accessed Oct. 17, 2006].

Jones, J., J. Ehrhardt, L.H.J. Goossens, R.M. Cooke, F. Fischer, Hasemann, and B.C.P. Kraan. 2001e. Probabilistic Accident Consequence Uncertainty Assessment Using COSYMA: Uncertainty from the Atmospheric Dispersion and Deposition Module. EUR 18822. FZKA-6308. European Communities [online]. Available: ftp://ftp.cordis.europa.eu/pub/fp5-euratom/docs/eur18822_en.pdf [accessed Oct. 17, 2006].

Kang, S.H., R.L. Kodell, and J.J. Chen. 2000. Incorporating model uncertainties along with data uncertainties in microbial risk assessment. Regul. Toxicol. Pharmacol. 32(1):68-72.

Kemeny, J. 1979. Report of the President's Commission on the Accident at Three Mile Island. Report of the Public Health And Safety Task Force. Washington, DC: U.S. Government Printing Office. October 1979 [online]. Available: http://www.threemileisland.org/downloads//193. pdf [accessed Nov. 27, 2006].

Kithil, R. 1995. Lightning's Social and Economic Costs. Presentation at International Aerospace and Ground Conference on Lightning and Static Electricity, September 26-28, 1995, Williamsburg, VA [online]. Available: http://www.lightningsafety.com/nlsi_lls/sec.html [accessed Oct. 18, 2006].

IRIS (Integrated Risk Information System). 2006. IRIS Database for Risk Assessment, U.S. Environmental Protection Agency [online]. Available: http://www.epa.gov/iris/ [accessed Nov. 10. 2006].

Lewis, H.W., R.J. Budnitz, H.J.C. Kouts, W.B. Loewenstein, W.D. Rowe, F. von Hippel, and F. Zachanariasen. 1978. Risk Assessment Review

Group Report to the U.S. Nuclear Regulatory Commission. NUREG/CR-0400. Nuclear Regulatory Commission, Washington, DC. 76pp.

Lichtenstein, S., P. Slovic, B. Fischhoff, M. Layman, and B. Combs. 1978. Judged frequency of lethal events. J. Exp. Psychol. Learn. 4:551-578.

Little, M.P., C.M. Muirhead, L.H.J. Goossens, F.T. Harper, B.C.P. Kraan, R.M. Cooke, and S.C. Hora. 1997. Probabilistic Accident Consequence Uncertainty Analysis: Late Health Effects Uncertainty Assessment, Vols. 1 and 2. NUREG/CR-6555. EUR 16774. SAND97-2322. Prepared for Division of Systems Technology, Office of Nuclear Regulatory Research, U.S. Nuclear Regulatory Commission, Washington, DC, and Commission of the European Communities, Brussels. Luxembourg: Office for Publications of the European Communities [online]. Available: http://www.osti.gov/bridge/servlets/purl/291008-wV5DjS/web viewable/291008.pdf and http://www.osti.gov/bridge/servlets/purl/291 009-fM9p1b/webviewable/291009.pdf [accessed Oct. 18, 2006].

Lowrance, W.W. 1976. Of Acceptable Risk: Science and the Determination of Safety. Los Altos, CA: W. Kaufmann.

Morales, K.H, J.G. Ibrahim, C.J. Chen, and L.M. Ryan. 2006. Bayesian model averaging with applications to benchmark dose estimation for arsenic in drinking water. J. Am. Stat. Assoc. 101(473):9-17.

NASA (National Aeronautics and Space Administration). 2002. Probabilistic Risk Assessment Procedures Guide for NASA Managers and Practitioners, Version 1.1. Prepared for Office of Safety and Mission Assurance NASA Headquarters, Washington, DC [online]. Available: http://www.hq.nasa.gov/office/codeq/doctree/praguide.pdf [accessed Oct. 18, 2006].

NASA (National Aeronautics and Space Administration). 2004. Probabilistic Risk Assessment Procedures Guide for NASA Managers and Practitioners. NPR 8705.5. Office of Safety and Mission Assurance NASA Headquarters, Washington, DC [online]. Available: http://nodis3.gsfc.nasa.gov/npg_img/N_PR_8705_0005_/N_PR_8705_0005_.pdf [accessed Oct. 23, 2006].

NEI (Nuclear Energy Institute). 2000. Probabilistic Risk Assessment Peer Review Process Guidance, Revision A3. NEI-00-02. Washington, DC: Nuclear Energy Institute. March 20, 2000.

NOAA (National Oceanic and Atmospheric Administration). 1995. Natural Hazard Fatalities for the United States, 1994. National Oceanic and Atmospheric Administration, Washington, DC.

NRC (National Research Council). 1983. Risk Assessment in the Federal Government: Managing the Process. Washington, DC: National Academy Press.

NRC (National Research Council). 1989. Improving Risk Communication. Washington DC: National Academy Press.

NRC (National Research Council). 1991. Human Exposure Assessment for Airborne Pollutants. Washington DC: National Academy Press.

NRC (National Research Council). 1993. Issues in Risk Assessment, Volumes I, II and III Washington DC: National Academy Press.

NRC (National Research Council). 1994. Spacecraft Maximum Allowable Concentrations for Selected Airborne Contaminants, Vol. 1. Washington, DC: National Academy Press.

NRC (National Research Council). 1996a. Spacecraft Maximum Allowable Concentrations for Selected Airborne Contaminants, Vol. 2. Washington, DC: National Academy Press.

NRC (National Research Council). 1996b. Spacecraft Maximum Allowable Concentrations for Selected Airborne Contaminants, Vol. 3. Washington, DC: National Academy Press.

NRC (National Research Council). 2000a. Toxicological Effects of Methylmercury. Washington, DC: National Academy Press.

NRC (National Research Council). 2000b. Spacecraft Maximum Allowable Concentrations for Selected Airborne Contaminants, Volume 4. Washington, DC: National Academy Press.

NRC (National Research Council). 2002. Estimating the Public Health Benefits of Proposed Air Pollution Regulations. Washington, DC: National Academies Press.

NRC (National Research Council). 2004. Spacecraft Water Exposure Guidelines for Selected Contaminants, Vol. 1. Washington, DC: National Academies Press.

NRC (National Research Council). 2005. Health Implications of Perchlorate Ingestion. Washington, DC: National Academies Press.

OMB (U.S. Office of Management and Budget). 2003. Regulatory Analysis. Circular A-4 to the Heads of Executive Agencies and Establishments, September 17, 2003 [online]. Available: http://www.whitehouse.gov/omb/circulars/a004/a-4.pdf [accessed Oct. 12, 2006].

OMB (U.S. Office of Management and Budget). 2006. Proposed Risk Assessment Bulletin. Released January 9, 2006. Washington, DC: Office of Management and Budget, Executive Office of the President [online]. Available: http://www.whitehouse.gov/omb/inforeg/proposed_risk_ assessment_bulletin_010906.pdf [accessed Oct. 11, 2006].

Raftery, A.E. 1995. Bayesian model selection in social research. Sociol. Methodol. 25:111-163.

Regli, S., J.B. Rose, C.N. Haas, and C.P. Gerba. 1991. Modelling the risk from Giardia and viruses in drinking water. Am. Water Works Assoc. J. 83(11):76-84.

Rogovin, M., and G.T. Frampton. 1980. Three Mile Island: A Report to the Commissioners and the Public. Washington, DC: U.S. Government Printing Office [online]. Available: http://www.threemileisland.org/downloads//354.pdf [accessed Nov. 27, 2006].

Sheps, D.S., M.C. Herbst, A.L. Hinderliter, K.F. Adams, L.G. Ekelund, J.J.

O'Neil, G.M. Goldstein, P.A. Bromberg, J.L. Dalton, M.N. Ballenger, et al. 1990. Production of arrhythmias by elevated carboxyhemoglobin in patients with coronary artery disease. Ann. Intern. Med. 113(5):343-351.

Slovic, P. 2000. The Perception of Risk. London: Earthscan.

Tversky, A., and D. Kahneman. 1974. Judgment under uncertainty: Heuristics and biases. Science 185(4157):1124-1131.

U.S. NRC (U.S. Nuclear Regulatory Commission). 1975. Reactor Safety Study: An Assessment of Accident Risks in the U.S. Commercial Nuclear Power Plants. Wash-1400, NUREG-75/014. Washington, DC: U.S. Nuclear Regulatory Commission.

U.S. NRC (U.S. Nuclear Regulatory Commission). 1979. Nuclear Regulatory Commission Issues Policy Statement on Reactor Safety Study and Review by Lewis Panel: NRC Statement on Risk Assessment and the Reactor Safety Study Report (WASH-1400) in Light of the Risk Assessment Review Group Report, January 18, 1979. No. 79-19. Office of Public Affairs, U.S. Nuclear Regulatory Commission, Washington, DC.

U.S. NRC (U.S. Nuclear Regulatory Commission). 1983. PRA Procedures Guide: A Guide to the Performance of Probabilistic Risk Assessments for Nuclear Power Plants. NUREG/CR-2300. Washington, DC: U.S. Nuclear Regulatory Commission.

U.S. NRC (U.S. Nuclear Regulatory Commission). 1990. Severe Accident Risks: An Assessment for Five U.S. Nuclear Power Plants, Vol. 1. - Final Summary Report; Vol. 2, Appendices A, B & C; Vol. 3. Appendices D & E. NUREG-1150. Division of Systems Research, Office of Nuclear Regulatory Research, U.S. Nuclear Regulatory Commission, Washington, DC [online]. Available: http://www.nrc.gov/reading-rm/doc-collections/nuregs/staff/sr1150/ [accessed Oct. 20. 2006].

U.S. NRC (U.S. Nuclear Regulatory Commission). 2006. An Approach for Determining the Technical Adequacy of Probabilistic Risk Assessment Results for Risk-Informed Activities. Draft Regulatory Guide Dg-1161. Office of Nuclear Regulatory Research, U.S. Nuclear Regulatory Commission, Washington, DC [online]. Available: http://ruleforum.llnl.gov/cgi-bin/downloader/rg_lib/123-0198.pdf [accessed Oct. 20, 2006].

Vesely, W.E., F.F. Goldberg, N.H. Roberts, and D.F. Haasl. 1981. Fault Tree Handbook. NUREG-0492. Systems and Reliability Research, Office of Nuclear Regulatory Research, U.S. Nuclear Regulatory Commission, Washington, DC. January 1981 [online]. Available: http://www.nrc.gov/reading-rm/doc-collections/nuregs/staff/sr0492/sr0492.pdf [accessed Oct. 23, 2006].

Wallace, R.B., ed. 1998. Maxcy-Rosenau-Last Public Health and Preventive Medicine, 14th Ed. Stamford, CT: Appleton and Lange.

Wiggins, J. 1985. ESA Safety Optimization Study. HEI-685/1026. Hernandez Engineering, Houston, TX.

Wittenberg, E., S.J. Goldie, B. Fischhoff, and J.D. Graham. 2003. Rationing decisions and individual responsibility in illness: Are all lives equal? Med. Decis. Making 23(3):194-221.

5

Omissions from the Bulletin

Omissions and incomplete information limit the utility of the proposed Office of Management and Budget (OMB) bulletin as balanced and comprehensive risk assessment guidance. Specifically, while prescribing standards to promote quality in a broad array of analyses, the bulletin is silent on several relevant topics and incomplete on others. As documented in comments from affected agencies to the committee, some omissions are related to substantive aspects of the risk assessment process, others to implementation issues.

The committee identified several risk assessment topics not discussed in the OMB bulletin and not discussed in this report. Examples include gene-environment interactions, the problem of mixtures, and cumulative exposure, among others. It would be impractical and inappropriate for this committee to attempt to address all risk assessment issues that might be relevant to one or more federal agencies. Guidance on those and other issues, however, is important, and their importance led to the recommendation that OMB encourage federal agencies to develop individual guidelines tailored to their own needs and practices (see Chapter 7).

ENGINEERED SYSTEMS

The proposed bulletin acknowledges the multiplicity of disciplines involved in the risk assessment process, including "engineering" (OMB 2006, p. 5). It also acknowledges the diversity of risk assessments conducted within the federal government, including "failure analysis of physical structures" (OMB 2006, p. 7), and it is clearly intended to cover such assessments. Despite these introductory statements, the bulletin focuses mainly on biologic systems, with an emphasis on human health risk assessment, and provides little guidance related to physical (engineered) systems.

In fact, the bulletin gives only minimal attention to risk assessments for which the end point is major failure of an engineered system. The vast majority of examples presented (and authorities cited) apply to toxicologic and other human health end points without corresponding attention to the failure of engineered systems. Moreover, it is unclear whether the bulletin's occasional mention of such failures refers mainly to human health consequences (for example, death or injury from a nuclear power plant accident) or includes the probability and consequences of the engineered failure itself (for example, bridge collapse or toxic release from a chemical plant without estimating the extent of related human health effects).

The bulletin fails to take advantage of the concepts and methods developed through the engineering community's investment of hundreds of millions of dollars in quantitative risk assessment for physical systems. Specifically, in referencing the risk studies, the bulletin is deficient in not recognizing the extensive and often effective efforts of the private sector in risk assessment of such subjects as off-shore oil platforms, chemical plants, nuclear reactors, and waste sites. Those studies have influenced positively risk assessment in the federal government. The incomplete and unbalanced approach to engineering risk assessment (as well as ecologic and other types of risk assessment) belies the bulletin's stated objective of improving the quality of risk assessment across the federal government.

SENSITIVE SUBPOPULATIONS

The bulletin has multiple standards and requirements related to "populations" and "subpopulations" (OMB 2006, Section IV[2], V[6]), but these standards are incomplete in relation to sensitive subpopulations. Specifically, the only reference to *sensitive* subpopulations, such as "children or the elderly," appears not in the bulletin, but in the supplementary information (OMB 2006, p. 19). Moreover, the strong emphasis on central estimates in the standards themselves means that the most vulnerable people in a population—who, almost by definition, lie in the tails of the probability distribution—might be underrepresented, depending on the characterization of the central estimate.

The bulletin's emphasis on central estimates (OMB 2006, Section V[3]), standards calling for a "range of plausible risk estimates" (OMB 2006, Section IV[3]), and cautions against exaggeration and overstatement (OMB 2006, Section IV[4]) could be viewed as restricting use of data from the tails of the probability distribution on the grounds that such information might generate risk estimates considerably higher than central tendency or general population estimates. If federal agencies interpret (or possibly misinterpret) the bulletin in that way, decision-makers could be deprived of risk-related information on vulnerable segments of the population and the potential impacts of measurable exposures that have not been identified as adverse (OMB 2006, Section V[7]).

Such information on the variability of effects across potentially affected populations—due to differences in sensitivity, exposure, or both—is essential to decision-making. With that in mind, experienced risk assessors characterize uncertainty (OMB 2006, p. 17) and variability (OMB 2006, p. 19) as calling not only for the *quantitative* estimates required by the bulletin but also for *qualitative* evaluation of hazard and exposure to identify special populations, such as infants, children, the elderly, subsistence subpopulations, environmental-justice subpopulations, and the like, for which risk estimates may be appropriate. However, if implemented literally and in the absence of clarifying language, the bulletin may be interpreted as requiring only quantitative analyses and only for the general population. Both approaches are clearly contrary to prior NRC guidance (NRC 1994).

EXEMPTIONS, WAIVERS, AND DEFERRALS

Unless an agency determines otherwise, the bulletin expressly excludes from its coverage assessments related to "licensing, approval and registration processes for specific product development activities," "inspections relating to health, safety, or environment," and an "individual product label" (OMB 2006, p. 10). Those provisions appear to exempt a broad set of risk assessments, including some Food and Drug Administration (FDA) assessments related to pharmaceuticals, assessments required under the Federal Insecticide, Fungicide, and Rodenticide Act for registering pesticides, and U.S. Department of Agriculture inspection of products destined for the food supply.[1]

Without providing reasons, the bulletin excludes from its requirements assessments submitted by manufacturers seeking product approvals or registrations—an exclusion that appears to apply to such substances as pesticides. As noted in Chapter 2, the recommendations set forth in the various expert studies apply generally to all risk assessments, and the committee finds no basis in the bulletin for blanket exclusion of assessments related to product approvals and registrations from standards designed to improve the quality of agency assessments. Responding to a committee question in that regard, OMB explained that the Information Quality Guidelines (67 Fed. Reg. 8460 [2002]) do not apply to adjudicatory matters. That is not consistent with the overarching objective of seeking higher-quality risk assessment, and the committee's concerns remain.

In written comments to the committee, several agencies noted omissions in the provisions related to exemptions, waivers, and deferrals. For example, although the bulletin allows an agency head to waive or defer some or all of the requirements (OMB 2006, Section VIII), the Centers for Disease Control and Prevention (CDC) notes that "the Bulletin provides little or no insight as to how an agency would justify a deferral or waiver, and it is unclear who decides whether an agency's rationale is 'compelling' or whether agencies may be challenged on this issue" (see Appendix E, p. HHS-21). Similarly, EPA notes that the bulletin "does not outline any roles and responsibilities for…resolution of disagreements between agencies and OMB, certifications, waivers, exemptions, and other areas. The document should describe how interactions between OMB and the agencies will work in implementing the Bulletin.…The proposed Bulletin does not describe any criteria for granting a waiver or for providing for exemptions" (see Appendix E, pp. EPA-13-14). FDA points out that the bulletin "omits a 'time sensitive' health or

---

[1]Agency comments on the exemptions were mixed. For example, the Department of the Interior (DOI) expressed concern that the exemption for single-product toxics labeling "might lead to human health and environmental risks that could be foreseen if the exemption was not in place" (see Appendix E, p. DOI-3). In contrast, EPA not only agreed with the exemptions for the program for registering (licensing) and reregistering pesticides but also urged extending the exemption to risk assessments in support of food tolerances (see Appendix E, p. EPA-16).

safety exception and provides only a weak agency deferral and waiver authority that requires the agency to comply with Bulletin requirements as soon as practicable" (see Appendix E, p. HHS-25). The committee finds that the bulletin's credibility depends partly on the extent to which affected agencies can expect even-handed and predictable administration of provisions that create exceptions, waivers, or deferrals of general policies. Agency comments suggest that the bulletin provides little confidence in that regard.

THE ROLE OF RISK ASSESSMENT POLICY
AND DEFAULT OPTIONS

The bulletin and the supplementary information acknowledge the role of "choice" and "professional judgment" in the risk assessment process (OMB 2006, pp. 3, 19, 20, 21, 25) but omit discussion and guidance on the role of such judgments in the selection of defaults for risk assessment. That omission is particularly striking in view of frequent citations of the 1994 National Research Council (NRC) report *Science and Judgment in Risk Assessment*, which, as the title indicates, gives special attention to the role of professional judgment in making risk assessment decisions in the absence of relevant experimental or field data—a circumstance common to many risk assessments.

At the outset, the committee stresses that relevant data are always preferred and are to be used when available. However, as described in Chapter 2, default options and inference judgments have a legitimate role in the risk assessment practice of many federal agencies. The 1994 NRC report explains that such default options "are used in the absence of convincing scientific knowledge on which of several competing models and theories is correct....The choice of such principles *goes beyond science and inevitably involves policy choices* on how to balance such criteria" (NRC 1994, p. 7, emphasis added). As a result, that report emphasizes two related but distinct components in its recommendation that an agency "clearly state the scientific *and the policy basis* for each default option" (NRC 1994, p. 8, emphasis added).

Informed in the first instance by the available data and analyses, risk assessment policies can have a strong, sometimes pivotal influence on the choices and judgments identified in the bulletin. Familiar examples include choices regarding use or nonuse of data from animal models, uncertainty defaults (for example, one vs 100 vs 1,000), and identification of populations of interest for any particular risk assessment (for example, general population vs sensitive subpopulation vs maximally exposed individuals) and among alternative dose-response models based on more or less conservative assumptions.

EPA notes that omission in its comments: "Scientific 'defaults' or 'inference guidelines' play an important role for EPA in providing a consistent and peer reviewed means of addressing recurring, fundamental issues of science policy in its risk assessments. The proposed Bulletin does not address this aspect of risk assessment practice" (see Appendix E, p. EPA-14). The Fish and Wildlife Service (FWS) offers a specific example: "The Service is concerned that the Bulletin appears to favor 'central tendencies' or expected outcomes as the best approach or the best science. It is the view of the Service that the best science is that which is objective, explicit and complete and the end or parts of the distribution that we focus on is guided by policy and social values" (see Appendix E, p. DOI-2).

Policy considerations are particularly important for assessments based on data from the biologic sciences but may also be important for other categories of risk assessment. For example, DOI recommends "expanding the discussion of risk assessments for physical structures to include . . . expert elicitation (where expert elicitation provides probabilistic valuation integrating data, analysis, experience and professional judgment when statistical data is not readily available)" (see Appendix E, p. DOI-2).

Although the bulletin stresses the importance of describing and analyzing variability and uncertainty, those discussions focus on quantitative factors without recognizing that, in the absence of data, any choice of defaults for use in risk assessment requires policy judgments. The bulletin thus emphasizes completeness and transparency as to the technical aspects of risk assessment but omits any requirements for comparable completeness and transparency regarding an agency's reasons for selecting from among the available default options.

EXTERNALLY GENERATED RISK ASSESSMENTS

Public participation in and contribution to risk assessment and decision-making are hallmarks of the regulatory process. It takes many forms, from one-page letters urging consideration of a constituent's view of a risk assessment issue to manuscripts for new yet-to-be-published studies to peer-reviewed alternative assessments developed by highly regarded academics and other science professionals. By law and practice, the agencies consider the external submissions with data, information, and analyses developed in or commissioned by the agencies.

Although Congress authorizes designated federal agencies, such as FDA and EPA, to require specific data related to product approvals and registrations, the bulletin does not make its proposed standards applicable to externally generated assessments, such as alternative assessments submitted to federal agencies as comment on risk assessments underlying proposed regulations. However, because externally generated assessments or conclusions from them are routinely submitted for agency consideration and use, a question arises as to the entity—submitter or agency—responsible for ensuring attention to and compliance with the requirements in the bulletin.

The bulletin does not address that question. It is important because of potential impacts on time and resources (staffing and funding). Generally, external assessments are submitted when the risk assessment and rulemaking are under way in line with previously established budgets and schedules. If an agency is responsible for determining whether information received from the public and used as part of a risk assessment complies with OMB requirements, additional time and resources would be required. Alternatively, if the submitter is responsible, the agency would know when the information is received whether it meets the standards and thus whether it can be considered without additional analysis and delay.

In a best-case situation in which the submitter is responsible for ensuring compliance with the bulletin, useful information conforming to the requirements could be immediately woven into a risk assessment (for example, see Appendix E, p. DOD-12). In a worst-case situation in which the agency is responsible, an agency could devote staff and time to conducting an analysis of information that proved to be nonconforming and possibly incur substantial delays in completing the overall assessment.

Recognizing that the bulletin's requirements apply only within the government, many agencies nevertheless responded to an NRC question on the issue. CDC indicated that "it would be helpful if quantitative assessments conducted by external groups met the same requirements when those assessments are used by a government agency" (see Appendix E, p. HHS-24). The Department of Defense noted that "it would be beneficial if contractors and private industry met the OMB Proposed Bulletin requirements" (see Appendix E, p. DOD-12). EPA noted that "the Agency has relied upon assessments conducted by external groups, including NRC panels, the World Health Organization, the Canadian government, ATSDR, and CAL-EPA. In general, their conformity with the requirements of the Bulletin, as feasible and appropriate, would be a laudable goal" (see Appendix E, p. EPA-16). Similar comments were received from several other agencies (see Appendix E, pp. FWS-12, OSHA-7, DOT-10, DOD-11-12, CPSC-6, and HUD-2).

Responding to a committee question on the issue, OMB contends that it is the responsibility of the federal government to make certain that such assessments meet relevant standards. The committee does not dispute that externally generated assessments and related risk information incorporated into the agency assessment process should conform to standards related to scientific quality and objectivity. The issue is whether the agency or the submitter is responsible for the initial evaluation of conformity to standards of quality and objectivity. For the same reasons that federal agencies are responsible for conforming to standards in proposing any risk assessment, it seems incumbent on external submitters to evaluate and document as part of their submission—that is, to assure the agencies and the public—that risk assessment information offered for use in decision-making conforms to the same relevant standards. If federal agencies are themselves responsible for the initial evaluation of all public submissions of risk assessment information (as defined in the bulletin) for conformity with the bulletin's standards, the risk assessment process and related regulation development could be brought to a standstill.

RISK COMMUNICATION

The supplementary information says that "it does not address in any detail the important processes of ... risk communication" (OMB 2006, p. 3).[2] That omission is inconsistent with reports issued by the NRC (1983, 1989, 1996), the Institute of Medicine (IOM 1999), the Presiden-

---

[2]Note that the supplementary information does address an aspect of risk communication in that it instructs the agencies always to communicate risk qualitatively, to communicate risk quantitatively whenever possible, to give a range of plausible estimates and their associated limitations when communicating risk quantitatively, and, to the extent feasible, to follow the Safe Drinking Water Act "quality standard for the dissemination of public information about risks of adverse health effects." A requirement is also included that instructs the agencies to compare the risks that are the subject of agency risk assessments with other familiar risks (see Chapter 4).

tial/Congressional Commission on Risk Assessment and Risk Management (PCCRARM 1997), the Canadian Standards Association (CSA
1997), the Royal Commission for Environmental Pollution (RCEP 1998),
HM Treasury (2005), and others. In the view of those reports, risk assessment is inseparable from risk communication.

The bulletin reflects a simple but incomplete view of risk communication as the last step in a competent risk assessment. Once the technical work has been completed, analysts have a duty to inform those with a
stake in the results. That sharing is essential to a democratic society, as
well as to the credibility of any regulatory process that depends on the
consent of the governed. The relevant scientific research has found that
citizens are poorly informed about many of the myriad risks currently or
potentially in their lives and about the costs and benefits of possible ways
to reduce the risks. It has also found that scientifically developed risk
communication can often bring citizens to the level of understanding
needed for decision-making purposes. By neglecting the obligation for
risk communication, the bulletin is incompatible with NRC and other
reports in a way that threatens the credibility of the methodology that it
seeks to support.

The accepted view of risk communication is, however, that it constitutes an essential element of all stages of risk assessment, not just the
last step. As discussed in the 1996 NRC report *Understanding Risk*, the
primary purpose of risk communication is to share information between
interested and affected parties with the aim of improving the quality and
relevance of risk assessments; the goal is not to persuade, as indicated by
OMB (OMB 2006, p. 11). Those affected by the results of an analysis
need an opportunity to provide information on issues based on their experience. For example, regarding exposure analysis, residents of a community or workers in an industry can provide information essential for
agencies to use in developing exposure scenarios critical to the risk assessment process. Stakeholders from all points on the spectrum of interested parties—other state and federal agencies, advocacy groups from
industry, and affected communities—can be expected to offer perspectives on the risk assessment policies under discussion. In the hazard stage
of the assessment, are animal studies reliable predictors of human risk?
Regarding the dose-response analysis, what constitutes an adequate margin of safety in a particular situation? Agency decisions on such policy
issues influence the course of any assessment, and stakeholder input—
that is, communication to an agency—is relevant.

Achieving more transparent analyses as emphasized in the bulletin
depends partly on effective risk communication. However, without de-

tailed attention to the broader risk communication principles outlined above, the bulletin is unlikely to accomplish its objective.

IMPACTS

As developed in the next chapter, the bulletin omits expected analyses of baseline information, cost-benefit considerations associated with implementing the bulletin, and the potential for adverse impacts on the practice of risk assessment in the federal government.

REFERENCES

CSA (Canadian Standards Association). 1997. Risk Management: Guidelines for Decision-Makers. CAN/CSA-Q850-97. Toronto, Canada: Canadian Standards Association.

HM Treasury (Her Majesty's Treasury). 2005. Managing Risks to the Public: Appraisal Guidance. London: HM Treasury. June 2005 [online]. Available: http://www.hm-treasury.gov.uk/media/8AB/54/Managing_risks_to_the_ public.pdf [accessed Oct. 18, 2006].

IOM (Institute of Medicine). 1999. Toward Environmental Justice. Research, Education, and Health Policy Needs. Washington, DC: National Academy Press.

NRC (National Research Council). 1983. Risk Assessment in the Federal Government: Managing the Process. Washington, DC: National Academy Press.

NRC (National Research Council). 1989. Improving Risk Communication. Washington, DC: National Academy Press.

NRC (National Research Council). 1994. Science and Judgment in Risk Assessment. Washington, DC: National Academy Press.

NRC (National Research Council). 1996. Understanding Risk, Informing Decisions in a Democratic Society. Washington, DC: National Academy Press.

OMB (U.S. Office of Management and Budget). 2006. Proposed Risk Assessment Bulletin. Released January 9, 2006. Washington, DC: Office of Management and Budget, Executive Office of the President [online]. Available: http://www.whitehouse.gov/omb/inforeg/proposed_risk_as-sessment_bulletin_010906.pdf [accessed Oct. 11, 2006].

PCCRARM (Presidential/Congressional Commission on Risk Assessment and Risk Management). 1997. Risk Assessment and Risk Management in Regulatory Decision-Making, Vol. 2. Washington, DC: U.S. General Printing Office [online]. Available: http://www.riskworld.com/Nreports/1997/risk-rpt/volume2/pdf/v2epa.PDF [accessed October 3, 2006].

RCEP (Royal Commission for Environmental Pollution). 1998. Setting Environmental Standards, the Royal Commission for Environmental Pollution 21st Report. London: The Stationary Office [online]. Available: http://www.rcep.org.uk/standardsreport.htm [accessed Oct. 25, 2006].

6

Impact on the Practice of Risk Assessment in the Federal Government

The committee was asked to comment in general terms on how the guidance in the proposed Office of Management and Budget (OMB) bulletin would affect the practice of risk assessment in the federal government. That task was interpreted by the committee as including the following questions: First, how would implementation of the OMB bulletin improve the practice of risk assessment from a scientific perspective? That is, what benefits would accrue from implementation of the bulletin? Second, what are the costs in staff resources that would be necessary to implement the bulletin? Third, how would implementation of the bulletin affect the timeliness of completing risk assessments in the federal government? Fourth, can the bulletin be integrated smoothly into the agencies' current practices? Fifth, overall, what are the expectations as to whether implementation of the bulletin would improve the practice of risk assessment in federal agencies and achieve the stated objective "to enhance the technical quality and objectivity of risk assessments prepared by federal agencies" (OMB 2006, p. 3)?

On the basis of the committee's general experience, information generated during its review of the bulletin, and the comments received from federal agencies (see Appendix E), the committee concludes that, although variable and uncertain to some extent, the potential for adverse impacts of the bulletin on the practice of risk assessment in the federal government is high. The bases of that conclusion are discussed below and include the likely drain on agency resources, the extended time necessary to complete risk assessments that are undertaken, and the highly likely disruptive effect on many agencies of implementing the bulletin. Moreover, if some of the provisions discussed in earlier chapters and below were ultimately interpreted in a rigid one-size-fits-all way, the overall adverse impact would be substantially greater.

As a starting point, the committee addresses OMB's failure to undertake—or at least provide to the public—an evaluation of the likely benefits and costs of implementing the bulletin for agency risk assessment practices and the consequences of that omission for the committee's work.

THE ABSENCE OF INFORMATION TO EVALUATE THE IMPACT OF THE BULLETIN ON AGENCY RISK ASSESSMENT PRACTICES

OMB, the champion of benefit-cost analysis for decision-making, requires agencies that propose major regulations to provide quantitative, or at least qualitative, information regarding the anticipated consequences of their proposals. It was therefore surprising that OMB did not include such information in its proposed bulletin.

For example, to gauge the benefits to be achieved from implementing the bulletin, it is essential to specify the baseline—in this case, the agencies' current practices with respect to risk assessment. Although OMB has implied that the agencies do not now meet the standards it seeks to establish, it has not constructed a baseline specifying risk assessment proficiency for each agency (or even each of the major regulatory agencies), including the extent to which a few, some, or many agencies produce generally satisfactory and high-quality risk assessments or the reasons why those or other agencies fall short of the specified standards. Specifically, OMB has not established which agencies do not know what good practices are and which agencies do not have the ability, resources, or incentives to meet those standards.

Similarly, OMB has not identified the costs that could be incurred by implementing the bulletin. The extent of the changes in the agencies will generally depend on the extent to which they are not currently meeting the standards set forth in the bulletin—again, a baseline issue. Beyond that, however, OMB has not identified the costs, such as the staff resources necessary to meet the bulletin's standards, the additional time that would be required to meet the standards, and the disruption that would result from changing established practices. Nor has OMB indicated what weight it gave to those factors in its decision to propose the bulletin.

Given the importance of such information for an evaluation of the impact of the bulletin, the committee has attempted on its own to analyze the various likely effects of the bulletin on the practice of risk assessment in the federal government.

BENEFITS

OMB anticipates that implementation of the bulletin would raise all agency risk assessment practices to consistently higher levels and that that would translate into better information for decision-makers and hence better decisions. The committee accepts (indeed, applauds) that goal but finds that the proposed bulletin cannot achieve that result.

In evaluating potential benefits, it is essential to understand that not all agencies are the same and that they deal with different types of hazards or risks. Indeed, there are substantial disparities among agencies (and even among components of the same agency) in sophistication with respect to risk assessment, expertise and experience with risk assessments, and resources available to devote to risk assessments. Some agencies have spent considerable time and resources in developing internal risk assessment guidelines (for example, EPA 1996, 1998, 2005; NASA 2002), others have taken the first few steps toward staffing up and are making some progress, and still others appear to rely almost completely on outsourcing for their risk assessments.

The agencies also have different missions, which require different types of risk assessments. There are risk assessments involving engineered systems, risk assessments involving ecologic science, and risk assessments dealing with public-health issues (perhaps those on which the bulletin is most focused) and involving biologic sciences. Although those assessments have features in common, they differ substantially in many ways.[1]

---

[1] See, for example, Appendix E, p. DOT-2 ("the operating administrations employ varied risk assessment practices that range from informed judgment to probabilistic risk assessments"); p. DOD-1 ("risk assessment methods and characterization of uncertainty are dependent upon and tailored to the specific purpose or function being assessed"); pp. HHS-1 and -2 ("FDA and CDC use very similar conceptual approaches to risk assessment although the different contexts

The bulletin would thus affect different agencies in vastly different ways, and the potential for benefits would be highly varied across agencies. In general, the introduction and implementation of standards and guidelines where none exist or where existing standards are inadequate could lead to improvements. The people responsible for the expanded range of risk assessments covered by the bulletin would undoubtedly benefit from having an explicit statement of what is expected of them[2]— and this is true even for those in the agencies that contract out most of their risk assessment work. Implementation of the bulletin might enable agency managers (particularly political appointees who may not have extensive experience with the scientific or technical work of the agency) to ask more pertinent questions of risk assessors and to demand compliance with the new standards.[3] And availability of the bulletin might diminish delays caused by having to start anew or make major revisions near the end of the process. Therefore, the committee expects that if the proposed bulletin were implemented, at best, some agency risk assessments might be slightly improved from a scientific or technical perspective.

One important committee concern is that imposing all the bulletin's provisions on all agency risk assessments would not improve their scientific quality. That is so because broad scientific consensus does not exist for some provisions, such as uncertainty and variability (discussed in Chapter 4). Another potential problem is that the bulletin specifies that the quality standard for the dissemination of public information in the 1996 amendments to the Safe Drinking Water Act "should be met, where feasible, in all risk assessments which address adverse health effects" (OMB 2006, p. 13). The committee was unable to identify any information regarding the implementation of that statute, and although it includes a number of scientifically valid suggestions, it represents a proposal at the edge of risk assessment science rather than one of general scientific acceptance.[4] In these circumstances, to impose across the board a legisla-

---

(e.g., food, environmental, and occupation) necessitate differences in these agencies approaches. ... FDA's efforts include probabilistic risk assessments, safety assessments and qualitative risk assessments"); and p. EPA-2.

[2]See, for example, Appendix E, p. DOD-10.

[3]See, for example, Appendix E, p. NASA-9 ("being able to cite an external requirement reinforces the existing risk assessment requirements established within NASA").

[4]See Appendix E, pp. EPA-16 and -17 ("EPA has *adapted* these requirements in

tive provision enacted for one specific statute as though it represents mainstream scientific thought seems premature and would produce uncertain results.

Moreover, if the goal is consistently high-quality risk assessments across the federal government, it means that federal agencies farthest behind would have to be brought up to the agencies doing a generally respectable job, and there is no indication that the agencies behind the curve will be able to improve if only they are told what they need to do.[5] In fact, many deficiencies in the technical quality of current risk assessments and risk assessment programs can be traced, not to inadequate guidance, but to inadequate resources, including inadequate budgets and inadequate staffing (qualitatively in relevant expertise or quantitatively in number of qualified experts).

Many agencies will require more and better data to satisfy the specific risk assessment requirements described in the bulletin.[6,7] That in turn will depend in part on future federal budgets for research and data-gathering,[8] whether that work is undertaken by agency personnel or

---

its implementation of the Information Quality Guidelines...'in light of our numerous statutes, regulations, guidance and policies'...and [to] accommodate the range of real world situations that EPA confronts in its implementation of our diverse programs.")

[5]Appendix E, pp. DOD-6 and -7, is not to the contrary; DOD asks for more guidance, but it is looking not for general statements but for specific implementation or policy clarifications to flesh out the general guidance.

[6]The committee notes that talented risk assessors can produce high-quality risk assessments (that is, risk assessments that capture the state of the knowledge concerning the hazard, describe uncertainties, and explain how the uncertainties affect the interpretation of the risk assessment results) with minimal or poor data. However, risk assessments conducted with minimal or poor data will inevitably yield risk estimates with greater uncertainty, which will undermine acceptance.

[7]See, for example, Appendix E, p. DOT-3 ("the challenges...involve a lack of data relating to the nature of the risks at issue"); DOD at page 5 ("lack of scientifically defensible and/or agreed upon input information"); p. DOE-3 ("one of the technical difficulties is the paucity of data"); p. EPA-5 ("the principal scientific challenge relates to limited data"); and p. HUD-1 ("data are not amenable to aggressive statistical data manipulation").

[8]See, for example, Appendix E, p. HHS-4 ("most challenges that FDA faces in conducting risk assessments are related to funding or resource scarcity rather than substantial scientific or technical issues"); and p. HUD-1 ("Congressional

through outsourcing. For some individual assessments, funding requirements can be substantial.[9] Even small, local assessments can generate substantial costs for research and data-gathering.

In addition, informed use of data depends on staff expertise and experience in each of the areas identified as risk assessment in the bulletin. Without adequate staffing, scientific data cannot be responsibly interpreted and applied for risk assessment purposes. For example, some agencies—such as the Centers for Disease Control and Prevention and some offices in the Food and Drug Administration and the Environmental Protection Agency (EPA)—have epidemiologists on staff, but other risk assessing offices that will need fully qualified epidemiologists to meet the standards set forth in the bulletin do not have such experts on board.[10]

Given the current state of affairs with respect to funding and staffing, the committee finds that implementation of the bulletin, without concentrated attention on data and staffing needs in relation to the baseline, is unlikely to achieve the objective of enhancing the technical quality of risk assessments throughout the federal government.

COSTS

Staff Resources to Implement Guidance

Although the benefits associated with the changes in practices called for by the bulletin would be varied and uncertain, the costs can be expected to affect every agency and, in general, to be substantial. That should be considered in the current context of limited funding for risk assessment activities and the challenges already facing agencies.[11] Thus,

---

authority and appropriations may limit the scope of research to support the risk assessment").

[9]For example, EPA alone "has funded a total of $368 million on PM [particulate matter] research and related technical work for fiscal years 1998-2003, including $66.7 million for fiscal year 2003" (NRC 2004).

[10]See Appendix E, p. HUD-1 ("cannot support full time equivalent staff for the [required] analyses").

[11]See, for example, Appendix E, p. HHS-4 ("the logistics of supporting risk assessment activities remain difficult and involve issues such as availability of staff expertise and availability of funding").

adding mandates (for example, expanding the scope and complexity of risk assessments) would necessitate reallocation of resources and would probably negatively affect the number of risk assessments produced by federal agencies, the availability of advisory materials from federal agencies, and the ability of the agencies to complete non-risk-assessment work.

First, as discussed in Chapter 3, the definition of risk assessment in the bulletin goes well beyond what the agencies have consistently construed as risk assessments. In addition, with so many separate documents (defined as including not just traditional risk assessments but also analyses, such as margin-of-exposure estimates, hazard determinations, and toxicologic profiles) individually subject to the standards and related certification, additional resources would be required for agencies to ensure that their work products satisfy the requirements of the bulletin.[12]

Second, in many instances, additional research would have to be undertaken or additional data gathered to meet the provisions of the bulletin. Consider, for example, Section IV(3), requiring a range of plausible risk estimates whenever a quantitative characterization of risk is provided, and Section IV(7c), requiring "information on the timing of exposure and the onset of the adverse effect(s)." Section IV(7b)'s requirement to "assess, to the extent feasible, countervailing risks caused by alternative mitigation measures" could lead, for example, to having to evaluate occupational risks posed by environmental interventions or even the secondary effect of income on health; this could result in an extremely broad-based analysis much larger in scope than currently undertaken. Consider also the additional analysis that would have to be undertaken to satisfy Section V(4c)'s requirement that risk assessors "provide a quantitative distribution of the uncertainty" and Section V(6)'s requirement "to characterize...variability through a quantitative distribution, reflecting different affected population(s), time scales, geography, or other parameters relevant to the needs and objectives of the assessment." In general,

---

[12]See, for example, Appendix E, p. NASA-9 (applying the bulletin to "any internal risk assessment performed within NASA that is releasable under the Freedom of Information Act...could [result in] a substantial burden to meet all of the requirements contained within the Bulletin"); and p. DOL-4 and -5 (the Occupational Safety and Health Administration's exposure assessments and nonregulatory informational products (for example, perchloroethylene exposures) have not been treated as risk assessments and would therefore be subject to new requirements).

adherence to the provisions of the bulletin would be more labor- and resource-intensive than current practices.[13] As noted above, staff would
have to be added to provide for necessary expertise; even for agencies
that have an excellent corps of experts in other fields, the bulletin's emphasis on uncertainty analysis will require major qualitative and quantitative changes in their staffing profile to ensure the availability of adequate
numbers of person qualified to produce and interpret these complex
analyses.[14] Virtually all the existing staff and the new staff would also
have to undergo training, a costly and time-consuming process.

Third, the lack of flexibility and the lack of clarity of the bulletin
would probably result in some unnecessary use of resources with little
gain in quality because, as the bulletin reads now, a standard is to be applied whether or not it has scientific relevance in any particular case. For
example, applying a quantitative analysis to a qualitative discussion of
toxicity would have little value. Reanalyzing analyses previously rejected or evaluating the rigor of proffered studies developed by outside
parties on similar issues would not ordinarily improve the quality of the
risk assessment itself.[15] And subjecting peer-reviewed scientific journal
articles or Power Point presentations to the provisions of the bulletin
would add little scientific rigor to the assessment of risks by the agencies.[16]

There is also the possibility of squandering resources because the
bulletin is not clear as to what constitutes compliance, in the sense of
what is sufficient to satisfy the requirements. For example, Section IV(3)
states that "when a quantitative characterization of risk is provided, a
range of plausible risk estimates shall be provided." How large must the
range be? Section IV(4b) requires that the risk assessors shall give
"weight to both positive and negative studies in light of each study's

---

[13]See Appendix E, p. DOD-11. See also, for example, Appendix E, p. EPA-14
("if categorically adopted [the Bulletin's provisions] would mandate a high level
of analysis and development of characterization that goes beyond most current
EPA practice in risk assessment").

[14]See Appendix E, p. DOD-11 ("increased the level of expertise needed to perform quantitative uncertainty analyses").

[15]See Appendix E, p. HHS-15. See also p. OMB-3 ("If third-party submissions
are to be used and made publicly available by Federal agencies, it is the responsibility of the Federal Government to make sure that such information meets
relevant standards").

[16]See Appendix E, pp. HHS-7 and -8.

technical quality." Apart from the possibility that affected entities could use this provision to further drain staff resources by requiring an agency to respond to unconventional or largely irrelevant studies,[17] how serious must a study be to qualify? How much discussion of the weight given is necessary? Section IV(5) requires that for "critical assumptions in the assessment…a quantitative evaluation of reasonable alternative assumptions and their implications for the key findings of the assessment" be included. How many alternative assumptions must be considered, and how detailed should the discussion of the implications be?[18] Given the likelihood of challenges to controversial risk assessments, agencies may feel compelled to reallocate even more resources to particularly important risk assessments, lest there be any question about their compliance with the bulletin.[19] These are clearly wasted costs that could be substantial as the stakes are raised.

Moreover, as discussed in Chapter 4, it is not always clear at the outset of a risk assessment whether it would ultimately fall under the general standards, the regulatory standards, or the special standards for influential risk assessments.[20] If the risk were considered influential and the most exacting standards were applied only to find little impact, substantial resources would have been used needlessly.

Although these new obligations would be imposed, there is no indication that any additional funds are being requested or appropriated. If current budgetary conditions continue for the indefinite future, it appears unlikely that additional resources will be made available. As a result, funding will have to come from within the agencies and presumably

---

[17]See Appendix E, p. HHS-20 ("There may be instances where parties (particularly competitors) may disagree over the 'science' to be applied…or even whether conventional scientific concepts are applicable or recognizable. In the latter case, individuals or firms advocating the use of 'unconventional' or 'alternative' therapies may…argue that individuals trained in 'conventional' science or medicine are either biased or not qualified to evaluate the merits of their products").

[18]See Appendix E, p. DOE-3 ("there is always one more scenario, or one more approach that someone feels deserves assessment").

[19]See, for example, Appendix E, p. EPA-14 ("while…the Bulletin does not create legal rights…, challenges that claim that the risk assessment or supporting analyses have not fully carried out the practices established by the Bulletin come in many other fora. Such claims could pose an additional burden").

[20]See also, for example, Appendix E, p. HHS-13 ("It is not always clear…at the outset of a risk assessment that it will be influential").

from funds otherwise targeted for risk assessments. The committee is concerned about two possibilities. Some agencies may try to meet the new requirements on some risk assessments, leaving them with inadequate resources to undertake other (already started or planned) risk assessments, so fewer risk assessments would be done, fewer risks would be identified (and the extent of the risks understood), and fewer solutions would be proposed for problems that need consideration. The alternative is for agencies to continue to do all the risk assessments they are now doing (indeed, in some cases, statutorily required to do) and the additional ones that are now covered by the bulletin but cut corners wherever they can, so the overall level of quality will decline.

Timeliness in Completing Risk Assessments

Many risk assessments take considerable time, some several years.[21] The bulletin obviously would add to the timeline of existing risk assessments, sometimes—for example, the requirements for gathering additional data or doing additional research or analysis discussed above—a great deal of time.[22] There would be additional demands from

---

[21]See Appendix E, p. DOT-5 ("the time…varies widely from days to years, depending on the complexity of the issue"); p. DOD-8 ("Health hazard assessments…take 30 to 90 days…Human health risk assessments for the Defense Environmental Restoration Program sites can vary from months…to 5 years or greater for complex sites"); p. DOE-4 ("the range may be from a few months to several years for extremely complex or controversial projects"); p. DOI-9 (time "varies, contracted risk assessments may take up to 2 years from problem identification to delivery"); p. EPA-9 ("assessments vary widely in their complexity and in the time needed for their production and completion…ninety days [for TOSCA]…few weeks or few months [for Superfund sites]…one to five years [for IRIS]…and some of the most complex assessments…in which there is significant controversy and significant new data, the time needed may extend well beyond five years"); pp. HHS-6 ("the Report on Carcinogens takes approximately 2.5 years for each agent under review") and -22 (surgeon general reports on smoking "varied from less than a year to over 5 years"); p. HUD-2 ("the period to complete an original risk assessment is usually two years"); p. NASA-7 ("the completion of nuclear mission safety analyses require about 3-5 years"); and p. DOL-4 ("most recently completed risk assessment…required about 2.5 years").

[22]See Appendix E, p. NASA-7 (applying the standards for influential risk as-

its application to documents not customarily considered risk assessments.[23] At a minimum, effective implementation of the bulletin would require agency management to add to already full workloads far more time for risk assessment planning at the front end of the process and for interpretation and use of the risk assessment at the end of the process.[24] An agency must also be mindful that, in some circumstances, the full scope of data needs may be identified only during the course of an assessment when data gaps appear; at that point, the assessment may be put on hold for additional data development to augment the assessment or require additional time and staffing to complete. Finally, delays in completing risk assessments, again as defined by the bulletin, may result in untimely responses to "unsafe conditions,"[25] urgent public-health needs,[26] untimely release of public alerts about serious risks,[27] or disease investigations, such as anthrax deaths, mumps outbreaks, or SARS.[28]

One element of the current timeline for completing risk assessments is the OMB requirement establishing minimum standards for peer review of scientific information disseminated by the federal government (70 Fed. Reg. 2664-2677 [2005]).[29] The requirement for peer review is re-

---

sessments to determine whether an internal policy or directive was required could "dramatically impact the time to develop, implement, and modify the internal controls"); p. DOL-6 ("deriving quantitative distributions of model uncertainty and variability…could add significant time…where such analyses are not critical to fully inform regulatory decisionmakers"); p. DOD-12 (giving "weight to both positive and negative studies in site-specific risk assessments…may significantly increase the time and resources needed to conduct the assessment"); and p. EPA-14 (describing the many problems with the standards calling for multiple analyses).

[23]See, for example, Appendix E, pp. HHS-21 and -22 and p. EPA-14.
[24]See, for example, Appendix E, p. HUD-3 ("the time course would have to be extended to make sure the procedures are properly followed"); p. DOD-11 ("some organizations…believe that adherence to [certain] provisions may impact the ability to meet critical and/or regulatory prescribed deadlines"); and p. EPA-15 ("if EPA followed all of the procedures described in the twenty standards, assessments could take considerably longer").
[25]See Appendix E, p. DOT-8.
[26]See Appendix E, p. HHS-21.
[27]See Appendix E, p. HHS-15.
[28]See Appendix E, p. HHS-10.
[29]OMB there stated that "peer review is one of the important procedures used to ensure that the quality of published information meets the standards of the scien-

peated in this bulletin.[30] As a practical matter, if the risk assessment bulletin were issued as is, agencies might add to the task of the peer reviewers that they determine whether the risk assessment they are reviewing meets the bulletin's guidance. If so, that will add another ingredient to the peer review process and possibly extend the time needed.[31] There is also concern that the call for peer review, with the call for public participation, in the bulletin goes beyond previously stated requirements.[32] More important, additional time would be added if, in addition to the peer review process, OMB were to review anew the work product even where there is an existing well-done peer review.[33]

In this connection, the committee notes that it supports the call for peer review of risk assessments because that is the standard course for ensuring good scientific standards on such work. The committee is therefore troubled by OMB's repeated references to the Information Quality Act (IQA) and its invocation as the legal authority for OMB to issue this bulletin (OMB 2006, p. 7), that suggest that challenges to a particular risk assessment—and almost every risk assessment is open to challenge on one ground or another—will be handled through the process designed for the IQA, a process that is more a legal or policy process than a scientific one.[34] Specifically, the committee is concerned that to the extent that the implementation of the technical aspects of risk assessment will be

---

tific and technical community" (p. 2665).

[30]Section III(5): "The agency shall follow appropriate procedures for peer review and public participation in the process of preparing the risk assessment."

[31]See, for example, Appendix E, p. DOE-5.

[32]See, for example, Appendix E, p. EPA-15 ("this section goes beyond [existing] guidelines by calling for a response to comment package for all influential risk assessments, and also in its call not only to explain the basis for the agency position, but also to explain why other approaches were not taken, and why"); and p. HHS-22 discussing surgeon general reports and noting that "adding the requirement for public participation and comment to this process likely would add a large volume of comments, which would affect the timeliness of the reports without adding improvements in the scientific quality to the report." See also Appendix E, p. DOT-8.

[33]See Appendix E, p. OMB-3 ("under existing authorities and procedures, OMB might review a risk assessment [that has been peer reviewed in accordance with established peer review procedures]").

[34]IQA gives the right to private groups to file administrative challenges to data disseminated by federal agencies, with an appeal to OMB (67 Fed. Reg. 8452 [2002]).

overseen by OMB and not by the peer-review process or by agency technical managers, scientific issues may be superseded by policy considerations.[35]

The bulletin also includes a number of requirements concerning presentation, such as Sections IV (1), (2), and (4c). Some—like providing "a clear statement of the...objectives of the risk assessment," a clear summary of "the scope of the assessment," "presenting the information about risk in an accurate, clear, complete and unbiased manner," and "describing the data, methods and assumptions used in the assessment with a high degree of transparency"—are fairly straightforward and should be part of any well-written risk assessment, although there may be matters of dispute as to how complete is "complete" and how transparent is "a high degree of transparency."[36] The bulletin also requires an executive summary (Section IV[6]) that includes among other things "information that places the risk in context/perspective with other risks familiar to the target audience" (see Chapter 4). The apparent purpose of this recommendation is to remedy a presumed inability of the readers of risk assessments to understand the numbers as written. That makes it an aspect of risk communication—a process that the bulletin specifically disclaims addressing (OMB 2006, p. 3). As discussed in Chapter 5, the bulletin's exclusion of risk communication is at variance with accepted practice, which holds that two-way risk communication is essential to sound assessment. If additional one-way communication is undertaken at the end of an assessment process, to make the results available to a wider (or less knowledgeable) audience, additional resources and time will be necessary to ensure that the materials are prepared in a scientifically sound way.[37] Here, as elsewhere in this discussion, committee reserva-

---

[35]This concern is greatly increased by public comments requesting that judicial review be considered a component of this process, further converting the scientific process into a legal one. OMB does not address the issue of enforcement in the bulletin, but in light of the many public comments on this issue, some clarification of OMB's position would be desirable.

[36]But see Appendix E, p. HHS-17 ("excessive characterization of every possible uncertainty or extensive evaluation of each assumption could make the risk assessment more confusing and less transparent").

[37]See, for example, Appendix E, p. DOD-11 ("additional labor will be required to...communicate the results to people unfamiliar with the risk assessment process"). See also Appendix E, p. DOT-8 ("requiring the risk assessment to contain a range of risk estimates so that the public is aware of whether the nature of the

tions and concerns are related to broad-brush application of all standards to all agencies; concerns regarding specific standards themselves are discussed elsewhere.

A slightly different problem arises from the bulletin's requirement that risk assessments used for regulatory analysis include a variety of evaluations of alternative mitigation measures (see Sections IV [7a], [7b], and [7c]). Although risk assessors contribute information for use in risk management, this standard goes well beyond the job description of the scientist or technical person assessing the risk onto the path of risk management, another subject that the bulletin said it would not address (OMB 2006, p. 3). Not only will these requirements be resource-intensive and time-consuming, but the committee is also concerned that if they were incorporated at the primary stage of the risk assessment process (for example, identifying a hazard and determining the extent of the risk), risk assessors may be greatly delayed in completing their work.

Another example of the burden that would be imposed by the bulletin is the provision that for every risk assessment document (again, defined to include not just complete risk assessments but also individual components), an agency will have to "include a certification explaining that the agency has complied" with the bulletin and the information-quality guidelines (OMB 2006, p. 25). That is not only getting a signature of an official or a check-the-boxes form; it apparently would require a serious explanation of each step of the process and how it constitutes compliance with the bulletin—a substantial time demand, even assuming that everything is in order, not only for the scientific or technical staff that performed the risk assessment but also for agency managers and presumably the general counsel's office.

Time, like funds in the federal government, is a limited commodity, even apart from the statutory or court-imposed deadlines that are so problematic for some agencies. Time spent by staff on one project, whether it is doing additional work to comply with the terms of the bulletin or to document that it has complied with the bulletin, is time not spent on another, potentially more important project. Again, the committee is concerned about two possibilities: fewer risk assessments (with the attendant consequences) or the same number of risk assessments but of lower quality.

---

risk is conservative…is time consuming, not always necessary, and could deter the DOT operating administrations from employing such assessments").

Integrating the Bulletin into Current Practices

In addition to the costs identified above, there would probably be substantial costs attributable to integrating the bulletin into current risk assessment practices in the federal government. As noted above, many agencies have devoted substantial resources over the last several decades to developing risk assessment guidelines appropriate for their missions. Some, like those at EPA, have been developed with substantial input from stakeholders, consultants, congressional staff, the National Research Council, and other experts and interested parties. If the bulletin were viewed not merely as technical guidance for the less proficient in the field but rather (as it appears to be) as the standards to be applied for all risk assessments, each of the "mismatches" would have to be identified, the causes for the differences in approach documented, and substantial negotiations conducted with OMB to arrive at a decision as to what is most appropriate for a particular agency.[38]

It is beyond dispute that what works for EPA is not the same as what works for the Department of Transportation or the National Aeronautics and Space Administration. One size does not fit all, particularly where the agencies come to the issue with such disparate expertise and experience and, more important, dramatically different risk assessment responsibilities and resources. As developed above, risk assessments in the federal government include those involving statistical analyses, those evaluating the strength of bridges or levees with engineering and the physical sciences, those involving ecologic science, and those involving public-health matters. Those call for very different types of analyses, and imposing one set of standards on the lot is likely to be wasteful, if not counterproductive to good science.

The committee notes that this is not just an up-front, one-time-only cost. Another of the bulletin's requirements is to have procedures in place to ensure that agencies are "aware of new, relevant information that

---

[38]See Appendix E, p. NASA-6 (where "a risk assessment evolves and is updated over the life of the project or program, it can be considered as a 'living' risk model with no fixed dates for their final delivery." See also Appendix E, p. DOL-2, noting that the Occupational Safety and Health Administration (OSHA) generally bases its regulatory decisions on a range of central estimates of risk derived from the best supported models and that it is unclear how quantitative uncertainty distributions would be taken into account in OSHA's regulatory framework.

might alter a previously conducted influential risk assessment" (OMB 2006, p. 21). That is a desirable provision and scientifically valid if there are resources available to monitor the scientific literature for any research associated with an agent for which an influential risk assessment has been conducted and there is a prospect that changes in the science can be reflected contemporaneously in the decision-making process. But, such advances in the science might produce other ways of considering a scientific issue, so the agencies would have to renegotiate with OMB as to how they should do their work.

ARE THE GOALS OF ENHANCING TECHNICAL QUALITY AND OBJECTIVITY OF RISK ASSESSMENT MET BY THE PROPOSED BULLETIN?

The committee was asked to determine whether the bulletin achieves its stated purpose to "enhance the technical quality and objectivity of risk assessments." The committee finds that it fails to achieve that purpose. The committee has identified a number of ways in which implementation of the overarching risk assessment principles can improve risk assessment practices but finds that the potential for benefits will vary widely among agencies and that, although salutary in some respects, the proposed bulletin will probably not achieve the objective of raising all agency risk assessment practices to consistently higher levels. In addition, the committee has identified some of the costs associated with the changes that would be brought about—in staff resources, timeliness of risk assessments, and other factors—and finds them to be substantial. Moreover, in earlier chapters, the committee identified various issues of interpretation; if these are not resolved in a way that provides flexibility to the agencies, the costs will be significantly increased.

Overall, the committee concludes that, although varied and uncertain to some extent, the potential for adverse impacts on the practice of risk assessment in the federal government if the proposed bulletin were implemented is very high. For that reason, the committee does not accept OMB's view that implementing the bulletin would enhance the technical quality and objectivity of risk assessments in the federal government.

REFERENCES

EPA (U.S. Environmental Protection Agency). 1996. Guidelines for Reproductive Toxicity Risk Assessment. EPA/630/R-96/009. Risk Assessment Forum, U.S. Environmental Protection Agency, Washington, DC [online]. Available: http://www.epa.gov/ncea/raf/pdfs/repro51.pdf [accessed July 27, 2006].

EPA (U.S. Environmental Protection Agency). 1998. Guidelines for Ecological Risk Assessment. EPA/630/R-95/002F. Risk Assessment Forum, U.S. Environmental Protection Agency, Washington, DC [online]. Available: http://cfpub.epa.gov/ncea/cfm/recordisplay.cfm?deid=12460 [accessed July 27, 2006].

EPA (U.S. Environmental Protection Agency). 2005. Guidelines for Carcinogen Risk Assessment. EPA/630/P-03/001B. Risk Assessment Forum, U.S. Environmental Protection Agency, Washington, DC [online]. Available: http://www.epa.gov/iris/cancer032505.pdf [accessed July 27, 2006].

NASA (National Aeronautics and Space Administration). 2002. Probabilistic Risk Assessment Procedures Guide for NASA Managers and Practitioners, Version 1.1. Prepared for Office of Safety and Mission Assurance NASA Headquarters, Washington, DC [online]. Available: http://www.hq.nasa.gov/office/codeq/doctree/praguide.pdf [accessed Oct. 18, 2006].

NRC (National Research Council). 2004. Research Priorities for Airborne Particulate Matter: IV. Continuing Research Progress. Washington, DC: The National Academies Press.

OMB (U.S. Office of Management and Budget). 2006. Proposed Risk Assessment Bulletin. Released January 9, 2006. Washington, DC: Office of Management and Budget, Executive Office of the President [online]. Available: http://www.whitehouse.gov/omb/inforeg/proposed_risk_ assessment_bulletin_010906.pdf [accessed Oct. 11, 2006].

7

Conclusions and Recommendations

For the reasons presented in this report, the committee concludes that the bulletin proposed by the Office of Management and Budget (OMB 2006) is fundamentally flawed and recommends that it be withdrawn. Although the committee fully supports the goal of increasing the quality and objectivity of risk assessment in the federal government, it agrees unanimously that the OMB bulletin would not facilitate federal agencies in reaching this goal. The committee also agrees that OMB should encourage the federal agencies to describe, develop, and coordinate their own technical risk assessment guidance. Therefore, the committee recommends that after additional study of current agency practices and needs, a different type of risk assessment bulletin be issued by OMB. It should outline goals and general principles of risk assessment designed to enhance the quality, efficiency, and consistency of risk assessment in the federal government. It should direct the agencies to develop technical guidance that would implement the general principles, be consistent with each agency's legislative mandates and missions, and draw on the expertise that exists in federal agencies and other organizations. The technical guidance developed or identified by the agencies should be peer-reviewed and contain procedures for ensuring agency compliance with the guidance. Although OMB should determine whether the technical guidance fully addresses the general principles, it should not be involved in the development or peer review of agency technical guidance. The committee strongly recommends that agencies addressing similar hazards or risks work together to develop common technical guidance for risk assessment. In that way, the appropriate consistency would be achieved in the federal government in risk assessment practices.

The committee arrived at its position after extensive discussion and deliberate consideration of many factors, including primarily the great variations in risk assessments among and within federal agencies and the fact that the expertise in risk assessment in the federal government resides, for the most part, in the agencies or with those with whom the agencies work.

Risk assessment is not a monolithic process or a single method. All risk assessments share some common principles, but their application varies widely among domains. Different technical issues arise in assessing the probability of exposure to a given dose of a chemical, of a malfunction of a nuclear power plant or air-traffic control system, or of the collapse of an ecosystem or a dam. And different technical issues arise in assessing the consequences of an accidental release from a nuclear power facility and an accidental release of a pesticide.

Risk assessment is not a field peopled with all-purpose experts. There are some with expertise in toxicology, decision analysis, dose-response assessment, ecologic risk assessment, engineering, and exposure assessment. In industry, some firms that specialize in one domain would not take on work in another. Federal agencies have staff familiar with the issues that are relevant to their missions; agencies without resident expertise have contractors with whom they have been working or associations to which they can turn.

One size does not fit all, nor can one set of technical guidance make sense for the heterogeneous risk assessments undertaken by federal agencies. Although the bulletin reflects that diversity and attempts to meet it with frequent references to "where appropriate" or "where feasible," the committee concludes that this approach is not workable for the agencies. As stated above, the committee strongly recommends that technical guidance be produced by the agencies and that agencies dealing with the same or similar hazards work together to produce common guidance to ensure an appropriately consistent approach.

As noted above, the committee agrees that there is room for improvement in risk assessment practices in the federal government and that additional guidance would help "to enhance the technical quality and objectivity of risk assessments prepared by federal agencies." However, the bulletin conveys the impression that risk assessments can and should achieve total objectivity. Although any scientific work should be free of bias, scientifically accurate, and based on reliable evidence, risk assessments cannot be wholly objective, because some important assumptions and judgments are based on policy or statutes. The committee strongly concludes that OMB should limit its efforts to stating goals and general principles of risk assessment and to directing the agencies to develop technical guidance consistent with the goals and principles. The committee has not provided suggestions for specific goals and principles in this report, because that was beyond the scope of its task.

CONCLUSIONS

Other conclusions that led to the committee's position that the OMB bulletin should be withdrawn are provided below. Three overarching conclusions are especially important.

- In view of the diversity of risk assessment responsibilities and proficiencies in the federal government, it would be difficult, if not impossible, to produce a single detailed technical guidance document that would be applicable to all federal agencies.
- New guidance that departs from established risk assessment principles and practices and is not supported by the current state of the science is unlikely to achieve the goals stated in the bulletin.
- Without baseline assessments of current risk assessment practices, needs, and capacities for improvement in the federal agencies, neither OMB nor the committee can make informed judgments on the kinds of guidance needed to reach the goals set forth in the bulletin and the related resources required to achieve that end.

Conclusions that are related to specific aspects of the proposed bulletin are provided below.

- In some general respects, the bulletin's requirements for risk assessments (for example, the call for balanced presentations of data and for explicit justification of scientific conclusions) are consistent with previous reports, including those cited in the bulletin. However, other aspects of the bulletin are inconsistent with previous reports in important ways. For example, it adopts a new definition of risk assessment and ignores, without explaining, the important impact that risk assessment policies have on the process, such as the need for consistent defaults and for clear criteria for moving away from the defaults. Without explicit and clear direction on such matters, agency risk assessments are more susceptible to being manipulated to achieve a predetermined result. The bulletin's call for formal analyses of uncertainties and for undefined "central or expected estimates" may, in the absence of adequate peer-reviewed technical guidance on the evaluation and expression of uncertainties, result in risk characterizations of reduced, rather than enhanced, quality. Those are serious concerns because any attempt to advance the practice of risk assessment that does not reflect the state of the art on these topics is likely to produce the opposite effect.

• The proposed definition of risk assessment in the OMB bulletin departs without justification from long-established concepts and practices, including those developed by National Research Council (NRC) and other expert committees and endorsed in existing peer-reviewed guidelines. In particular, the proposed definition broadens the definition of risk assessment to include components of risk assessment, such as hazard assessment and exposure assessment. Such a broadening, which treats different procedures under the same name, is needlessly confusing. More important, several of the standards proposed in the bulletin are not applicable to individual components of risk assessment. The committee also disagrees with defining risk assessment as a document; risk assessment is a process from which documents can result.

• The dominating theme of the bulletin and its supplementary information is improving the quality of risk assessments undertaken by federal agencies, but the stated goals do not all support this theme. The goals stated in the bulletin and the supplementary information emphasize *efficiency* in the conduct of risk assessment activities more than *quality*.

• The discussion of the range of risk estimates and central estimates in the proposed bulletin is incomplete and confusing. A central estimate and risk range might be misleading when sensitive populations are of primary concern. Those numerical quantities are meaningful only in the context of some distribution characterizing variable traits or uncertainties. The choice of summary statistics cannot be a blanket prescription but must reflect the specific context.

• The description of uncertainty and variability in the bulletin is simplistic. It does not recognize the complexities of different types of risk assessments or the need to tailor uncertainty analysis to an agency's particular needs. There is no scientific consensus to support the bulletin's universal prescriptions for how uncertainty should be evaluated.

• The bulletin's treatment of adverse effects is simplistic and too restrictive. Effects chosen for risk assessment may be adverse effects, precursor effects, or nonadverse effects. The point of departure to be chosen in a risk assessment depends on a number of factors, such as the questions being addressed, the scientific information available, and an understanding of the underlying mechanisms for the effect of interest.

• The bulletin is silent on several important aspects of the risk assessment process. Specifically, it gives little attention to risk assessments for which the end point is major failure of engineered systems, to sensitive populations, to the often decisive role of risk assessment policy in choices regarding default options, to the integral role of risk communication, and to risk assessment standards for stakeholder assessments submitted for use in the rule-making process. The bulletin also fails to explain the basis for exempting risk assessments associated with licensing and approval processes.

• Although risk assessment and risk management are closely related and it is desirable to build links between them, the committee agrees with accepted practice that they are distinct. The bulletin blurs the important distinction between them by setting risk assessment standards related to risk mitigation and comparative-risk activities usually regarded as risk management. Risk assessors should not be required to undertake what have been traditional risk management functions, such as identifying alternative mitigation strategies.

• The bulletin claims that it avoids addressing risk communication in any detail, but it includes quite specific guidance on this topic. The guidance provided is not well informed or consistent with previous expert panel reports. In general, the bulletin takes the outmoded view that risk communication is mainly a matter of disseminating key findings after a risk assessment has been completed and not the contemporary view that it is a continuing discussion among risk assessors, risk managers, and stakeholders from start to finish. The more objectionable risk communication guidance in the bulletin includes instructions to the agencies always to communicate ranges of plausible estimates and always to compare assessed risks with other familiar risks—guidance that is not consistent with relevant research literature.

• Although OMB has not constructed a baseline reflecting current agency risk assessment practices, the committee concludes on the basis of agency comments and its own knowledge of risk assessment practices that there are aspects of the bulletin that could be beneficial but that the cost—in staff resources, timeliness of completing risk assessments, and other factors—are likely to be substantial. Overall, the committee concludes that, while varied and uncertain to some extent, the potential for negative impacts on the practice of risk assessment in the federal government is very high if the currently proposed bulletin were to be implemented.

RECOMMENDATIONS

The committee offers OMB the following recommendations to consider in developing a new risk assessment bulletin.

- After withdrawing the current bulletin and before proceeding further, OMB should produce a description of current agency risk assessment practices and resources and the likely effects (both benefits and costs) of changing those practices.
- Before mandating substantial changes in agency risk assessment practices, OMB should ensure that sufficient funds and staffing are available on a continuing basis to support the agencies in their risk assessment responsibilities. Adequate staffing and funding are prerequisites to the kind of risk assessment envisioned in the bulletin.
- OMB should ensure that any government-wide risk assessment bulletin takes full account of and makes allowance for variations among agencies with respect to the types of risk assessments they engage in, the resources they have to devote to risk assessments, and their proficiency in risk assessment generally.
- Any guidance on risk assessment should provide a definition of risk assessment that is compatible with previous NRC documents and guidelines of other expert organizations; does not include information documents or individual components of risk assessment, such as hazard or exposure assessment; preserves the clear conventional distinctions between risk assessment and risk management; and refers to a process, not a document.
- OMB should develop goals for risk assessment that emphasize the central objective of enhanced scientific quality and the complementary objectives of efficiency and consistency among agencies evaluating the same or similar risks. The goals should support the production of risk assessments that provide clear, relevant, and scientifically sound information for policy-makers.
- OMB should develop general principles for risk assessment that are fully consistent with the recommendations provided by previous committees of NRC and those of other expert organizations. The committee recommends that the affected federal agencies develop their own

technical risk assessment guidelines that are consistent with the OMB general principles.

• The committee strongly recommends that discussion of uncertainty and variability, presentation of risk results, definition of adversity, and other similar topics be reserved for the technical guidance to be developed by the agencies.

REFERENCES

OMB (U.S. Office of Management and Budget). 2006. Proposed Risk Assessment Bulletin. Released January 9, 2006. Washington, DC: Office of Management and Budget, Executive Office of the President [online]. Available: http://www.whitehouse.gov/omb/inforeg/proposed_risk_assessment_bulletin_010906.pdf [accessed Oct. 11, 2006].

Appendix A

Biographical Information on the Committee to Review the OMB Risk Assessment Bulletin

John F. Ahearne *(Chair)* is the director of the Ethics Program for Sigma Xi, the Scientific Research Society, and an adjunct scholar at Resources for the Future. He was elected to the National Academy of Engineering in 1996. His professional interests are risk analysis, reactor safety, energy issues, resource allocation, and public-policy management. He has served as commissioner and chair of the U.S. Nuclear Regulatory Commission, system analyst for the White House Energy Office, deputy assistant secretary of energy, and principal deputy assistant secretary of defense. Dr. Ahearne currently serves on the Department of Energy's Nuclear Energy Research Advisory Committee. In addition, he has been active in several National Research Council committees examining issues in risk assessment and is a past president of the Society for Risk Analysis. He is a fellow of the American Physical Society, Society for Risk Analysis, American Association for the Advancement of Science, and American Academy of Arts and Sciences. Dr. Ahearne received his PhD in physics from Princeton University.

George V. Alexeeff is deputy director for scientific affairs in the Office of Environmental Health Hazard Assessment (OEHHA) of the California Environmental Protection Agency. He oversees a staff of over 80 scientists in multidisciplinary evaluations of the health impacts of pollutants and toxicants in air, water, soil, and other media. Activities include reviewing epidemiologic and toxicologic data to identify hazards and derive risk-based assessments, developing guidelines to identify chemicals hazardous to the public, recommending air-quality standards, identifying toxic air contaminants, developing public-health goals for water contaminants, preparing evaluations for carcinogens and reproductive toxins (Proposition 65), issuing sport-fish advisories, training health personnel on pesticide-poisoning recognition, reviewing hazardous-waste site risk assessments, and conducting multimedia risk assessments. Previously, he was chief of the Air Toxicology and Epidemiology Section of OEHHA from October 1990 through February 1998. Dr. Alexeeff has over 50 publications in the fields of toxicology and risk assessment. He earned his PhD in pharmacology and toxicology from the University of California, Davis.

Gregory B. Baecher is a professor in the civil engineering program at the University of Maryland. He was elected to the National Academy of Engineering in 2006. Previously, Dr. Baecher served on the faculty of civil engineering at the Massachusetts Institute of Technology and as the CEO of ConSolve Incorporated in Lexington, Massachusetts. His expertise includes risk analysis, water-resources engineering, and statistical methods. Dr. Baecher has served on numerous National Research Council committees and panels. He earned his PhD in civil engineering from the Massachusetts Institute of Technology.

A. John Bailer is distinguished professor in the Department of Mathematics and Statistics and a senior researcher in the Scripps Gerontology Center at Miami University in Oxford, Ohio. His research interests include the design and analysis of environmental- and occupational-health studies and quantitative risk estimation. Dr. Bailer is a fellow of the American Statistical Association (ASA), a fellow of the Society for Risk Analysis, and a recipient of the ASA Statistics and the Environment Distinguished Achievement Medal. He has served on a number of National Research Council committees. He also has served as a member of subcommittees of the Board of Scientific Counselors of the National Toxicology Program. He received his PhD in biostatistics from the University of North Carolina at Chapel Hill.

Roger M. Cooke is the Chauncey Starr Senior Fellow at Resources for the Future (RFF). His research interests include the mathematical modeling of risk and uncertainty, structured expert-judgment methods, and the implementation of uncertainty analysis in policy-related decision-making. Recent research activities include assessing health risks posed by oil fires in Kuwait after the first Gulf War, chemical-weapons disposal, nuclear risk, nitrogen oxide emissions, and microbiologic risk. Before joining RFF, Dr. Cooke was professor of applied decision theory at the Department of Mathematics of Delft University of Technology in the Netherlands. He earned his PhD at Yale University.

Charles E. Feigley is professor of environmental health sciences at the Arnold School of Public Health at the University of South Carolina (USC). His current research is primarily in exposure assessment and occupational-hygiene engineering with an emphasis on developing innovative exposure-assessment and exposure-control methods in health-care and school environments. He is principal investigator of the USC Center for Public Health Preparedness funded by the Centers for Disease Control and Prevention. He has served on a number of National Research Council committees. He received his PhD in environmental sciences and engineering from the University of North Carolina.

Baruch Fischhoff is Howard Heinz University Professor in the Department of Social and Decision Sciences and Department of Engineering and Public Policy of Carnegie Mellon University, where he is head of the decision-sciences major and the Center for Integrated Study of Human Dimensions of Global Change. He was elected to the Institute of Medicine in 1993. Dr. Fischhoff's research includes risk perception and communication, risk analysis and management, adolescent decision-making, medical informed consent, and environmental protection. He has been a co-author or editor of four books: *Acceptable Risk* (1981), *A Two-State Solution in the Middle East: Prospects and Possibilities* (1993), *Preference Elicitation* (1999), and *Risk Communication: The Mental Models Approach* (2001). Dr. Fischhoff has served on numerous Institute of Medicine and National Research Council committees. He is a fellow of the American Psychological Association and recipient of its Early Career Awards for Distinguished Scientific Contribution to Psychology and for Contributions to Psychology in the Public Interest. He is a past president of the Society for Risk Analysis and recipient of its Distinguished Achievement Award. He is a member of the Department of Homeland Security's Science and Technology Advisory Committee, the World Federation of Scientists Permanent Monitoring Panel on Terrorism, and the Environmental Protection Agency's Scientific Advisory Board, where he chairs the Subcommittee on Homeland Security. Dr. Fischhoff earned a PhD in psychology from the Hebrew University of Jerusalem.

Charles P. Gerba is professor of environmental microbiology in the Departments of Microbiology and Immunology and Soil, Water and Environmental Science at the University of Arizona. He actively conducts research on the development of new disinfectants and drinking-water treatment processes, new methods for the detection of waterborne pathogens, occurrence and fate of pathogens in the environment, and microbial risk assessment. Dr. Gerba has written more than 400 articles and several textbooks in environmental microbiology and quantitative microbial risk assessment. He previously served as a member of the U.S. Environmental Protection Agency's Science Advisory Board Committee on Drinking Water and Research Strategies. He is a member of the American Academy of Microbiology. He received a PhD in microbiology from the University of Miami.

Rose H. Goldman is associate professor of medicine at Harvard Medical School and associate professor in the Department of Environmental Health at the Harvard School of Public Health. She is also chief of occupational and environmental medicine at Cambridge Health Alliance. Dr. Goldman's research interests include repetitive strain injuries, neurotoxicology, pediatric environmental health, and environmental and occupational medicine. She is a co-project director of the Pediatric Environmental Health Specialty Unit at Cambridge Hospital and Children's Hospital Boston. Dr. Goldman has served on numerous Institute of Medicine and National Research Council committees. She earned her MPH from the Harvard School of Public Health and her MD from the Yale School of Medicine and is board-certified in internal and preventive medicine (occupational medicine).

Robert Haveman is professor emeritus of economics and public affairs and research affiliate at the Institute for Research on Poverty at the University of Wisconsin-Madison. His research interests and publications focus on public finance, economics of environmental and natural-resources policy, benefit-cost analysis, and economics of poverty and social policy. Dr. Haveman's current projects include work on the discrepancy in reported earnings in surveys compared with administrative records, on the adequacy of savings of older workers beginning retirement, and on the effects of Section 8 housing assistance on employment and earnings. He was director of the Institute for Research on Poverty from 1971 to 1975 and of the La Follette School of Public Affairs from 1988 to 1991. Dr. Haveman has served as senior economist for the Subcommittee on Economy in Government, Joint Economic Committee, U.S. Congress. Dr. Haveman earned his PhD in economics from Vanderbilt University.

William E. Kastenberg is the Daniel M. Tellep Distinguished Professor in Engineering at the University of California, Berkeley. He was elected to the National Academy of Engineering in 1997. His research interests include the development and application of risk-assessment and risk-management methods for complex technologic, natural, and social systems. He has examined a broad array of technical and social issues regarding nuclear and nonnuclear risks, including severe accidents at commercial nuclear-power plants, the spatial and temporal persistence of pesticides, incinerator emissions, contaminated groundwater, malicious human acts, and cost-benefit considerations for severe accident mitigation. More recently, he has focused on ethical issues concerning the development of new technologies. He is the author or coauthor of over 150 published papers and conference proceedings related to nuclear-reactor safety, risk assessment, risk management, public health, environmental risk assessment, ethics, and multistakeholder decision-making. Dr. Kastenberg was elected a fellow of the American Association for the Advancement of Science in 1990 and of the American Nuclear Society in 1978. He has served on numerous National Research Council committees. Dr. Kastenberg earned his PhD in nuclear engineering from the University of California, Berkeley.

Sally Katzen is visiting professor of law at George Mason University. Previously, she taught administrative law and information-technology policy at the University of Michigan Law School. She has taught administrative law at the University of Pennsylvania Law School and the Georgetown Law Center. She has also taught American government courses to undergraduates at Smith College, Johns Hopkins University, and the University of Michigan (Washington Program). Before her teaching positions, she served as the administrator of the Office of Information and Regulatory Affairs in the Office of Management and Budget (OMB) (1993-1998), as the deputy director of the National Economic Council in the White House (1998-1999), and as the deputy director for management in OMB (1999-2001). Before her government service, she was a partner in the Washington, DC, law firm of Wilmer, Cutler, and

Pickering, specializing in administrative law and legislative matters. She earned her JD from the University of Michigan Law School.

Eduardo Miranda is an assistant professor in the Department of Civil and Environmental Engineering at Stanford University. Before joining Stanford, Dr. Miranda worked as a consulting structural engineer specializing in risk analysis and earthquake engineering. His research interests include the development of fragility functions for structural and nonstructural components, performance-based engineering, the simulation and visualization of construction operations, computer-based design automation of structures, the development of advanced structural systems, and the application and development of new sensing technology to civil engineering structures. Dr. Miranda earned his MS and PhD from the University of California, Berkeley.

Michael Newman is professor of marine science at the Virginia Institute of Marine Science at the College of William and Mary. His research interests include ecotoxicology, general and applied aquatic ecology, contaminant effects on populations, bioaccumulation, factors modifying inorganic-contaminant toxicity, fate of inorganic contaminants in aquatic systems, quantitative methods for ecologic risk assessment, toxicity models, and water quality. He earned his MS and PhD in environmental sciences from Rutgers University.

Dorothy E. Patton (retired) was previously adjunct professor at the Georgetown (University) Public Policy Institute and is a consultant with the Risk Science Institute of the International Life Sciences Institute. Dr. Patton has over 24 years of experience with the Environmental Protection Agency (EPA), where she served as the director of the Office of Science Policy, the executive director of the Science Policy Council, and the executive director of the Risk Assessment Forum. In those positions, her responsibilities included developing and implementing risk assessment policies and practices, environmental research planning and priority-setting, and long-range strategic planning in line with congressional mandates. She began her EPA career as an attorney in the Office of General Counsel, where she worked on air, pesticide, and toxic-substances issues. Dr. Patton has served on numerous National Research Council committees. She earned a PhD in biology from the University of Chicago and a JD from Columbia University School of Law.

Charles Poole is an associate professor in the Department of Epidemiology at the University of North Carolina School of Public Health. Previously, he was with the Boston University School of Public Health. Dr. Poole's work focuses on the development and use of epidemiologic methods and principles, including problem definition, study design, data collection, statistical analysis, and the interpretation and application of research results, such as systematic review and meta-analysis. His research experience includes studies in environmental and occupational epidemiology. Dr. Poole was an epidemiologist in the Office of Pesticides and Toxic Substances of the Environmental Protection Agency for 5 years and worked for a decade as an epidemiologic consultant with a firm and independently. Dr. Poole has been a member of a number of National Research Council and Institute of Medicine committees. He received his MPH in health administration from the University of North Carolina School of Public Health and his ScD in epidemiology from the Harvard School of Public Health.

Danny D. Reible is the Bettie Margaret Smith Chair of Environmental Health Engineering at the University of Texas at Austin and codirector of the Environmental Protection Agency's Hazardous Substance Research Center/South and Southwest. Dr. Reible was elected to the National Academy of Engineering in 2005. His research focuses on transport phenomena and their application to environmental mechanics, especially contaminant fate and transport in sediments. He directs projects to develop process understanding and tools for the assessment and management of risks posed by contaminated sediments and dredged materials. He has served on a number of National Research Council committees and boards. Dr. Reible earned his PhD in chemical engineering from the California Institute of Technology.

Joseph V. Rodricks is a founding principal of ENVIRON International, a technical consulting firm founded in 1982. He is an internationally recognized expert in toxicology and risk analysis and in their uses in regulation. He has consulted for hundreds of manufacturers, government agencies, and the World Health Organization. He has more than 150 publications on toxicology and risk analysis, and he has lectured nationally and internationally on these topics. Dr. Rodricks was formerly deputy associate commissioner for health affairs, and toxicologist for the Food and Drug Administration (1965-1980), and he is now a visiting professor at the Johns Hopkins University School of Public Health. He has been certified as a diplomate by the American Board of Toxicology since 1982.

Dr. Rodricks's experience includes chemical products and contaminants in foods, food ingredients, air, water, hazardous wastes, the workplace, consumer products, and medical devices and pharmaceutical products. He has served on numerous National Research Council and Institute of Medicine committees. He earned his PhD in biochemistry from the University of Maryland and did postdoctoral work at the University of California, Berkeley.

Appendix B

OMB Proposed Risk Assessment Bulletin

OFFICE OF MANAGEMENT AND BUDGET

Proposed Risk Assessment Bulletin

SUMMARY: As part of an ongoing effort to improve the quality, objectivity, utility, and integrity of information disseminated by the federal government to the public, the Office of Management and Budget (OMB), in consultation with the Office of Science and Technology Policy (OSTP), proposes to issue new technical guidance on risk assessments produced by the federal government.

DATES: Interested parties should submit comments to OMB's Office of Information and Regulatory Affairs on or before June 15, 2006.

ADDRESSES: Because of potential delays in OMB's receipt and processing of mail, respondents are strongly encouraged to submit comments electronically to ensure timely receipt. We cannot guarantee that comments mailed will be received before the comment closing date. Electronic comments may be submitted to: OMB_RAbulletin@omb.eop.gov. Please put the full body of your comments in the text of the electronic message and as an attachment. Please include your name, title, organization, postal address, telephone number and e-mail address in the text of the message. Please be aware that all comments are available for public inspection. Accordingly, please do not submit comments containing trade secrets, confidential or proprietary commercial or financial information, or other information that you do not want to be made available to the public. Comments also may be submitted via facsimile to (202) 395-7245.

FOR FURTHER INFORMATION CONTACT: Dr. Nancy Beck, Office of Information and Regulatory Affairs, Office of Management and Budget, 725 17th Street, N.W., New Executive Office Building, Room 10201, Washington, DC, 20503. Telephone (202) 395-3093.

SUPPLEMENTARY INFORMATION:

Introduction

Risk assessment is a useful tool for estimating the likelihood and severity of risks to human health, safety and the environment and for informing decisions about how to manage those risks. For the purposes of this Bulletin, the term "risk assessment" refers to a document that assembles and synthesizes scientific information to determine whether a potential hazard exists and/or the extent of possible risk to human health, safety or the environment.

The acceptance of risk assessment in health, safety, and environmental policy was enhanced by the seminal report issued by the National Academy of Sciences (NAS) in 1983: *Risk*

This proposed bulletin is being released for peer review and public comment. It should not be construed to represent the official policy of the U.S. Office of Management and Budget.

Assessment in the Federal Government: Managing the Process. The report presented a logical approach to assessing environmental, health and safety risk that was widely accepted and used by government agencies.

Over twenty years after publication of the NAS report, there is general agreement that the risk assessment process can be improved. The process should be better understood, more transparent and more objective. Risk assessment can be most useful when those who rely on it to inform the risk management process understand its value, nature and limitations, and use it accordingly.

Many studies have supported the use of risk assessment and recommended improvements. For example, in 1993 the Carnegie Commission on Science, Technology, and Government issued "Risk and the Environment: Improving Regulatory Decision-making."[1] In 1994, the NAS issued "Science and Judgment in Risk Assessment" to review and evaluate the risk assessment methods of EPA.[2] In 1995, the Harvard Center for Risk Analysis issued "Reform of Risk Regulation: Achieving More Protection at Less Cost."[3] In 1997, the Presidential/Congressional Commission on Risk Assessment and Risk Management issued "Risk Assessment and Risk Management in Regulatory Decision-Making."[4] A series of NAS reports over the past 10 years have made useful recommendations on specific aspects and applications of risk assessment.[5] The findings in these reports informed the development of this Bulletin.

OMB, in collaboration with OSTP, has a strong interest in the technical quality of agency risk assessments because these assessments play an important role in the development of public policies at the national, international, state and local levels. The increasing importance of risk assessment in the development of public policy, regulation, and decision making requires that the

---

[1]Carnegie Commission on Science, Technology and Government, *Risk and the Environment: Improving Regulatory Decision Making*, New York, NY, June 1993.
[2]National Research Council *Science and Judgment in Risk Assessment*, Washington DC: National Academy Press, 1994.
[3]Harvard Group on Risk Management Reform, *Reform of Risk Regulation: Achieving More Protection at Less Cost*, Human and Ecological Risk Assessment, vol. 183, 1995, pp. 183-206.
[4]Presidential/Congressional Commission on Risk Assessment and Risk Management, Vol. 2, *Risk Assessment and Risk Management in Regulatory Decision-Making,* hereinafter *"Risk Commission Report,"* 1997.
[5]See, e.g., National Research Council, *Health Implications of Perchlorate Ingestion,*, Washington DC: National Academy Press, 2005; National Research Council, *Arsenic in Drinking Water 2001 Update*, Washington DC: National Academy Press, 2001; National Research Council, *Toxicological Effects of Methylmercury*, Washington DC: National Academy Press, 2000; National Research Council, *Health Effects of Exposure to Radon, BEIR VI*, Washington DC: National Academy Press, 1999; National Research Council, *Science and the Endangered Species Act*, Washington, DC: National Academy Press, 1995; National Research Council, *Science and Judgment in Risk Assessment*, Washington DC: National Academy Press, 1994; National Research Council, *Issues in Risk Assessment I: Use of the Maximum Tolerated Dose in Animal Bioassays for Carcinogenicity*, Washington DC: National Academy Press, 1993; National Research Council, *Issues in Risk Assessment II: The Two Stage Model of Carcinogenesis*, Washington DC: National Academy Press, 1993; National Research Council, *Issues in Risk Assessment III: A Paradigm for Ecological Risk Assessment*, Washington DC: National Academy Press, 1993; National Research Council, *Pesticides in the Diet of Infants and Children*, Washington DC: National Academy Press, 1993; National Academy of Engineering, *Keeping Pace with Science and Engineering: Case Studies in Environmental Regulation*, Washington DC: National Academy Press, 1993; National Research Council, *Risk Assessment in the Federal Government: Managing the Process*, Washington DC: National Academy Press, 1983.

This proposed bulletin is released for peer review and public comment. It should not be construed to represent the official policy of the U.S. Office of Management and Budget.

technical quality and transparency of agency risk assessments meet high quality standards. Moreover, a risk assessment prepared by one federal agency may inform the policy decisions of another federal agency, or a risk assessment prepared by one or more federal agencies may inform decisions made by legislators or the judiciary. This Bulletin builds upon the historic interest that both OMB and OSTP have expressed in advancing the state of the art of risk assessment.[6]

The purpose of this Bulletin is to enhance the technical quality and objectivity of risk assessments prepared by federal agencies by establishing uniform, minimum standards. Federal agencies should implement the technical guidance provided in this Bulletin, recognizing that the purposes and types of risk assessments vary. The Bulletin builds on OMB's Information Quality Guidelines and Information Quality Bulletin on Peer Review and is intended as a companion to OMB Circular A-4 (2003), which was designed to enhance the technical quality of regulatory impact analyses, especially benefit-cost analysis and cost-effectiveness analysis. Like OMB Circular A-4, this Bulletin will need to be updated periodically as agency practices and the peer-reviewed literature on risk assessment progress.

The audience for the Bulletin includes analysts and managers in federal agencies with responsibilities for assessing and managing risk or conducting research on improved approaches to risk assessment. The Bulletin should also be of interest to the broad range of specialists in the private and public sectors involved in or affected by risk assessments and/or decisions about risk and safety.

Although this Bulletin addresses certain technical aspects of risk assessment, it does not address in any detail the important processes of risk management and risk communication.[7] The technical guidance provided here addresses the development of the underlying documents that may help inform risk management and communication, but the scope of this document does not encompass how federal agencies should manage or communicate risk.

Uses of Risk Assessments

Risk assessment is used for many purposes by the Federal Government. At a broad level, risk assessments can be used for priority setting, managing risk, and informing the public and other audiences. The purpose of the assessment may influence the scope of the analytic work, the type of data collected, the choice of analytic methods, and the approach taken to reporting the findings. Accordingly, the purpose of an assessment should be made clear before the analytical work begins.

---

[6]See U.S. Office of Science and Technology Policy, *Chemical Carcinogens: A Review of the Science and Its Associated Principles,* 50 FR10371 (1985); and, U.S. Office of Management and Budget, Memorandum for the Regulatory Working Group, *Principles for Risk Analysis,* Jan 12, 1995.

[7]National Research Council *Understanding Risk: Informing Decisions in a Democratic Society,* Washington DC: National Academy Press, 1996; Risk Commission Report, Volume 2, 1997; National Research Council, *Improving Risk Communication,* Washington DC: National Academy Press, 1989.

This proposed bulletin is being released for peer review and public comment. It should not be construed to represent the official policy of the U.S. Office of Management and Budget.

Priority Setting

Risk assessment is sometimes used as a tool to compare risks for priority-setting purposes.[8] For example, in 1975 the Department of Transportation prepared a comparative assessment of traffic safety hazards related to highway and vehicle design as well as driver behavior.[9] A wide range of countermeasures were compared to determine which measures would be most effective in saving lives and reducing injuries. Similarly, risk assessment models relating to food safety and agricultural health concerns may be used to rank relative risks from different hazards, diseases, or pests. In 1987 and again in 1990, the Environmental Protection Agency (EPA) prepared a comparative assessment of environmental hazards – both risks to human health and the environment – to inform the Agency's priority setting.[10] This work demonstrated that the environmental risks of greatest concern to the public often were not ranked as the greatest risks by agency managers and scientists.

Screening-level risk assessments are sometimes used as a first step in priority setting. The purpose of the "screen" is to determine, using conservative (or worst-case) assumptions, whether a risk could exist, and whether the risk could be sufficiently serious to justify agency action. If the screening-level assessment indicates that a potential hazard is not of concern, the agency may decide not to undertake a more comprehensive assessment. If the screening-level assessment indicates that the potential hazard may be of concern, then the agency may proceed to undertake a more comprehensive assessment to estimate the risk more accurately.[11]

Informing Risk Management Decisions

Often, a risk assessment is conducted to help determine whether to reduce risk and, if so, to establish the appropriate level of stringency. A wide set of standards derived from statutes, regulations, and/or case law guide regulatory agencies in making risk management decisions. In such situations, the risk management standard is known a priori based on "acceptable risk" considerations.[12]

Risk assessments may be used to look at risk reduction under various policy alternatives to determine if these alternatives are effective in reducing risks. In some agency programs, the

---

[8]Davies, J. C. (ed), *Comparing Environmental Risks: Tools for Setting Government Priorities*, Resources for the Future, Washington, DC, 1996; Minard, R, *State Comparative Risk Projects: A Force for Change*, Northeast Center for Comparative Risk, South Royalton, Vermont, March 1993.

[9]U.S. Department of Transportation, *National Highway Safety Needs Report*, Washington, DC, April 1976.

[10]U.S. Environmental Protection Agency, Unfinished Business: A Comparative Assessment of Environmental Protection, Washington, DC, 1987; U.S. Environmental Protection Agency, Reducing Risk: Setting Priorities and Strategies for Environmental Protection, Science Advisory Board, Washington, DC, 1990.

[11]National Research Council, *Science and Judgment in Risk Assessment*, Washington DC: National Academy Press, 1994.

[12]Douglas, M, *Risk Acceptability According to the Social Sciences*, Russell Sage Foundation, New York, NY, 1985; Fischhoff, B, S Lichtenstein, P Slovic, SL Derby, RL Keeney, *Acceptable Risk*, Cambridge University Press, UK, 1981.

This proposed bulletin is released for peer review and public comment. It should not be construed to represent the official policy of the U.S. Office of Management and Budget.

results of risk assessments are an important technical input to benefit-cost analyses, which are then used to inform risk management decisions in rulemakings.[13]

Informing the Public

In some circumstances, risk assessments are undertaken to inform the public through education and informational programs.[14] Such programs can help citizens make informed decisions in their personal lives. For example, Federal agencies alert the public about the risks of living in a home with elevated levels of radon gas, of purchasing a sport utility vehicle with a certain height-to-width ratio, and taking long-term estrogen therapy. The dissemination of public risk information, even if it is not accompanied by a regulation, can induce changes in the behavior of consumers, patients, workers, and businesses.

Sometimes, Federal agencies undertake large-scale risk assessments that are designed to inform multiple audiences. For example, the Surgeon General's Report on Smoking and Health has, over the years, contained a wide variety of health risk estimates. These estimates have been adopted in programs and documents disseminated by local and state governments, Federal agencies, private companies, and the public at large. In some cases, Federal scientists participate in an international effort to develop risk models that can be used to educate the public and inform decisions throughout the world.[15]

Types of Risk Assessments

Risk assessment is a broad term that encompasses a variety of analytic techniques that are used in different situations, depending upon the nature of the hazard, the available data, and needs of decision makers.[16] The different techniques were developed by specialists from many disciplines, including toxicology, epidemiology, medicine, chemistry, biology, engineering, physics, statistics, management science, economics and the social sciences. Most risk assessments are performed by teams of specialists representing multiple disciplines. They are often prepared by government scientists or contractors to the government.

---

[13] Breyer, S., *Breaking the Vicious Circle: Toward Effective Risk Regulation*, Harvard University Press, Cambridge, MA 1993; Hahn, RW (ed), *Risks, Costs and Lives Saved: Getting Better Results from Regulation*, Oxford University Press, New York, NY, 1996; Viscusi, WK, *Rational Risk Policy*, Clarendon Press, Oxford, UK, 1998; National Research Council, *Valuing Health Risks, Costs, and Benefits for Environmental Decisionmaking*, Washington, DC: National Academy Press, 1990.

[14] Fischhoff, B, S Lichtenstein, P Slovic, SL Derby, RL Keeney, *Acceptable Risk*, Cambridge University Press, UK, 1981; Douglas, M, *Risk Acceptability According to the Social Sciences*, Russell Sage Foundation, New York, NY, 1985; Wilson, R, EAC Crouch, *Risk-Benefit Analysis*, Harvard University Press, Cambridge, MA, 2001.

[15] Renn, O, *White Paper on Risk Governance: Towards an Integrative Approach*, International Risk Governance Council, Geneva, Switzerland, September 2005.

[16] Haimes, YY, *Risk Modeling, Assessment, and Management*, John Wiley and Sons, New York, New York, 1998; Wilson, R, EAC Crouch, *Risk-Benefit Analysis*, Harvard University Press, Cambridge, MA, 2001.

This proposed bulletin is being released for peer review and public comment. It should not be construed to represent the official policy of the U.S. Office of Management and Budget.

Actuarial Analysis of Real-World Human Data

When large amounts of historic data from humans are available, an actuarial risk assessment may be performed using classical statistical tools. For example, the safety risks associated with use of motor vehicles, including the risks of a vehicle's design features, may be estimated by applying statistical tools to historic data on crashes, injuries and/or fatalities. When sufficient numbers of people have been exposed to large doses of chemicals and radiation, it may be feasible to estimate risks using health data and statistical methods. The field of epidemiology, a branch of public health and medicine, performs such assessments by combining actuarial analyses with biologic theory and medical expertise.[17] The field of radiation risk assessment has been informed by epidemiology, including studies of the World War II bombings at Hiroshima and Nagasaki and more recently the experiences of workers who were exposed to radiation on the job. Estimates of the health risks of tobacco products have been generated primarily on the basis of epidemiology.

Dose-Response Analysis Using Experimental Data

Special techniques of risk assessment have been developed for settings where humans and/or animals are exposed – intermittently or continuously – to various doses of substances.[18] The adverse effects of concern may range from different types of cancer to developmental, reproductive or neurological effects. Real-world data on adverse effects in humans or wildlife may not be available because (a) adequate data have not been collected, (b) the adverse effects (e.g., certain types of leukemia) are too rare to analyze directly, (c) the exposures of concern are associated with a new technology or product, or (d) adverse effects may occur only after a long period (e.g., several decades) of exposure.

When direct real-world data on toxicity are unavailable or are inadequate, risk assessments may be performed based on data from toxicity experiments with rodents, since rats and mice have relatively short lifetimes and are relatively inexpensive to house and feed. Toxicity experiments involving rodents, although controversial to some, have three important advantages: (1) the doses, whether administered by injection, in feed or by inhalation, can be measured precisely, (2) different doses can be applied to different groups of rodents by experimental design, and (3) pathology can be performed on rodents to make precise counts of tumors and other adverse events.

When dose-response data are available from a rodent experiment, the assessor usually faces two critical extrapolation issues: how effects observed in rodents are relevant to people or wildlife and how effects observed at the high doses used in experiments are relevant to the low doses typically found in the environment. Techniques have been developed to perform such extrapolations and to portray the resulting uncertainty in risk estimates associated with extrapolation.

---

[17]Monson, R, *Occupational Epidemiology, Second Edition*, CRC Press, Boca Raton, Florida, 1990.

[18]Rodricks, JV, *Calculated Risks: The Toxicity and Human Health Risks of Chemicals in Our Environment*, Cambridge, University Press, New York, NY, 1992.

This proposed bulletin is released for peer review and public comment. It should not be construed to represent the official policy of the U.S. Office of Management and Budget.

Infectious Disease and Epidemic Modeling

Risk assessments of infectious agents pose special challenges since the rate of diffusion of an infectious agent may play a critical role in determining the occurrence and severity of an epidemic. Risk assessments of the spread of the HIV virus, and the resulting cases of AIDs, were complicated by the different modes of transmission (e.g., sexual behavior, needle exchange and blood transfusion) and the analyst's need to understand the relative size and degree of mixing of these populations.[19] Scientific understanding of both biology and human behavior are critical to performing accurate risk assessments for infectious agents.

Failure Analysis of Physical Structures

One of the best known types of risk assessments addresses low-probability, high-consequence events associated with the failure of physical structures.[20] Since these events are exceedingly rare (e.g., bridge failure or a major core meltdown at a nuclear reactor), it may not be feasible to compute risks based on historic data alone. Engineers have developed alternative techniques (e.g., fault-tree analysis) that estimate both the probability of catastrophic events and the magnitude of the resulting damages to people, property and the environment. Such "probabilistic" risk assessments are now widely used in the development of safety systems for dams, nuclear and chemical plants, liquefied natural gas terminals, space shuttles and other physical structures.

Legal Authority

This Bulletin is issued under statutory authority and OMB's general authorities to oversee the quality of agency analyses, information and regulatory actions.

In the "Information Quality Act," Congress directed OMB to issue guidelines to "provide policy and procedural guidance to Federal agencies for ensuring and maximizing the quality, objectivity, utility and integrity of information" disseminated by Federal agencies. Pub. L. No. 106-554, § 515(a). The Information Quality Act was developed as a supplement to the Paperwork Reduction Act, 44 U.S.C. § 3501 et seq., which requires OMB, among other things, to "develop and oversee the implementation of policies, principles, standards, and guidelines to . . . apply to Federal agency dissemination of public information." Moreover, Section 624 of the Treasury and General Government Appropriations Act of 2001, often called the "Regulatory Right-to-Know Act," (Public Law 106-554, 31 U.S.C. § 1105 note) directs OMB to "issue guidelines to agencies to standardize . . . measures of costs and benefits" of Federal rules.

---

[19]Turner, CF., et al., *AIDS: Sexual Behavior and Intravenous Drug Use*, National Research Council, Washington, D.C., 1989, pp. 471-499.

[20]Pate-Cornell, ME, *Uncertainties in Risk Analysis: Six Levels of Treatment*, Reliability Engineering and System Safety, vol. 54(2-3), 1996, pp. 95-111; Haimes, YY, *Risk Modeling, Assessment, and Management*, John Wiley and Sons, New York, New York, 1998.

This proposed bulletin is being released for peer review and public comment. It should not be construed to represent the official policy of the U.S. Office of Management and Budget.

Executive Order 12866, 58 Fed. Reg. 51,735 (Oct. 4, 1993), establishes that OIRA is "the repository of expertise concerning regulatory issues, including methodologies and procedures that affect more than one agency," and it directs OMB to provide guidance to the agencies on regulatory planning. E.O. 12866, § 2(b). The Order requires that "[e]ach agency shall base its decisions on the best reasonably obtainable scientific, technical, economic, or other information." E.O. 12866, § 1(b)(7). The Order also directs that "[i]n setting regulatory priorities, each agency shall consider, to the extent reasonable, the degree and nature of risks posed by various substances or activities within its jurisdiction." E.O. 12866, § 1(b)(4). Finally, OMB has additional authorities to oversee the agencies in the administration of their programs.

All of these authorities support this Bulletin.

The Requirements of This Bulletin

This bulletin addresses quality standards for risk assessments disseminated by federal agencies.

Section I: Definitions

Section I provides definitions that are central to this Bulletin. Several terms are identical to or based on those used in OMB's government-wide information quality guidelines, 67 Fed. Reg. 8452 (Feb. 22, 2002), and the Paperwork Reduction Act, 44 U.S.C. § 3501 et seq.

The term "Administrator" means the Administrator of the Office of Information and Regulatory Affairs in the Office of Management and Budget (OIRA).

The term "agency" has the same meaning as in the Paperwork Reduction Act, 44 U.S.C. § 3502(1).

The term "Information Quality Act" means Section 515 of Public Law 106-554 (Pub. L. No. 106-554, § 515, 114 Stat. 2763, 2763A-153-154 (2000)).

The term "risk assessment" means a scientific and/or technical document that assembles and synthesizes scientific information to determine whether a potential hazard exists and/or the extent of possible risk to human health, safety, or the environment. For the purposes of this Bulletin, this definition applies to documents that could be used for risk assessment purposes, such as an exposure or hazard assessment that might not constitute a complete risk assessment as defined by the National Research Council.[21] This definition includes documents that evaluate baseline risk as well as risk mitigation activities.

---

[21] National Research Council *Risk Assessment in the Federal Government: Managing the Process*, Washington DC: National Academy Press, 1983.

This proposed bulletin is released for peer review and public comment. It should not be construed to represent the official policy of the U.S. Office of Management and Budget.

The term "influential risk assessment" means a risk assessment the agency reasonably can determine will have or does have a clear and substantial impact on important public policies or private sector decisions. The term "influential" should be interpreted consistently with OMB's government-wide Information Quality Guidelines and the Information Quality Guidelines of the relevant agency. A risk assessment can have a significant economic impact even if it is not part of a rulemaking. For instance, the economic viability of a technology can be influenced by the government's characterization of the risks associated with the use of the technology. Alternatively, the federal government's assessment of risk can directly or indirectly influence the regulatory actions of state and local agencies or international bodies.

Examples of "influential risk assessments" include, but are not limited to, assessments that determine the level of risk regarding health (such as reference doses, reference concentrations, and minimal risk levels), safety and environment. Documents that address some but not all aspects of risk assessment are covered by this Bulletin. Specific examples of such risk assessments include: margin of exposure estimates, hazard determinations, EPA Integrated Risk Information System (IRIS) values, risk assessments which support EPA National Ambient Air Quality Standards, FDA tolerance values, ATSDR toxicological profiles, HHS/NTP substance profiles, NIOSH current intelligence bulletins and criteria documents, and risk assessments performed as part of economically significant rulemakings. Documents falling within these categories are presumed to be influential for the purposes of this Bulletin.

The term "available to the public" covers documents that are made available to the public by the agency or that are required to be disclosed under the Freedom of Information Act, 5 U.S.C. § 552.

Section II: Applicability

Section II states that, *to the extent appropriate*, all publicly available agency risk assessments shall comply with the standards of this Bulletin. This statement recognizes that there may be situations in which it is not appropriate for a particular risk assessment to comport with one or more specific standards contained in this Bulletin, including the general standards in Section IV, which apply to both influential and non-influential risk assessments. A rule of reason should prevail in the appropriate application of the standards in this Bulletin. For example, in a screening-level risk assessment, the analyst may be seeking to define an upper limit on the unknown risk that is not likely to be exceeded. Screening-level assessments, in this situation, would not have to meet the standard of "neither minimizing nor exaggerating the nature and magnitude of risk." On the other hand, it is expected that every risk assessment (even screening- level assessments) will comply with other standards in Section IV. For example, it is expected that every risk assessment shall describe the data, methods, and assumptions with a high degree of transparency; shall identify key scientific limitations and uncertainties; and shall place the risk in perspective/context with other risks familiar to the target audience. Similarly, every quantitative risk assessment should provide a range of plausible risk estimates, when there is scientific uncertainty or variability.

This Bulletin does not apply to risk assessments that arise in the course of individual agency adjudications or permit proceedings, unless the agency determines that: (1) compliance with the Bulletin is practical and appropriate and (2) the risk assessment is scientifically or technically novel or likely to have precedent-setting influence on future adjudications and/or permit proceedings. This exclusion is intended to cover, among other things, licensing, approval and registration processes for specific product development activities. This Bulletin also shall not apply to risk assessments performed with respect to inspections relating to health, safety, or environment.

This Bulletin also does not apply to any risk assessment performed with respect to an individual product label, or any risk characterization appearing on any such label, if the individual product label is required by law to be approved by a Federal agency prior to use. An example of this type of risk assessment includes risk assessments performed for labeling of individual pharmaceutical products. This Bulletin does apply to risk assessments performed with respect to classes of products. An example of this type of risk assessment is the risk assessment performed by FDA in their evaluation of the labeling for products containing trans-fatty acids.

Section III: Goals

For each covered risk assessment, this Bulletin lays out five aspirational goals.

1. Goals Related to Problem Formulation

As a risk assessment is prepared, risk assessors should engage in an iterative dialogue with the agency decision maker(s) who will use the assessment. There will be many choices regarding the objectives, scope, and content of the assessment, and an iterative dialogue will help ensure that the risk assessment serves its intended purpose and is developed in a cost-effective manner. For example, a risk manager may be interested in estimates of population and/or individual risk and an iterative dialogue would ideally bring this to the attention of a risk assessor early in the process.

2. Goals Related to Completeness

There is often a tension between the desire for completeness in the scientific sense and the desire for a well-defined scope that limits the inquiry to a set of practical, tractable, and relevant questions. The scope of an assessment should reflect a balance between the desire for scientific completeness and the need to provide relevant information to decision makers. The concept of considering the benefits and cost of acquiring further information (e.g., a broader scope or better data on a more narrow scope) is presented in the OMB Information Quality Guidelines, the OMB Information Quality Bulletin for Peer Review, and OMB Circular A-4.[22]

---

[22]US Office of Management and Budget, Guidelines for Ensuring and Maximizing the Quality, Objectivity, Utility, and Integrity of Information Disseminated by Federal Agencies, 67 FR 8452-8460 Feb. 22, 2002; US Office of Management and Budget, Final Information Quality Bulletin for Peer Review, 70 FR 2664-2677, Jan 14, 2005; and US Office of Management and Budget, Circular A-4, Sept 2003 available at: http://www.whitehouse.gov/omb/circulars/a004/a-4.pdf.

This proposed bulletin is released for peer review and public comment. It should not be construed to represent the official policy of the U.S. Office of Management and Budget.

3. Goals Related to Effort Expended

The level of effort should be commensurate with the importance of the risk assessment, taking into consideration the nature of the potential hazard, the available data, and the decision needs. For instance, if an agency is only interested in a screening-level assessment, then an assessment which explores alternative dose-response models may not be warranted.

4. Goals Related to Resources Expended

Agencies should take into account the importance of the risk assessment in gauging the resources, including time and money, required to meet the requirements of this Bulletin.[23]

5. Goals Related to Peer Review and Public Participation

Agencies should consider appropriate procedures for peer review and public participation in the process of preparing the risk assessment. When a draft assessment is made publicly available for comment or peer review, the agency is required to clarify that the report does not represent the official views of the federal government. Precise disclaimer language is recommended in OMB's Information Quality Bulletin on Peer Review. Public comments can play an important role in helping to inform agency deliberations.[24] When people are engaged early in the process, the public typically has an easier time concurring with government documents and decisions which may affect them.[25]

Section IV: General Risk Assessment and Reporting Standards

Each risk assessment disseminated by a Federal agency is subject to OMB's Information Quality Guidelines and the agency's Information Quality Guidelines. These guidelines require risk assessments to meet the three key attributes of utility, objectivity, and integrity.

---

[23] See Risk Commission Report, Vol. 2, at 63 ("Deciding to go forward with a risk assessment is a risk management decision, and scaling the effort to the importance of the problem, with respect to scientific issues and regulatory impact, is crucial."); id., at 21 ("The level of detail considered in a risk assessment and included in the risk characterization should be commensurate with the problem's importance, expected health or environmental impact, expected economic or social impact, urgency, and level of controversy, as well as with the expected impact and cost of protective measures."), 1997.

[24] Risk Commission Report, Vol. 2, at 21 ("Stakeholders play an important role in providing information that should be used in risk assessments and in identifying specific health and ecological concerns that they would like to see addressed." id., at 185, 1997.

[25] National Research Council, *Understanding Risk: Informing Decisions in a Democratic Society*, Washington DC: National Academy Press, 1996.

This proposed bulletin is being released for peer review and public comment. It should not be construed to represent the official policy of the U.S. Office of Management and Budget.

This Bulletin identifies six standards that apply to both influential and non-influential risk assessments. An additional seventh standard is also presented for risk assessments that are likely to be used in regulatory analysis.

1. Standards Relating to Informational Needs and Objectives

A risk assessment should clearly state the informational needs driving the assessment as well as the objectives of the assessment. This simple requirement will ensure that readers and users are able to understand the questions the assessment sought to answer and will help to ensure that risk assessments are used for their intended purposes. This is particularly important in cases where likely users of the risk assessment are not the original intended audience for the document. For example, an explicit statement of the ranges of chemical doses for which the assessment is relevant will inform other users as to whether or not the assessment is relevant their purposes.

2. Standards Relating to Scope

Every risk assessment should clearly summarize the scope of the assessment. The statement of scope may necessitate policy judgments made by accountable policy officials and managers as well as analysts. The scope of some assessments may be highly discretionary while others may be rigidly determined or influenced by statutory requirements, court deadlines or scarcity of available agency resources. In cases where the scope of an assessment has been restricted primarily due to external considerations beyond the agency's control, policy makers and other participants in the process should be made aware of those complicating circumstances and the technical limitations they have introduced in the agency's work product.

To begin framing the scope of a risk assessment, the first step should be to specify and describe the agent, technology and/or activity that is the subject of the assessment. The next step entails describing the hazard of concern. In order for an assessment to be complete, the assessment must address all of the factors within the intended scope of the assessment. For example, a risk assessment informing a general regulatory decision as to whether exposure to a chemical should be reduced would not be constrained to a one-disease process (e.g., cancer) when valid and relevant information about other disease processes (e.g., neurological effects or reproductive effects) are of importance to decision making.

The third step in framing the scope of the assessment entails identifying the affected entities. Affected entities can include populations, subpopulations, individuals, natural resources, animals, plants or other entities. If a risk assessment is to address only specific subpopulations, the scope should be very clear about this limitation. An analytic product may be incomplete when it addresses only risks to adults when there is information suggesting that children are more exposed and/or more susceptible to adverse effects than are adults.

Once the affected entities are defined, the assessment should define the exposure or event scenarios relevant to the purpose of the assessment as well as the type of event-consequence or dose-response relationship for the exposure or event ranges that are relevant to the objectives of the risk assessment. Although scientific completeness may entail analysis of different health effects and multiple target populations, the search for completeness will vary depending upon the nature of the assessment. In a fault-tree analysis of nuclear power accidents, an aspect of completeness may be whether pathways to accidents based on errors in human behavior have been addressed as well as pathways to accidents based on defects in engineering design or physical processes.

When agencies ask whether a particular chemical or technology causes or contributes to a particular disease, completeness in a scientific sense may entail consideration of evidence regarding the causative role of other factors in producing the disease of interest. For example, an assessment of radon exposure and lung cancer may need to consider the role of cigarette smoking as a potential confounding factor that influences the estimated risk of radon. Alternatively, the evidence on smoking may suggest that the risks of radon are larger for smokers than non-smokers, a so-called risk-modifying or synergistic factor. The scientific process of considering confounding and/or synergistic factors may assist policy makers in developing a broader sense of how risk can be reduced significantly and the range of decision options that need to be considered if maximum risk reduction is to be achieved.

3. Standards Related to Characterization of Risk

Every risk assessment should provide a characterization of risk, qualitatively and, whenever possible, quantitatively.[26] When a quantitative characterization of risk is provided, a range of plausible risk estimates should be provided.[27] Expressing multiple estimates of risk (and the limitations associated with these estimates) is necessary in order to convey the precision associated with these estimates.

In the 1996 amendments to the Safe Drinking Water Act (SDWA), Congress adopted a basic quality standard for the dissemination of public information about risks of adverse health effects. Under 42 U.S.C. 300g–1(b)(3)(B), the agency is directed "to ensure that the presentation of information [risk] effects is comprehensive, informative, and understandable." The agency is further directed "in a document made available to the public in support of a regulation [to] specify, to the extent practicable— (i) each population addressed by any estimate [of applicable risk effects]; (ii) the expected risk or central estimate of risk for the specific populations [affected]; (iii) each appropriate upper-bound or lower-bound estimate of risk; (iv) each significant uncertainty identified in the process of the assessment of [risk] effects and the studies that would assist in resolving the uncertainty; and (v) peer-reviewed studies known to the [agency] that support, are directly relevant to, or fail to support any estimate of [risk] effects and

---

[26]National Research Council, *Science and Judgment in Risk Assessment*, at 185, ("EPA should make uncertainties explicit and present them as accurately and fully as feasible and needed for risk management decision-making. To the greatest extent feasible, EPA should present quantitative, as opposed to qualitative, representations of uncertainty."), Washington DC: National Academy Press, 1994.

[27]See Carnegie Commission on Science, Technology and Government, *Risk and the Environment: Improving Regulatory Decision Making*, New York, NY, June 1993, at 87 ("Regulatory agencies should report a range of risk estimates when assessing risk and communicating it to the public. How risk estimates, whether derived from an inventory or not, are conveyed to the public significantly affects the way citizens perceive those risks. Single-value risk estimates reported to the public do not provide an indication of the degree of uncertainty associated with the estimate. Such numbers do not convey the conservative nature of some risk estimates.").

This proposed bulletin is being released for peer review and public comment. It should not be construed to represent the official policy of the U.S. Office of Management and Budget.

the methodology used to reconcile inconsistencies in the scientific data.'' These SDWA quality standards should be met, where feasible, in all risk assessments which address adverse health effects.

4. Standards Related to Objectivity

Risk assessments must be scientifically objective, neither minimizing nor exaggerating the nature and magnitude of the risks. On a substantive level, objectivity ensures accurate, reliable and unbiased information. When determining whether a potential hazard exists, weight should be given to both positive and negative studies, in light of each study's technical quality. The original and supporting data for the risk assessment must be generated, and the analytical results developed, using sound statistical and research methods.

Beyond the basic objectivity standards, risk assessments subject to this Bulletin should use the best available data and should be based on the weight of the available scientific evidence.[28] The requirement for using the best available scientific evidence was applied by Congress to risk information used and disseminated pursuant to the SDWA Amendments of 1996 (42 U.S.C. 300g-1(b)(3)(A)&(B)). Under 42 U.S.C. 300g–1(b)(3)(A), an agency is directed "to the degree that an agency action is based on science," to use "(i) the best available, peer-reviewed science and supporting studies conducted in accordance with sound and objective scientific practices; and (ii) data collected by accepted methods or best available methods (if the reliability of the method and the nature of the decision justifies use of the data)." Agencies have adopted or adapted this SDWA standard in their Information Quality Guidelines for risk assessments which analyze risks to human health, safety, and the environment. We are similarly requiring this as a general standard for all risk assessments subject to this Bulletin.

In addition to meeting substantive objectivity standards, risk assessments must be accurate, clear, complete and unbiased in the presentation of information about risk. The information must be presented in proper context. The agency also must identify the sources of the underlying information (consistent with confidentiality protections) and the supporting data and models, so that the public can judge for itself whether there may be some reason to question objectivity. Data should be accurately documented, and error sources affecting data quality should be identified and disclosed to users.

A risk assessment report should also have a high degree of transparency with respect to data, assumptions, and methods that have been considered. Transparency will increase the

---

[28]Risk Commission Report, Vol. 1, at 38 ("Because so many judgments must be based on limited information, it is critical that all reliable information be considered. Risk assessors and economists are responsible for providing decision-makers with the best technical information available or reasonably attainable, including evaluations of the weight of the evidence that supports different assumptions and conclusions.") The Risk Commission Report provides examples of the kinds of considerations entailed in making judgments on the basis of the weight of the scientific evidence in a toxicity study: quality of the toxicity study; appropriateness of the toxicity study methods; consistency of results across studies; biological plausibility of statistical associations; and similarity of results to responses and effects in humans. Vol. 2 at 20, 1997.

This proposed bulletin is released for peer review and public comment. It should not be construed to represent the official policy of the U.S. Office of Management and Budget.

credibility of the risk assessment, and will allow interested individuals, internal and external to the agency, to understand better the technical basis of the assessment.

5. Standards Related to Critical Assumptions

Risk assessments should explain the basis of each critical assumption and those assumptions which affect the key findings of the risk assessment. If the assumption is supported by, or conflicts with, empirical data, that information should be discussed. This should include discussion of the range of scientific opinions regarding the likelihood of plausible alternate assumptions and the direction and magnitude of any resulting changes that might arise in the assessment due to changes in key assumptions. Whenever possible, a quantitative evaluation of reasonable alternative assumptions should be provided. If an assessment combines multiple assumptions, the basis and rationale for combining the assumptions should be clearly explained.

6. Standards Related to the Executive Summary

Every risk assessment should contain an executive summary which discloses the objectives and scope, the key findings of the assessment, and the key scientific limitations and uncertainties in the risk assessment. Presentation of this information in a helpful and concise introductory section of the report will not only foster improved communication of the findings, but will also help ensure that the risk assessment is appropriately utilized by diverse end users. Major limitations are those that are most likely to affect significantly the determinations and/or estimates of risk presented in the assessment.

The executive summary should also place the estimates of risk in context/perspective with other risks familiar to the target audience. Due care must be taken in making risk comparisons. Agencies might want to consult the risk communication literature when considering appropriate comparisons. Although the risk assessor has considerable latitude in making risk comparisons, the fundamental point is that risk should be placed in a context that is useful and relevant for the intended audience.[29]

7. Standards Related to Regulatory Analysis

When a risk assessment is being produced to support or aid decision making related to regulatory analysis, there are additional standards that should be met. Risk assessors should consult OMB Circular A-4, which addresses requirements designed to improve the quality of regulatory impact analyses. For major rules involving annual economic effects of $1 billion or more, a formal quantitative analysis of the relevant uncertainties about benefits and costs is required.[30] In this Bulletin, we highlight important aspects of risk assessments useful for regulatory analysis:

---

[29] National Research Council, *Improving Risk Communication*, Washington DC: National Academy Press, 1989, at 165-79; see also Risk Commission Report, Volume 1, at 4, One of the key recommendations of the Risk Commission Report was that the problems a regulation is intended to address should be placed in their "public health and ecological context.", 1997.

[30] US Office of Management and Budget, *Circular A-4*, Sept, 2003, available at: http://www.whitehouse.gov/omb/circulars/a004/a-4.pdf.

This proposed bulletin is being released for peer review and public comment. It should not be construed to represent the official policy of the U.S. Office of Management and Budget.

1) The scope of the risk assessment should include evaluation of alternative options, clearly establishing the baseline risk analysis and the risk reduction alternatives that will be evaluated. When relevant, knowledge of the hazard and anticipated countermeasures should be understood in order to accurately capture the baseline risk.

2) The risk assessment should include a comparison of the baseline risk against the risk associated with the alternative mitigation measures being considered, and describe, to the extent feasible, any significant countervailing risks caused by alternative mitigation measures.[31]

3) The risk assessment should include information on the timing of exposure and the onset of the adverse effect(s) as well as the timing of control measures and the reduction or cessation of adverse effects.

4) When estimates of individual risk are developed, estimates of population risk should also be developed. Estimates of population risk are necessary to compare the overall costs and benefits of regulatory alternatives.

5) When a quantitative characterization of risk is made available, this should include a range of plausible risk estimates, including central estimates. A "central estimate" of risk is the mean or average of the distribution; or a number which contains multiple estimates of risk based on different assumptions, weighted by their relative plausibility; or any estimate judged to be most representative of the distribution.[32] The central estimate should neither understate nor overstate the risk, but rather, should provide the risk manager and the public with the expected risk.[33]

Section V: Special Standards for Influential Risk Assessments

In addition to the standards presented in section IV, all influential risk assessments should meet certain additional standards. When it is not appropriate for an influential risk assessment to adhere to one or more of the standards in this section of the Bulletin, the risk assessment should contain a rationale explaining why the standard(s) was (were) not met.

1. Standard for Reproducibility

Influential risk assessments should be capable of being substantially reproduced. As described in the OMB Information Quality Guidelines, this means that independent reanalysis of the original or supporting data using the same methods would generate similar analytical results, subject to an acceptable degree of precision. Public access to original data is necessary

---

[31] Graham, J.D., Jonathan B. Wiener (eds), *Risk Versus Risk: Tradeoffs in Protecting Health and the Environment*, Harvard University Press, Cambridge, MA, 1995.

[32] See, e.g., Holloway, CA, *Decision Making Under Uncertainty: Models and Choices* (1979), at 76, 214, 91-127 Theodore Colton, *Statistics in Medicine* (1974), at 28-31.

[33] National Research Council, *Science and Judgment in Risk Assessment*, at 170-75, Washington DC: National Academy Press, 1994.

This proposed bulletin is released for peer review and public comment. It should not be construed to represent the official policy of the U.S. Office of Management and Budget.

to satisfy this standard, though such access should respect confidentiality and other compelling considerations.[34] It is not necessary that the results of the risk assessment be reproduced. Rather, someone with the appropriate expertise should be able to substantially reproduce the results of the risk assessment, given the underlying data and a transparent description of the assumptions and methodology.

2. Standard for Comparison to Other Results

By definition, influential risk assessments have a significant impact. In such situations, it is appropriate for an agency to find and examine previously conducted risk assessments on the same topic, and compare these risk assessments to the agency risk assessment. A discussion of this comparison should be incorporated into the risk assessment.

3. Standard for Presentation of Numerical Estimates

When there is uncertainty in estimates of risk, presentation of single estimates of risk is misleading and provides a false sense of precision. Presenting the range of plausible risk estimates, along with a central estimate, conveys a more objective characterization of the magnitude of the risks. Influential risk assessments should characterize uncertainty by highlighting central estimates as well high-end and low-end estimates of risk. The practice of highlighting only high-end or only low-end estimates of risk is discouraged.

This Bulletin uses the terms "central" and "expected" estimate synonymously. When the model used by assessors is well established, the central or expected estimate may be computed using standard statistical tools. When model uncertainty is substantial, the central or expected estimate may be a weighted average of results from alternative models. Formal probability assessments supplied by qualified experts can help assessors obtain central or expected estimates of risk in the face of model uncertainty.[35]

4. Standard for Characterizing Uncertainty

Influential risk assessments should characterize uncertainty with a sensitivity analysis and, where feasible, through use of a numeric distribution (e.g., likelihood distribution of risk for a given individual, exposure/event scenario, population, or subpopulation). Where

---

[34] See US Office of Management and Budget, *Guidelines for Ensuring and Maximizing the Quality, Objectivity, Utility, and Integrity of Information Disseminated by Federal Agencies*, 67 FR 8456, ("However, the objectivity standard does not override other compelling interests such as privacy, trade secrets, intellectual property, and other confidentiality protections.") Feb. 22, 2002.

[35] National Research Council, *Estimating the Public Health Benefits of Proposed Air Pollution Regulations*, Washington, DC: National Academies Press, 2002; Cooke, RM, *Experts in Uncertainty: Opinion and Subjective Probability in Science*, Oxford University Press, New York, NY, 1991; Evans, JS, JD Graham, GM Gray, RL Sielken, *A Distributional Approach to Characterizing Low-Dose Cancer Risk*, Risk Analysis, vol. 14(1), 1994, pp. 25-34; Hoffman, O, S Kaplan, *Beyond the Domain of Direct Observation: How to Specify a Probability Distribution that Represents the State-of-the-Knowledge About Uncertain Inputs*, Risk Analysis, vol. 19(1), 1999, pp. 131-134; Morgan, MG, M Henrion, M Small, Uncertainty: *A Guide to Dealing with Uncertainty in Quantitative Risk and Policy Analysis*, Cambridge University Press, Cambridge, UK, 1990.

This proposed bulletin is being released for peer review and public comment. It should not be construed to represent the official policy of the U.S. Office of Management and Budget.

appropriate, this should include sufficient description so that the lower and upper percentiles and the median, mean, mode, and shape of the uncertainty distribution are apparent.

When one or more assumptions are used in a risk assessment, the assessor may evaluate how plausible changes in the assumptions influence the results of the assessment. An assumption may be used for a variety of reasons (e.g., to address a data gap or to justify the selection of a specific model or statistical procedure). Professional judgment is required to determine what range of assumptions is plausible enough to justify inclusion in the sensitivity analysis. Sensitivity analysis is particularly useful in pinpointing which assumptions are appropriate candidates for additional data collection to narrow the degree of uncertainty in the results. Sensitivity analysis is generally considered a minimum, necessary component of a quality risk assessment report.

A model is a mathematical representation -- usually a simplified one -- of reality. Where a risk can be plausibly characterized by alternative models, the difference between the results of the alternative models is model uncertainty. For example, when cancer risks observed at high doses of chemical exposure are extrapolated to low doses (i.e., doses below the range of empirical detection of cancer risk), a dose-response model must be employed to compute low-dose risks. Biological knowledge may be inadequate to predict the shape of the dose-response curve for cancer in the low-dose region. While it is common for risk assessors to use a model where cancer risk is proportional to dose (even at low doses), there are cases where it has been demonstrated, through huge epidemiological studies or detailed biologic data from the laboratory, that a non-linear dose-response shape is appropriate. When risk assessors face model uncertainty, they need to document and disclose the nature and degree of model uncertainty. This can be done by performing multiple assessments with different models and reporting the extent of the differences in results.[36] A weighted average of results from alternative models based on expert weightings may also be informative.[37]

When the model used by assessors is well established, the central or expected estimate may be computed using classical statistics. When model uncertainty is substantial, the central or expected estimate may be a weighted average of the results from alternative models.[38] Judgmental probabilities supplied by scientific experts can help assessors obtain central or

---

[36]Holland, CH, RL Sielken, *Quantitative Cancer Modeling and Risk Assessment*, Prentice-Hall, Englewood Cliffs, New Jersey, 1993; Olin, S, W Farland, C Park, L Rhomberg, R Scheuplein, T Starr, J Wilson (eds), *Low-Dose Extrapolation of Cancer Risks: Issues and Perspectives*, International Life Sciences Institute, Washington, DC, 1995.

[37]Morgan, MG, M Henrion, M Small, Uncertainty: *A Guide to Dealing with Uncertainty in Quantitative Risk and Policy Analysis*, Cambridge University Press, Cambridge, UK, 1990; Cooke, RM, *Experts in Uncertainty: Opinion and Subjective Probability in Science*, Oxford University Press, New York, NY, 1991; National Research Council, *Estimating the Public Health Benefits of Proposed Air Pollution Regulations*, Washington, DC: National Academies Press, 2002.

[38]Clemen, RT, *Making Hard Decisions: An Introduction to Decision Analysis*, Second Edition, Duxbury Press, Pacific Grove, CA, 1996; Morgan, MG, M Henrion, M Small, Uncertainty: *A Guide to Dealing with Uncertainty in Quantitative Risk and Policy Analysis*, Cambridge University Press, Cambridge, UK, 1990; Hoffman, O, S Kaplan, *Beyond the Domain of Direct Observation: How to Specify a Probability Distribution that Represents the State-of-the-Knowledge About Uncertain Inputs*, Risk Analysis, vol. 19(1), 1999, pp. 131-134.

This proposed bulletin is released for peer review and public comment. It should not be construed to represent the official policy of the U.S. Office of Management and Budget.

expected estimates of risk in the face of model uncertainty.[39] Central or expected estimates of risk play an especially critical role in decision analysis and cost-benefit analysis.[40]

Statistical uncertainty sometimes referred to as data uncertainty or parameter uncertainty occurs when some data exist on the value of an input, but the value of the input is not known with certainty. If a sample of data exists on an input, the degree of statistical uncertainty in the input value is influenced by the size of the sample and other factors. Risk assessors should document and disclose the nature and degree of statistical uncertainty.

5. Standard for Characterizing Results

Results based on different effects observed and/or different studies should be presented to convey how the choice of effect and/or study influences the assessment. Authors of the assessment have a special obligation to evaluate and discuss alternative theories, data, studies and assessments that suggest different or contrary results than are contained in the risk assessment. When relying on data from one study over others, the agency should discuss the scientific justification for its choice.

6. Standard for Characterizing Variability

A risk is variable when there are known differences in risk for different individuals, subpopulations, or ecosystems. In some cases variability in risk is described with a distribution. Where feasible, characterization of variability should include sufficient description of the variability distribution so that the lower and upper percentiles and the median, mean, and mode are apparent.[41] This section should also disclose and evaluate the most influential contributors to variation in risk. This characterization should reflect the different affected populations (e.g., children or the elderly), time scales, geography, and other parameters relevant to the needs and objectives of the risk assessment. If highly exposed or sensitive subpopulations are highlighted, the assessment should also highlight the general population to portray the range of variability.[42]

---

[39]Morgan, MG, M Henrion, M Small, Uncertainty: *A Guide to Dealing with Uncertainty in Quantitative Risk and Policy Analysis*, Cambridge University Press, Cambridge, UK, 1990; Cooke, RM, *Experts in Uncertainty: Opinion and Subjective Probability in Science*, Oxford University Press, New York, NY, 1991; Evans, JS , JD Graham, GM Gray, RL Sielken, *A Distributional Approach to Characterizing Low-Dose Cancer Risk*, Risk Analysis, vol. 14(1), 1994, pp. 25-34.

[40]Pate-Cornell, ME, *Uncertainties in Risk Analysis: Six Levels of Treatment*, Reliability Engineering and System Safety, vol. 54(2-3), 1996, pp. 95-111; Clemen, RT, *Making Hard Decisions: An Introduction to Decision Analysis*, Second Edition, Duxbury Press, Pacific Grove, CA, 1996; Viscusi, WK, *Rational Risk Policy*, Clarendon Press, Oxford, UK, 1998.

[41]Burmaster, DE, PD Anderson, *Principles of Good Practice for the Use of Monte Carlo Techniques in Human Health and Ecological Risk Analysis*, Risk Analysis, vol. 14(4), 1994, pp.477-481.

[42]Cullen, AC, HC Frey, Probabilistic Techniques in Exposure Assessment: A Handbook for Dealing with Variability and Uncertainty in Models and Inputs, Plenum Press, New York, NY, 1999; Hattis, D, DE Burmaster, *Assessment of Variability and Uncertainty Distributions for Practical Risk Analyses*, Risk Analysis, vol. 14(5), 1994, pp.713-730; National Research Council, *Human Exposure for Airborne Pollutants: Advances and Opportunities*, Washington, DC: National Academies Press 1991.

This proposed bulletin is being released for peer review and public comment. It should not be construed to represent the official policy of the U.S. Office of Management and Budget.

7. Standard for Characterizing Human Health Effects

Since the dictionary definition of "risk" refers to the possibility of an adverse consequence or adverse effect, it may be necessary for risk assessment reports to distinguish effects which are adverse from those which are non-adverse. Given that the capacity of science to detect effects is rapidly growing, sometimes faster than our ability to understand whether detected or predicted effects are adverse, the adversity determination is not always an obvious one.

Where human health effects are a concern, determination of which effects are adverse shall be specifically identified and justified based on the best available scientific information generally accepted in the relevant clinical and toxicological communities.

In chemical risk assessment, for example, measuring the concentration of a chemical metabolite in a target tissue of the body is not a demonstration of an adverse effect, though it may be a valid indicator of chemical exposure. Even the measurement of a biological event in the human body resulting from exposure to a specific chemical may not be a demonstration of an adverse effect. Adversity typically implies some functional impairment or pathologic lesion that affects the performance of the whole organism or reduces an organism's ability to withstand or respond to additional environmental challenges. In cases where qualified specialists disagree as to whether a measured effect is adverse or likely to be adverse, the extent of the differences in scientific opinion about adversity should be disclosed in the risk assessment report. In order to convey how the choice of the adverse effect influences a safety assessment, it is useful for the analyst to provide a graphical portrayal of different "safe levels" based on different effects observed in various experiments. If an unusual or mild effect is used in making the adverse-effect determination, the assessment should describe the ramifications of the effect and its degree of adversity compared to adverse effects that are better understood and commonly used in safety assessment.

Although the language in this section explicitly addresses human health endpoints, for other endpoints, such as ecological health, it is expected that the agency would rely upon information from a relevant group of experts, such as ecologists or habitat biologists, when making determinations regarding adversity of effects.

8. Standard for Discussing Scientific Limitations

Influential risk assessments should, to the extent possible, provide a discussion regarding the nature, difficulty, feasibility, cost and time associated with undertaking research to resolve a report's key scientific limitations and uncertainties.

9. Standard for Addressing Significant Comments

An agency is expected to consider all of the significant comments received on a draft influential risk assessment report. Scientific comments shall be presumed to be significant. In order to ensure that agency staff is rigorous in considering each significant comment, it is typically useful to prepare a "response-to-comment" document, to be issued with, or as part of, the final assessment report, to summarize the significant comments and the agency's responses to those comments. Agency responses may range from revisions to the draft report or an acknowledgement that the agency has taken a different position than the one suggested by the commenter. Where agencies take different positions than commenters, the agency response to comments should provide an explicit rationale for why the agency has not adopted the position suggested by the commenter (e.g., why the agency position is preferable or defensible).

Section VI: Updates

Influential risk assessments should provide information or analysis, within the intended scope of the assessment, which assists policy makers in determining whether more data needs to be gathered or whether the assessment can be based on the data and assumptions currently available. Since risk assessment is typically an iterative process, with risk estimates subject to refinement as additional data are gathered, it is useful for assessments to disclose how fast the relevant database and assumptions are evolving and how likely it is that the database and assumptions will be significantly different within several months or years. While risk assessments should offer insight into what additional scientific understanding might be achieved through additional data collection and/or analysis, the decisions about whether to invest in additional inquiry, whether to take interim protective steps while additional inquiry is underway, or whether to act promptly without additional inquiry are policy decisions that are beyond the scope of the risk assessment report.

Each agency should, taking into account the resources available, priorities, and the importance of the document, consider revising its influential risk assessments as relevant and scientifically plausible information becomes available. Each agency should (1) have procedures in place that would ensure it is aware of new, relevant information that might alter a previously conducted influential risk assessment, and (2) have procedures in place to ensure that this new, relevant information is considered in the context of a decision to revise its previously conducted assessment. In addition, as relevant and scientifically plausible information becomes available, each agency shall consider updating or replacing its assumptions to reflect new data or scientific understandings.[43]

Section VII: Certification

For each risk assessment subject to this Bulletin, the agency shall include a certification, as part of the risk assessment document, explaining that the agency has complied with the

---

[43] See National Research Council, *Science and Judgment in Risk Assessment*, at 90, Washington DC: National Academy Press, 1994, ("Over time, the choice of defaults should have decreasing impact on regulatory decision-making. As scientific knowledge increases, uncertainty diminishes. Better data and increased understanding of biological mechanisms should enable risk assessments that are less dependent on default assumptions and more accurate as predictions of human risk."); Risk Commission Report, Volume 2, at iv ("Agencies should continue to move away from the hypothetical . . . toward more realistic assumptions based on available scientific data."), 1997.

This proposed bulletin is being released for peer review and public comment. It should not be construed to represent the official policy of the U.S. Office of Management and Budget.

requirements of this Bulletin and the applicable Information Quality Guidelines, except as provided in Section VIII.

Section VIII: Deferral and Waiver

The agency head may waive or defer some or all of the requirements of this Bulletin where warranted by compelling rationale. In each such instance, the agency shall include a statement in the risk assessment document that the agency is exercising a deferral or waiver as well as a brief explanation for the deferral or waiver. If the agency head defers the risk assessment requirements prior to dissemination, the risk assessment requirements shall be complied with as soon as practicable. A compelling rationale might cover health and safety risk assessments which are time-sensitive or need to be released due to an emergency situation. It is expected that a need for such a deferral would be an infrequent event. In the rare case of a time-sensitive necessary release, a complete risk assessment, which meets the standards set out in this Bulletin, should be provided to the public as soon as is practicable.

Section IX: OIRA and OSTP Responsibilities

OIRA, in consultation with OSTP, is responsible for overseeing agency implementation of this Bulletin. OIRA and OSTP shall foster learning about risk assessment practices across agencies.

Section X: Effective Date

The requirements of this Bulletin apply to: (1) final public risk assessments disseminated after 12 months following the publication of this Bulletin in final form, and (2) draft risk assessments disseminated after six months following the publication of this Bulletin in final form. These dates are necessary to ensure Federal agencies have sufficient time to both (1) become familiar with these standards and (2) incorporate these standards into ongoing risk assessments.

Section XI: Judicial Review

This Bulletin is intended to improve the internal management of the Executive Branch and is not intended to, and does not create any right or benefit, substantive or procedural, enforceable at law or in equity, against the United States, its agencies or other entities, its officers or employees, or any other person.

RISK ASSESSMENT BULLETIN

I. Definitions.
      For purposes of this Bulletin, the term—
          1. "agency" has the same meaning as the Paperwork Reduction Act, 44 U.S.C. § 3502(1);
          2. "influential risk assessment" means a risk assessment the agency reasonably can determine will have or does have a clear and substantial impact on important public policies or private sector decisions;
          3. "risk assessment" means a scientific and/or technical document that assembles and synthesizes scientific information to determine whether a potential hazard exists and/or the extent of possible risk to human health, safety or the environment.

II. Applicability.
          1. To the extent appropriate, all agency risk assessments available to the public shall comply with the standards of this Bulletin.
          2. This Bulletin does not apply to risk assessments performed with respect to:
              a. inspections relating to health, safety, or environment;
              b. individual agency adjudications or permit proceedings (including a registration, approval, or licensing) unless the agency determines that
                  i. compliance with this Bulletin is practical and appropriate and
                  ii. the risk assessment is scientifically or technically novel or likely to have precedent-setting influence on future adjudications and/or permit proceedings; and
              c. an individual product label, or a risk characterization appearing on any such label, if the individual product label is required by law to be approved by a Federal agency prior to use.

III. Goals.
          1. The objectives of the assessment shall be a product of an iterative dialogue between the assessor(s) and the agency decisionmaker(s).
          2. The scope and content of the risk assessment shall be determined based on the objectives of the assessment and best professional judgment, considering the benefits and costs of acquiring additional information before undertaking the assessment.
          3. The type of risk assessment prepared shall be responsive to the nature of the potential hazard, the available data, and the decision needs.
          4. The level of effort put into the risk assessment shall be commensurate with the importance of the risk assessment.
          5. The agency shall follow appropriate procedures for peer review and public participation in the process of preparing the risk assessment.

IV. General Risk Assessment and Reporting Standards.
      Each agency risk assessment shall:
          1. Provide a clear statement of the informational needs of decision makers, including the objectives of the risk assessment.
          2. Clearly summarize the scope of the assessment, including a description of:
              a. the agent, technology and/or activity that is the subject of the assessment;

This proposed bulletin is being released for peer review and public comment. It should not be construed to represent the official policy of the U.S. Office of Management and Budget.

　　b. the hazard of concern;

　　c. the affected entities (population(s), subpopulation(s), individuals, natural resources, ecosystems, or other) that are the subject of the assessment;

　　d. the exposure/event scenarios relevant to the objectives of the assessment; and

　　e. the type of event-consequence or dose-response relationship for the hazard of concern.

　3. Provide a characterization of risk, qualitatively and, whenever possible, quantitatively. When a quantitative characterization of risk is provided, a range of plausible risk estimates shall be provided.

　4. Be scientifically objective:

　　a. as a matter of substance, neither minimizing nor exaggerating the nature and magnitude of risks;

　　b. giving weight to both positive and negative studies in light of each study's technical quality; and

　　c. as a matter of presentation:

　　　i. presenting the information about risk in an accurate, clear, complete and unbiased manner; and

　　　ii. describing the data, methods, and assumptions used in the assessment with a high degree of transparency.

　5. For critical assumptions in the assessment, whenever possible, include a quantitative evaluation of reasonable alternative assumptions and their implications for the key findings of the assessment.

　6. Provide an executive summary including:

　　a. key elements of the assessment's objectives and scope;

　　b. key findings;

　　c. key scientific limitations and uncertainties and, whenever possible, their quantitative implications; and

　　d. information that places the risk in context/perspective with other risks familiar to the target audience.

　7. For risk assessments that will be used for regulatory analysis, the risk assessment also shall include:

　　a. an evaluation of alternative options, clearly establishing the baseline risk as well as the risk reduction alternatives that will be evaluated;

　　b. a comparison of the baseline risk against the risk associated with the alternative mitigation measures being considered, and assess, to the extent feasible, countervailing risks caused by alternative mitigation measures;

　　c. information on the timing of exposure and the onset of the adverse effect(s), as well as the timing of control measures and the reduction or cessation of adverse effects;

　　d. estimates of population risk when estimates of individual risk are developed; and

　　e. whenever possible, a range of plausible risk estimates, including central or expected estimates, when a quantitative characterization of risk is made available.

V. Special Standards for Influential Risk Assessments.
　　All influential agency risk assessments shall:
　　　1. Be "capable of being substantially reproduced" as defined in the OMB Information Quality Guidelines.
　　　2. Compare the results of the assessment to other results published on the same topic from qualified scientific organizations.
　　　3. Highlight central estimates as well as high-end and low-end estimates of risk when such estimates are uncertain.
　　　4. Characterize uncertainty with respect to the major findings of the assessment including:
　　　　　a. document and disclose the nature and quantitative implications of model uncertainty, and the relative plausibility of different models based on scientific judgment; and where feasible:
　　　　　b. include a sensitivity analysis; and
　　　　　c. provide a quantitative distribution of the uncertainty.
　　　5. Portray results based on different effects observed and/or different studies to convey how the choice of effect and/or study influences the assessment.
　　　6. Characterize, to the extent feasible, variability through a quantitative distribution, reflecting different affected population(s), time scales, geography, or other parameters relevant to the needs and objectives of the assessment.
　　　7. Where human health effects are a concern, determinations of which effects are adverse shall be specifically identified and justified based on the best available scientific information generally accepted in the relevant clinical and toxicological communities.
　　　8. Provide discussion, to the extent possible, of the nature, difficulty, feasibility, cost and time associated with undertaking research to resolve a report's key scientific limitations and uncertainties.
　　　9. Consider all significant comments received on a draft risk assessment report and:
　　　　　a. issue a "response-to-comment" document that summarizes the significant comments received and the agency's responses to those comments; and
　　　　　b. provide a rationale for why the agency has not adopted the position suggested by commenters and why the agency position is preferable.

VI. Updates.
　　As relevant and scientifically plausible information becomes available, each agency shall, considering the resources available, consider:
　　　1. revising its risk assessment to incorporate such information; and
　　　2. updating or replacing its assumptions to reflect new data or scientific understandings.

VII. Certification.
　　For each risk assessment subject to this Bulletin, the agency shall include a certification explaining that the agency has complied with the requirements of this Bulletin and the applicable Information Quality Guidelines, except as provided in Section VIII.

This proposed bulletin is being released for peer review and public comment. It should not be construed to represent the official policy of the U.S. Office of Management and Budget.

VIII. Deferral and Waiver.

The agency head may waive or defer some or all of the requirements of this Bulletin where warranted by compelling rationale. In each such instance, the agency shall include a statement in the risk assessment document that the agency is exercising a deferral or waiver as well as a brief explanation for the deferral or waiver. If the agency head defers the requirements prior to dissemination, the agency shall comply with them as soon as practicable.

IX. OIRA and OSTP Responsibilities.

OIRA, in consultation with OSTP, shall be responsible for overseeing agency implementation of this Bulletin. OIRA and OSTP shall foster better understanding about risk assessment practices and assess progress in implementing this Bulletin.

X. Effective Date.

The requirements of this Bulletin apply to: (1) final public risk assessments disseminated after twelve months following the publication of this Bulletin in final form, and (2) draft risk assessments disseminated after six months following the publication of this Bulletin in final form.

XI. Judicial Review.

This Bulletin is intended to improve the internal management of the Executive Branch and is not intended to, and does not create any right or benefit, substantive or procedural, enforceable at law or in equity, against the United States, its agencies or other entities, its officers or employees, or any other person.

Appendix C

Statement of Task

The Board on Environmental Studies and Toxicology (BEST) will conduct a scientific review of the *Proposed Risk Assessment Bulletin* recently released by the Office of Management and Budget (OMB). Specifically, the committee will determine whether the application of the proposed guidance will meet OMB's stated objective to "enhance the technical quality and objectivity of risk assessments prepared by federal agencies." In performing its task, the committee will comment, in general terms, on how the guidance will affect the practice of risk assessment in the federal government. The committee will identify critical elements that might be missing from the guidance. The committee will also determine whether OMB appropriately incorporated recommendations from previous reports of the NRC and other organizations into the proposed risk assessment guidance. In addition, the committee will assess whether there are scientific or technical circumstances that might limit applicability of the guidance.

Appendix D

National Research Council Committee to Review the OMB Risk Assessment Bulletin

Public Meeting: May 22, 2006
The National Academy of Sciences Building, Auditorium
2100 C Street, NW
Washington, DC

PUBLIC AGENDA

9:00   Purpose of Public Session and Introduction of Committee Members
John Ahearne, *Chair*

9:10   OMB Perspective on Risk Assessment Bulletin
Nancy Beck, Toxicologist/Risk Assessor, Office of Information &
Regulatory Affairs, Office of Management and Budget

9:25   Reflections on the Rationale for Improved Risk Assessment
    Practices
John Graham, Dean, RAND Graduate School

9:55   Impact of OMB Bulletin on Current Agency Risk Assessment Standards
    and Practices

Agency Presentations:
                USDA   Linda Abbott
                             Senior Scientist for Risk Modeling

	Office of Risk Assessment and Cost-Benefit Analysis
DOL	William Perry Acting Deputy Director Directorate of Standards and Guidance Occupational Safety and Health Administration
EPA	George Gray Science Advisor and Assistant Administrator Office of Research and Development

10:35   Break

10:50   Impact of OMB Bulletin on Current Agency Risk Assessment Standards and Practices (*continued*)

Agency Presentations:

DOD	Shannon Cunniff Director of Emerging Contaminants Environment, Safety, and Occupational Health
DOE	Al Cobb Senior Policy Advisor Office of Policy and International Affairs
NASA	Homayoon Dezfuli Manager for System Safety Office of Safety and Mission Assurance

HHS	Christopher Portier
	Associate Director, NIEHS
	Director, Office of Risk Assessment
	National Institute of Environmental Health
	   Sciences
	National Institutes of Health
	
	Steve Galson
	Director, Center for Drug Evaluation and
	   Research
	Food and Drug Administration
	
	Christine Sofge
	Chief, Risk Evaluation Branch
	Education and Information Division
	National Institute for Occupational Safety
	   and Health
	Centers for Disease Control and
	   Prevention

11:50	Comments or Questions from NAS Committee
12:05	Comments or Questions from the Public
12:15	Break for Lunch
1:00	Panel Presentations and Discussion on OMB Definition of Risk Assessment, Usefulness of Proposed Standards, and Possible Omissions from the OMB Bulletin

Presentations:

Gilbert Omenn
Professor of Medicine, Genetics and Public Health
University of Michigan Medical School

Alan Krupnick
Senior Fellow and Director, Quality of the Environment
Resources for the Future

Stephen Heinig
Senior Research Fellow
Association of American Medical Colleges

Lorenz Rhomberg
Principal
Gradient Corporation

Judith Graham
Managing Director, Long-Range Research Initiative Team
American Chemistry Council

Robert Shull
Director of Regulatory Policy
OMB Watch

Jennifer Sass
Senior Scientist, Health and Environment
Natural Resources Defense Council

2:45	Break
3:00	Comments and Questions from the Committee for Presenters
3:20	Comments and Questions from the Agencies for Presenters
3:40	Comments and Questions from the Public for Presenters
4:00	Open Microphone
5:00	Adjourn/End of Public Session

Appendix E

Questions for Federal Agencies from the Committee and Agency Responses to Questions

BACKGROUND INFORMATION ON NRC REVIEW
OF THE OMB RISK ASSESSMENT BULLETIN

The National Research Council's Committee to Review the OMB Risk Assessment Bulletin has been tasked with conducting a scientific review of the proposed Risk Assessment Bulletin released by the Office of Management and Budget (OMB). More specifically, the committee was asked to determine whether the application of the proposed guidance will meet OMB's stated objective to "enhance the technical quality and objectivity of risk assessments prepared by federal agencies." The committee will evaluate generally the impact of the Bulletin on risk practices, identify possible omissions from the Bulletin, and determine whether there are circumstances that might limit applicability. To address its charge, the committee is hoping that the agencies will assist it by responding to the questions below.

QUESTIONS FOR ALL AGENCIES POTENTIALLY
AFFECTED BY THE OMB BULLETIN

General questions about current risk assessment practices

•   Please provide a brief overview of your current risk assessment practices. Specifically, do you conduct probabilistic risk assessment? Is there a common approach to both risk assessments and uncertainty analysis? How do you currently address uncertainty and variability in your agency's risk assessments?

•   Please identify any substantial scientific or technical challenges that you may encounter when conducting risk assessments for your agency.

•   What is your current definition of risk assessment, and what types of products are covered by that definition?

•   About how long (that is, from initiation of the risk assessment to delivery to the regulatory decision maker) does it take to produce the various types of risk assessments?

Questions about OMB's definition of risk assessment and applicability

•   Using the definition of risk assessment described in the OMB Bulletin, are there work products that would now be considered risk assessments that were not previously considered risk assessments? If so, what are they?

Questions about type of risk assessment (tiered structure)

•   In your agency, is there currently a clear demarcation between risk assessments used for regulatory analysis and those not used for regulatory analysis? Is this clear at the outset of the risk assessment?

•   In your agency, is there currently a clear demarcation between "influential risk assessment" used for regulatory purposes and other risk assessments used for regulatory purposes? Is this clear at the outset of the risk assessment?

Questions about impact of the Bulletin on agency risk assessment practices

•   If applicable, please specify provisions in the Bulletin that can be expected to have a <u>substantial positive effect</u> on the quality, conduct, and use of risk assessments undertaken by your agency.

•   If applicable, please specify provisions in the Bulletin that can be expected to have a <u>substantial negative effect</u> on the quality, conduct, and use of risk assessments undertaken by your agency.

•   If your agency followed the procedures described in the Bulletin, would it affect the time course for production of the risk assessment (that is, the time required from initiation of the risk assessment to delivery to the regulatory decision maker)? If so, please explain why?

•   One of the Bulletin's reporting standards states the need to be scientifically objective by "giving weight to both positive and negative studies in light of each study's technical quality." Please give an example of how this would be implemented by your agency or department.

•   Does your agency use risk assessments conducted by external groups? Would it be helpful to you if risk assessments submitted to your agency by external groups, such as consultants and private industry, met the requirements proposed in the OMB Bulletin?

ADDITIONAL QUESTIONS FOR SPECIFIC AGENCIES

DOE

•   What are DOE's current overall challenges regarding risk assessment? Specifically, please address DOE sites that have to be remediated (e.g., Hanford); DOE facilities (e.g., research and test reactors and processing plants); special projects (e.g., Yucca Mountain); and other sites (e.g., Pantex). How will the OMB Bulletin impact the quality, conduct, and use of risk assessments in these cases?

EPA

•   Regarding pesticides specifically, what risk-assessment activities will be covered by the Bulletin and what risk-assessment activities will be exempted?

•   Does EPA have any examples of the application of the 1996 requirements of the Safe Drinking Water Act, as described on page 13 of the Bulletin? Can any examples be provided to the committee? If none are available, can EPA provide an explanation?

•   Does EPA have a working definition of "expected risk" or "central estimate?" The agency indicated in its 1986 cancer guidelines (51 FR 33992-34003) that central estimates of low-dose risk, based on "best fit" of the observed dose-response relationship, were meaningless—that "fit" in the high-dose region provided no information about "best fit" in the region of extrapolation. The newer cancer guidelines appear to adopt the same thinking. Has the Agency changed its view on this point? If so, why?

FDA

•   Dr. Galson indicated at the public meeting that there were problems with the application of OMB requirements to certain types of assessments. Can FDA suggest specific language to exclude those problematic assessments from OMB requirements, rather than just offering examples of those assessments? In other words, how would FDA describe in general terms the types of assessments it would like to see excluded?

QUESTIONS FOR OMB

• Dr. Graham discussed the recent perchlorate evaluation as an example that would have benefited from this Bulletin. Does the Bulletin support using a "precursor" of an adverse effect or other mechanistic data as the basis of a risk assessment, as was recommended in the National Academies' perchlorate review.

• Is it correct that those submitting data and risk assessments to the government to obtain product registrations, approvals, and licenses are excluded from the requirements of the Bulletin?

• Will the Bulletin require further review by OMB staff of risk assessments that have been peer reviewed in accordance with established peer review procedures and standards, including publication in a reputable peer reviewed journal?

• Public participants in the risk assessment and rulemaking processes —industry groups, environmental groups, other governmental entities, individual scientists—often provide risk assessments for agency consideration. Will these outside assessments be held to the same standards as agency-generated assessments, that is, to the requirements in the Bulletin?

• The 1983 NRC report Risk Assessment in the Federal Government: Managing the Process treats "risk assessment" as a term of art that covers four distinct analyses (hazard identification, dose-response assessment, exposure analysis, and risk characterization), each typically based on a number of separate studies and analyses. The OMB Bulletin defines "risk assessment" to apply to "any document" that "could be used for risk assessment purposes, such as an exposure or hazard assessment that might not constitute a complete risk assessment as defined by the National Research Council." What is the advantage of defining risk assessment in this way?

• The Bulletin discusses the importance of risk assessors interacting with decision-makers. What safeguards will be built into the process to protect the scientific process from being framed by the decision-maker instead of the science?

Appendix E

Agency Responses to Questions*

- Consumer Product Safety Commission
- Department of Defense
- Department of Energy
- Department of Health and Human Services
- Department of Housing and Urban Development
- Department of Interior
- Department of Labor
- Department of Transportation
- Environmental Protection Agency
- National Aeronautics and Space Administration
- Office of Management and Budget

*Agencies that were sent the committee's questions but did not provide responses:

- Department of Homeland Security
- Nuclear Regulatory Commission
- Department of Agriculture

Below are responses developed by the U.S. Consumer Product Safety Commission's (CPSC) staff to the questions posed by the National Research Council in its scientific review of the proposed Risk Assessment Bulletin released by the Office of Management and Budget. (Note: These comments are those of the CPSC staff, have not been reviewed or approved by, and may not necessarily represent the view of, the Commission.)

General questions about current risk assessment practices

•   Question: Please provide a brief overview of your current risk assessment practices. Specifically, do you conduct probabilistic risk assessment? Is there a common approach to both risk assessments and uncertainty analysis? How do you currently address uncertainty and variability in your agency's risk assessments?

CPSC Staff Response

In general, the CPSC staff performs risk assessments addressing a variety of hazards, including toxicity, electrical, fire and burn, and mechanical hazards. Depending on staff and agency needs, CPSC staff conducts all manner of analyses, both qualitative and quantitative. Some analyses constitute complete risk assessments, while others deal with one or more individual steps of risk assessment, *e.g.*, hazard identification or exposure assessment.

The toxicological risk assessment practices used by the CPSC staff are described in the CPSC Chronic Hazard Guidelines (FR 57: 46626-46653, 1992). The guidelines include sections on cancer, neurotoxicity, reproductive-developmental toxicity, exposure, bioavailability, and acceptable risk. The staff uses either probabilistic methods or sensitivity analysis to assess uncertainty or variability. The approach to evaluating uncertainty and variability is determined by the analyst on a case-by-case basis, based on the purpose of the risk assessment and availability of data.

•   Question: Please identify any substantial scientific or technical challenges that you may encounter when conducting risk assessments for your agency.

CPSC Staff Response

When performing toxicological risk assessments staff may encounter a variety of technical and scientific challenges, such as the lack of complete toxicity or exposure data, or the lack of methodologies to develop such data. These challenges are addressed on a case-by-case basis, and may include performing exposure assessment studies, such as migration and emissions studies, and developing novel laboratory methods. The staff also nominates chemicals for further toxicological testing by the National Toxicology Program.

Consider, for example, the CPSC staff's risk assessment of diisononyl phthalate (DINP), which is a plasticizer used in teethers and toys made from polyvinyl chloride. CPSC convened a Chronic Hazard Advisory Panel (CHAP)[1] to address the toxicity and potential

---

[1] Convening a CHAP is a statutory mandate before CPSC can regulate products based on chronic toxicity of a substance, 15 U.S.C. 2077 and 2080(b).

risks from DINP, especially the human relevance of rodent tumors induced by perox-isome proliferation. Lack of exposure data for DINP in children's products led to the conduct of observational studies of children's mouthing behavior, as well as the development of methods to measure the mitigation of DINP from certain toys, and laboratory analysis of toys in the market to determine the proportion that contained DINP.

•   Question: What is your current definition of risk assessment, and what types of products are covered by that definition?

CPSC Staff Response

The staff defines risk assessment following the definition of the National Research Council (1983), in which a risk assessment encompasses hazard identification, dose-response assessment, exposure assessment, and risk characterization. Depending on the agency's needs, the staff may complete one or more of these steps for a particular task, but a risk assessment generally consists of all four steps.

The definition applies to all consumer products under CPSC jurisdiction, and includes a variety of toxicological and physical hazards. However, the CPSC's Chronic Hazard Guidelines (57:46626-46653, 1992) were developed primarily to address chronic toxicity.

•   Question: About how long (that is, from initiation of the risk assessment to delivery to the regulatory decision maker) does it take to produce the various types of risk assessments?

CPSC Staff Response

The length of the risk assessment process is highly variable, depending on the intended use of the assessment, *e.g.*, for screening or priority setting, or regulatory analysis; the needs of the decision maker; factors such as the availability of data and the amount, quality, and complexity of available data; and the need for public comment and peer review. The simplest assessments may be completed in a matter of days, while more involved analyses take months or years, especially if the agency must perform extensive studies to assess exposure or convene a CHAP.

Questions about OMB's definition of risk assessment and applicability

•   Question: Using the definition of risk assessment described in the OMB Bulletin, are there work products that would now be considered risk assessments that were not previously considered risk assessments? If so, what are they?

CPSC Staff Response

Using the definition in the OMB Bulletin, almost every work product prepared by the CPSC staff could be considered a risk assessment. This would include:

•   Injury or fatality reports;

•   The agency budget, which employs "risk-based" decision making;

•   Product Safety Assessments—short-turnaround assessments of specific products;

•   Toxicity reviews; and

•   Routine testing of products, such as toys and fireworks, for compliance with standards.

Work products from the CPSC's Directorate for Epidemiology might especially be affected by the expanded definition of risk assessment contained in the Bulletin. For the most part, these work products provide information on injuries and fatalities associated with consumer products and, under the Bulletin's definitions, would be considered either risk assessments or work products that contain data that are used in risk assessments. Examples include hazard sketches (estimates of the number of product-related injuries and descriptions of injury scenarios), estimates of consumer product-related injuries and deaths as part of Product Safety Assessments, and analyses supporting Commission briefing packages that are associated with regulatory activities.

Some of these work products contain estimates of risk in the form of injuries or deaths per unit exposure. Exposure may be defined as products in use or per unit population possibly subdivided by age group. Exposure-based analyses are more commonly found in staff work products where there are a large number of injuries or deaths. They are less common when there are relatively few casualties and/or valid exposure measures are not available. In those cases, it is likely that most readers would conclude that the risk is small regardless of the exposure measure selected.

Questions about type of risk assessment (tiered structure)

•   Question: In your agency, is there currently a clear demarcation between risk assessments used for regulatory analysis and those not used for regulatory analysis? Is this clear at the outset of the risk assessment?

CPSC Staff Response

There is no clear demarcation between risk assessments used for regulatory analysis and those not used for regulatory analysis. Moreover, the importance to the agency of a specific risk assessment is not necessarily determined only by whether it is used to support a regulation. For example, in the staff risk assessment of DINP in children's products, it was determined that the risk was low and no regulations were pursued. Nonetheless, it was important to perform the best risk assessment possible to be reasonably certain that the products (soft plastic toys) were not hazardous.

The intended use of a staff risk assessment is usually clear at the outset, *e.g.*, responding to public petitions, evaluating the impact of a regulation, or supporting the development of voluntary standards. In the event that staff objectives or agency needs change during the process, adjustments are made.

- Question: In your agency, is there currently a clear demarcation between "influential risk assessment" used for regulatory purposes and other risk assessments used for regulatory purposes? Is this clear at the outset of the risk assessment?

CPSC Staff Response

There is currently no clear demarcation between "influential risk assessments" and other risk assessments used for regulatory purposes. Additionally, staff believes that the *a priori* determination of whether a risk assessment is influential is problematic since the impact of the action may not be easily predicted. For example, a determination that something is an "influential risk assessment" may depend upon both the magnitude of the risk and the eventual scope of the regulatory action.

Because of the practical difficulties in distinguishing between influential and non-influential risk analyses at the outset of a project, and because of the additional resources that would be required to prepare influential risk assessments, it would be useful for OMB to provide clarification on how agencies should make this determination.

Questions about impact of the Bulletin on agency risk assessment practices

- Question: If applicable, please specify provisions in the Bulletin that can be expected to have a <u>substantial positive effect</u> on the quality, conduct, and use of risk assessments undertaken by your agency.

CPSC Staff Response

It is unclear whether the provisions of the Bulletin will have a <u>substantial positive effect</u>. As a matter of routine, the CPSC staff strives to perform risk assessments that are scientifically defensible and of the highest quality by using the CPSC's Chronic Hazard Guidelines that clearly define how risk assessments should be performed and by having significant CPSC staff risk assessments peer-reviewed in accordance with OMB guidelines. The staff believes that it appropriately applies the best practices in risk assessment consistent with agency needs and resources.

- Question: If applicable, please specify provisions in the Bulletin that can be expected to have a <u>substantial negative effect</u> on the quality, conduct, and use of risk assessments undertaken by your agency.

CPSC Staff Response

The staff believes a number of provisions in the Bulletin could have a negative effect on the quality, conduct, and use of risk assessments undertaken by the CPSC. Several examples follow.

1. While many of the proposed requirements seem reasonable, meeting the standards could come at significant cost in terms of time and other resources. For example, while the proposed Bulletin addresses the need to consider resources in *Section III: Goals*, it is

not clear that the flexibility implied in this section is reflected in the language elsewhere in the Bulletin. CPSC staff believes that lack of flexibility would result in unnecessarily applying requirements that will not actually improve assessments in all cases (i.e., a one size fits all approach is likely not possible or desirable). Further, staff expects that during the process of planning a risk assessment, there will be discussions about which Bulletin standards will be applicable. Such discussions will be *a priori*, i.e., before the risk assessment has been conducted. Because the applicability of Bulletin standards is ultimately made on the basis of the risk findings and potential regulatory action, it is entirely possible that the standards chosen at the design stage and those required subsequently based on the findings (or potential regulatory action implied by the findings) may be different. This can have serious resource implications.

2. The Bulletin's general requirement (Section IV, 6) that Executive Summaries should "place the estimates of risk in context/perspective with other risks familiar to the target audience" could have three negative effects. First, staff resources will be needed for the analysis of other risk assessments to determine (a) comparability and (b) validity of the analysis. In some cases, the comparable risk may be in areas outside the expertise of CPSC staff and outside assistance may be necessary. Second, we expect that there will be challenges to the selection of comparable risks, especially when the choice of appropriate comparisons is limited. Third, putting comparative risk information in an Executive Summary, without an explanation of the context in which it was derived, could mislead the reader.

If this requirement is implemented, it would be useful for OMB to provide more information on how this requirement might be met.

3. The requirement to revise each risk assessment as new information becomes available could have a negative impact. CPSC staff agrees that some risk assessments remain a source of information years after they are conducted, and such important assessments should be updated as information becomes available. However, many CPSC risk assessments are conducted for specific purposes, *e.g.*, preliminary assessments conducted to support decisions on the disposition of petitions, and may never again be used for informational or regulatory purposes. While the proposed Bulletin states that resources should be considered in meeting this requirement, CPSC staff believes that the flexibility implied in this statement would not necessarily be realized and that scarce resources would be spent on inconsequential, outdated, assessments.

4. Section VII of the Bulletin says that the agency shall include a certification as part of the risk assessment document, explaining that the agency has complied with the requirements of the Bulletin and the applicable Information Quality Guidelines. This requirement needs clarification since the method of certification, which is unspecified in the Bulletin, could have resource implications.

• Question: If your agency followed the procedures described in the Bulletin, would it affect the time course for production of the risk assessment (that is, the time required from initiation of the risk assessment to delivery to the regulatory decision maker)? If so, please explain why?

CPSC Staff Response

CPSC staff believes that the effect of the proposed Bulletin on the time course of a risk assessment would in part depend on the level of flexibility afforded the assessor. If, for example, the Bulletin requires certain steps that the assessor previously might have determined to be unnecessary, then the time course might be lengthened significantly. This would be especially applicable to many routine work products, such as screening level risk assessments and other tasks not normally considered risk assessments.

• Question: One of the Bulletin's reporting standards states the need to be scientifically objective by "giving weight to both positive and negative studies in light of each study's technical quality." Please give an example of how this would be implemented by your agency or department.

CPSC Staff Response

This issue is addressed in the Chronic Hazard Guidelines. CPSC staff considers "all of the available data" in performing risk assessments.

• Question: Does your agency use risk assessments conducted by external groups? Would it be helpful to you if risk assessments submitted to your agency by external groups, such as consultants and private industry, met the requirements proposed in the OMB Bulletin?

CPSC Staff Response

The CPSC issued Chronic Hazard Guidelines in 1992, in part, to guide manufacturers in complying with the requirements of the Federal Hazardous Substances Act. CPSC staff generally does not use risk assessments performed by outside groups, but sometimes it will consider an external risk assessment if it is applicable and if it provides information that the staff does not have. To the extent that such externally-derived assessments would then be used by staff in performing its work, the staff believes that it would be appropriate that such assessors follow accepted risk assessment practices, including the CPSC Chronic Hazard Guidelines, as well as other requirements of the federal government.

Department of Defense Response to Questions for All Agencies Potentially Affected by the Draft OMB Risk Assessment Bulletin – July 2006

1. The Department of Defense (DoD) appreciates the opportunity to respond to the questions posed by the National Research Council's Committee chartered to review the Office of Management and Budget's (OMB's) proposed Risk Assessment Bulletin. The Committee was tasked to determine if the proposed guidance will meet OMB's stated objective to "enhance the technical quality and objectivity of risk assessments prepared by federal agencies."

2. A wide variety of risk and hazard assessments are performed by many different offices and organizations across DoD with varying missions ranging from basic research to civil works. These include risk assessments performed for:

- Developing DOD environment, safety and occupational health (ESOH) standards.
- Assessing site-specific human health and ecological risks from environmental contamination.
- Assessing ESOH risks from operating weapons systems and military platforms (*e.g.*, community noise level from aircraft operations; risks to military personnel from weapons firing).
- Assessing materials being considered for use in weapons systems and platforms.
- Assessing the risks of infectious diseases to DoD's operating forces.

3. The responses below focus primarily on risk assessments performed in the functional areas of environmental protection, human safety and health and facilities/civil works. Due to time constraints for developing responses and the sensitive or classified nature of certain national defense programs, the responses do not cover such areas as military operations/threat assessments, munitions, or all areas of weapons systems development and acquisition.

<u>**DoD Responses to Questions**</u>

1. <u>**General questions about current risk assessment practices**</u>

    a. Please provide a brief overview of your current risk assessment practices.

    Risk assessment methods and characterization of uncertainty are dependent upon and tailored to the specific purpose or function being assessed. There are some common approaches prescribed within functional areas, but no over-arching approach for all types of risk assessments.

    The following provides some examples of the types of risk assessments performed by DoD and the approach used.

Occupational Health Risk Assessments:

    DoD develops internal exposure limits for occupational hazards when a regulatory standard is not available, or when DoD determines the regulatory standard does not sufficiently reduce the risk to DoD personnel or operations. In the development of such internal standards, a comprehensive health risk assessment would normally be prepared.

Environmental Risk Assessments:

Site-specific risk assessments for releases of hazardous substances, pollutants, and contaminants resulting in environmental contamination are conducted under the Defense Environmental Restoration Program following the process set forth in the Comprehensive Environmental Response, Compensation, and Liability Act (CERCLA) and the Resource Conservation and Recovery Act (RCRA). The majority of the human health assessments conducted by DoD follow the methodology outlined in the Environmental Protection Agency's (EPA's) *Risk Assessment Guidance for Superfund (RAGS), Volume I, Human Health Evaluation Manual, Parts A through E.* The EPA's *Ecological Risk Assessment Guidance for Superfund* (ERAGS) is used for conducting ecological risk assessments. The Department is currently developing a methodology to assess the hazards associated with military munitions and explosives of concern in collaboration with EPA.

The Department occasionally conducts risk assessments pursuant to RCRA authorities. For example, at installations that have hazardous waste combustion facilities or activities, RCRA assessments are usually conducted. The human health portion of RCRA assessments follow the methodology outlined in the *Human Health Risk Assessment Protocol for Hazardous Waste Combustion Facilities.* These types of risk assessments are almost exclusively screening in nature, but often the results are used to make permitting decisions.

Health Hazard Assessments:

Health hazard assessments are conducted following a formal approach or standard operating procedure for various programs within the DoD. The assessments are completed by a team of professional subject matter experts (*e.g.*, industrial hygienists, toxicologists, acoustic engineers, physicians, epidemiologists, etc.) as warranted by the specific assessment. The results of these assessments are documented in a formal health hazard assessment report.

A hazard assessment may use multiple inputs to assess the significance of a hazard including:

• Benchmark system design standards (*e.g.*, military standards, industry standards, consensus standards);
• Established risk criteria (*e.g.*, Occupational Safety and Health Administration's Permissible Exposure Limits, American Conference of Governmental Industrial Hygienists Threshold Limit Values, other military unique criteria); or
• Experience from previous systems, safety assessments, human factor assessments, operational requirement documents, management documents, test documents, user manuals, and field observations.

Examples of the application of health hazard assessments follow:

- The control of health hazards associated with the life cycle management of new and modified equipment to identify potential hazards early in the life cycle and eliminate hazards in the design phase.

- The evaluations of materials being considered for various applications, such as use aboard submarines.

Civil Works:

The Army Corps of Engineers (COE) is expanding the use of risk assessment in dam safety including a screening level portfolio risk assessment. Currently, the Louisiana Coastal Protection and Restoration (LaCPR) study is proposed to include a multifaceted risk assessment, the incorporation of large uncertainty scenario drivers, and a risk-informed decision process. The National Research Council (NRC) reviewed the Army Corps of Engineers risk assessment approach to flood damage reduction and published their findings in 1999. Generally, NRC thought the approach was a great improvement but identified some issues for further consideration. The continuing need for risk assessments was reinforced by the events surrounding hurricane Katrina.

The COE also uses risk assessments in evaluating the appropriate options for the disposal of dredged material during the maintenance and construction of the nation's waterways. The COE has developed a variety of guidance manuals and procedures for the evaluation and testing of dredged material. Some of the COE work in this area was reviewed previously by the NRC (*e.g.*, Contaminated Sediments in Ports and Waterways: Cleanup Strategies and Technologies, 1997).

b. Specifically, do you conduct probabilistic risk assessment?

Probabilistic risk assessments may be performed within DoD for past or predictive effects on health, although rarely in support of baseline risk assessments conducted for the Defense Environmental Restoration Program. Probabilistic techniques have been explored but dismissed in a number of cases because of lack of scientifically defensible technical information; lack of acceptance by the regulatory community; difficulty in communicating the results to the public; and/or significant time, resource, and cost restraints. Probabilistic risk assessments are not always needed to adequately inform the decision-makers and stakeholders about the risks and hazards present and should be performed if necessary to aid decision making.

Markov Chain Monte Carlo Analysis has been used for chemical specific risk assessments in conjunction with the development of pharmacokinetic models.

c.   Is there a common approach to both risk assessments and uncertainty analysis? How do you currently address uncertainty and variability in your agency's risk assessments?

There is a common approach to the conduct of DoD risk assessments depending on the functional area and purpose for which the assessment is being done (*e.g.*, environmental site assessments follow EPA RAGS and ERAGS guidance as addressed above).

There is not a common approach for uncertainty analysis for the diversity of risk assessments that DoD conducts. Typically, uncertainty and variability are addressed in risk assessments either qualitatively or quantitatively. The uncertainty analyses performed in individual risk assessments vary by the type of assessment produced and time/resource constraints. Levels of effort are not consistent; some uncertainty sections in some risk documents are very detailed, others are not. Variability is often addressed by statistical approaches and spatial analyses.

Below are some specific comments related to uncertainty analyses found in DoD risk assessments:

- Within the uncertainty sections of the assessment, specific areas may be examined (*e.g.*, for ecological risk assessments, area use factors (AUFs) are typically considered).

- While cancer risks and hazard quotients are generally summed across chemicals and exposure pathways, there is usually no discussion regarding the underlying scientific uncertainty of this approach.

- It is common practice to direct environmental sampling in a biased manner (*e.g.*, directed to wastewater outfalls). This biased approach is consistent with most regulatory guidance and attempts to ensure human health protection. This practice incorporates a wide margin of safety to account for uncertainty as to the exact exposure point and variability in types of exposure. However, the uncertainty is not captured by current site attribution methods. It is common practice to use this type of biased sampling data in comparison to ambient/background for the purpose of attributing contamination to the entire site.

- In the face of scientific uncertainty associated with site characterization, it is common practice to use either the maximum detected concentration or if sufficient data are available, the 95th upper confidence limit (UCL) of the mean concentration as being representative of the site. The associated uncertainty and variability is rarely included in the risk characterization, although it is sometimes discussed in a qualitative manner.

- Although the scientific uncertainty associated with chemical-specific/ toxicological risk assessment (*e.g.*, IRIS risk assessment) is carried into each site-specific chemical risk assessment, risk characterizations rarely discuss the uncertainty associated with the safety and uncertainty factors assigned to toxicity criteria found in IRIS.

d.   Please identify any substantial scientific or technical challenges that you may encounter when conducting risk assessments for your agency.

Listed below are some of the substantial/scientific challenges DoD encounters when conducting risk assessments.

- Assigning Risk Assessment Codes (RACs) for health hazard assessments

  When assigning RACs for life cycle management of new and modified equipment and other safety analyses, variability is introduced because of the subjective, professional judgment used in assigning severity and probability values. While risk assessments may use state-of-the-art techniques, they have inherent limitations based on the capabilities of current technologies to predict ESOH effects (*e.g.*, limitations in laboratory toxicology studies to predict human health effects related to new materials).

- Consistency and satisfying the various regulatory agencies in regards to transparency

  The degree to which a risk assessment is considered minimally or not transparent to one agency may be considered efficient preparation to another. Setting a minimal standard for transparency would facilitate more efficient production of risk assessments. In addition, the various federal and state program offices with which we interact often have different interpretations of the same guidance documents or the same regulations. Consequently, the risk assessment "target" is constantly moving, making it difficult to effectively produce a risk assessment that meets all regulatory requirements.

- Effectively communicating complex and highly technical risk assessment information

  Stakeholders unfamiliar with the risk assessment process or individuals who have emotional attachment to the issue present a challenge for risk communication. Mandatory performance of even more complex risk assessments, such as probabilistic risk assessments, can amplify this challenge. Standardizing the types of risk assessments and more clearly defining when and how each type of risk assessment is to be conducted would be a significant improvement.

- A lack of scientifically defensible and/or agreed upon input information.

  Toxicity data, especially for the acute portion of the risk assessments and for the dermal pathways, is absent for many of the chemicals included in our risk assessments. Likewise, fate and transport data are often unavailable, as are scientifically defensible exposure inputs and statistical distributions for these exposure inputs. Consequently, this absence of information has hindered the use and performance of probabilistic risk assessments. Targeting research to fill these information gaps would allow risk assessors to produce more comprehensive and technically defensible products.

- Calculating risk for intermittent exposure(s)

  From an applied perspective, exposures being assessed may be intermittent and the risk assessment model and associated toxicity data are not sufficiently refined to account for intermittent exposures. Consequently, exposures may be averaged over some exposure duration, resulting in an underestimation or overestimation of risk, depending on the chemicals involved. Further development of the existing model or development of a new model, specific for intermittent exposures, would be a good first step to removing this challenge. Toxicity data representative of intermittent exposures would also need to be developed.

- Over-estimating risk

  The current approach to ensuring health protection in the face of scientific uncertainty was devised almost 30 years ago. That approach is to multiply a default factor of up to 10 for each of four types of uncertainty assumed to act independently. Uncertainty factors are applied for inter-human variability/sensitivity, animal to human extrapolation, LOAEL to NOAEL extrapolation, and sub-chronic to chronic extrapolation. Today, many health risk assessors believe that multiplying default uncertainty factors overestimates risk. When coupled with the use of non-peer reviewed toxicity values, the approach may lead to significantly overestimated risk values and thus overly conservative cleanup levels.

- Evaluating the vapor intrusion pathway

  Regulators frequently require DOD to evaluate the vapor intrusion pathway under residential scenarios. This is problematic because: 1) the methodology remains technically complex and controversial among risk assessors; 2) residential indoor air is not regulated; and, 3) standards for residential indoor air have not been established.

- Lack of toxicity values for emerging contaminants

  Regulators frequently request that DOD conduct risk assessments on contaminants for which toxicity values have not been established and for which inadequate toxicological information exists.

The following is a list of subjects identified by DoD risk assessment professionals as lacking policy or guidance, or consistency in policy or guidance.

- — Consistent and reasonable policies and practices on the use of background data (anthropogenic and naturally-occurring background) and quantifying and accounting for background.
- — Guidance for identifying and characterizing genetic polymorphisms (genotype-environment interactions) and inter-individual differences in susceptibility to toxicants.
- — Consistent policies and practices on evaluating ecological habitats.
- — Guidance for estimating exposure concentrations of contaminants in soil and groundwater in human-health risk assessments.
- — Policy or requirements for defining the extent of site characterization required to inform a risk management decision for a site.
- — Guidance for determining home ranges for receptors being evaluated in ecological risk assessments.

—   Guidance, policy, or requirements for selecting toxicity values from a range of possible values.

—   Guidance for determining the weight-of-evidence in carcinogen assessments.

—   Policy or requirements for the appropriate use of screening concentrations in risk assessments.

—   Guidance for addressing inconsistencies with statistical approaches for use in risk assessments.

—   Guidance or standards for assessing risks of contaminants when analytical limits of detection or analytical capability may not be developed/available to meet existing public health goals.

e. —— What is your current definition of risk assessment, and what types of products are covered by that definition?

For different programs and different agencies within DoD, there are slightly different definitions that relate specifically to the type of assessment being performed. Some of the definitions are presented below:

Occupational Health Program:

Risk assessment is defined as a structured process to identify and assess hazards. An expression of potential harm, described in terms of hazard severity, accident probability, and exposure to hazard. Sub-definitions follow:

•   Hazard Severity. An assessment of the expected consequence, defined by degree of injury or occupational illness that could occur from exposure to a hazard.

•   Accident Probability. An assessment of the likelihood that, given exposure to a hazard, an accident will result. An accident receives a specific classification based on an established criteria scheme.

•   Exposure to Hazard. An expression of personnel exposure that considers the number of persons exposed and the frequency or duration of the exposure.

Environmental Program:

Risk assessment is the collection and evaluation of scientific information for the purpose of determining potential adverse health impacts to human and/or ecological populations from exposure to substances (chemical or biological) released into the environment.

Health Hazard Assessment Program:

Risk assessment is an organized process used to describe and estimate the likelihood of adverse health outcomes from occupational or environmental exposures to hazards. It consists of four steps: hazard identification, toxicity assessment, exposure assessment and risk characterization.

In the Defense Environmental Restoration Program, a site-specific risk assessment is used in risk management decisions to determine the extent of risks at a site and the need for response actions.

Health hazard assessment is a methodical evaluation of the consequences of exposure to a hazard(s) with particular focus on potential adverse human effects. The HHA process may incorporate hazard identification, characterization, assessment and communication. It may be used to support a regulatory program or policy position and meet one or more of the following criteria:

-      Focus on significant emerging issues
-      Support major regulatory decisions or policy/guidance of major impact
-      Establish a significant precedent, model, or methodology
-      Support major regulatory decisions or policy/guidance of major impact
-      Have significant inter-agency implications
-      Consider an innovative approach for a previously defined problem, process, or methodology
-      Satisfy a statutory or other legal mandate for peer review

Civil Works

The COE does not have risk "terms of reference" nor overall risk assessment standards. As the COE explores an appropriate approach to implementing the OMB bulletin, the necessary Engineering Regulations will be revised in accordance with the requirements of Section IV of the bulletin.

f. About how long (that is, from initiation of the risk assessment to delivery to the regulatory decision maker) does it take to produce the various types of risk assessments?

The length of time to produce a risk assessment varies greatly depending on the complexity of the subject and the type of risk assessment. Health hazard assessments, as addressed in this response, typically take 30 to 90 days from receipt of a complete package for review. Human health risk assessments for the Defense Environmental Restoration Program sites can vary from months for simple sites to five years or greater for complex sites.

The time needed to produce a risk assessment depends greatly on the amount of information available at the initiation of the risk assessment and/or the specific requirements for conducting the assessment. The time required can be significant in situations where (1) no sampling has been performed, (2) risk communication is just beginning, (3) toxicological information does not exist or has to be developed, and/or (4) the exposure/health effects are not known or well understood. In urgent situations, there may be a need to provide as accurate an estimate of risk as possible in a very short timeframe. In these cases, a risk estimate may be made in as little as a few hours.

2. Questions about OMB's definition of risk assessment and applicability

Using the definition of risk assessment described in the OMB Bulletin, are there work products that would now be considered risk assessments that were not previously considered risk assessments? If so, what are they?

The term "risk assessment" is a very broad term that the OMB Bulletin correctly recognized can involve many different methodologies in the varied disciplines that utilize the assessment of risks as a decision making tool. However, we do not believe that it will significantly change what products we consider risk assessments at this time.

The applicability of the OMB Bulletin requirements to some DoD activities some projects is somewhat unclear. For example, the second paragraph of Section II states, "[t]his Bulletin does not apply to risk assessments that arise in the course of individual agency adjudications or permit proceedings…" Additional confusion arises from the sentence, "[t]his Bulletin also shall not apply to risk assessments performed with respect to inspections relating to health, safety, or environment." Therefore, it is possible that the Bulletin would not be applicable to some inspection work products.

3. Questions about type of risk assessment (tiered structure)

a. In your agency, is there currently a clear demarcation between risk assessments used for regulatory analysis and those not used for regulatory analysis? Is this clear at the outset of the risk assessment?

Typically, there is usually a clear distinction between risk assessments used for regulatory analysis and those that are not (i.e., used for internal DoD purposes). Many of the environmental risk assessments are site-specific and are performed to meet statutory (*e.g.*, CERCLA) and regulatory requirements. Whereas chemical-specific toxicological risk assessments are done to determine reference doses or concentrations and typically have the potential to impact the state of the science, the published values may be used by other agencies for regulatory purposes. These are typically done by DoD for military-specific chemicals.

Other risk assessments may be done to answer military-specific, force protection, or threat assessment questions.

b. In your agency, is there currently a clear demarcation between "influential risk assessment" used for regulatory purposes and other risk assessments used for regulatory purposes? Is this clear at the outset of the risk assessment?

There is no clear demarcation between "influential risk assessment" used for regulatory purposes and other risk assessments used for regulatory purposes.

4. Questions about impact of the Bulletin on agency risk assessment practices

a. If applicable, please specify provisions in the Bulletin that can be expected to have a substantial positive effect on the quality, conduct, and use of risk assessments undertaken by your agency.

The general framework provided by the Bulletin will be useful to DOD for improving scientific rigor for its risk assessment procedures. Below are some specific improvements that will likely be realized:

- Increased transparency of the science and assumptions in the risk assessment.

- Improving the scientific defensibility of risk assessments as a result of the provisions listed in Section IV: "General Risk Assessment and Reporting Standards."

- Defining the central tendency (CT) as an "expected effect" and the requirement to express risk as a range should produce more realistic risk management decisions. However, it would be beneficial if the OMB Bulletin provided examples of when it may be appropriate to regulate using the expected effect vice the most conservative estimate.

- A more comprehensive characterization of the sources of uncertainty via use of quantitative approaches will be included in risk assessments performed. We consider this extremely important and beneficial for chemical-specific risk assessments (whereas this may not be as necessary for more routine, site-specific risk assessments). Perhaps more importantly, is the recognition and use of this uncertainty information in risk management decisions.

- More detailed discussion(s) of the full range of uncertainty will be generated by modeling of data (the strengths and weaknesses associated with various assumptions/modeling). This is frequently lacking in health risk assessments. These modeling assumptions include those associated with dose-response curves and point-of-departure (POD); dose ranges and associated likelihood estimates for identified human health outcomes.

- More detailed discussions of variability (the range of risks reflecting true differences among members of the population due to, for example, differences in susceptibility) and uncertainty (the range of plausible risk estimates arising because of limitations in knowledge) will have a positive effect on the outcome of the risk assessment. Failure to characterize variability and uncertainty thoroughly can convey a false sense of precision in the conclusions of the risk assessment.

- For cancer health risk estimates, quantitative estimates of the POD corresponding to central, upper-bound, and lower-bound estimates; the use of different plausible POD values; different plausible mathematical functions fit to the observed epidemiological data, where available, and different assumptions for estimating historical exposures among human subjects (epidemiological data), when applicable, should significantly improve the risk assessments.

•   For non-cancer health risk estimates for chemical-specific risk assessments, characterization of the uncertainty associated with fitting a dose-response relationship to the available data and selection of a POD. Where applicable, it should be acknowledged that the information available remains insufficient to support a meaningful point estimate.

b.   If applicable, please specify provisions in the Bulletin that can be expected to have a substantial negative effect on the quality, conduct, and use of risk assessments undertaken by your agency.

The adherence to the provisions listed in Section V: "Special Standards for Influential Risk Assessment" and in Section IV: "General Risk Assessment and Reporting Standards", the performance of risk assessments will be more labor and resource intensive.

Additional labor will be required to:

•   Collect the necessary information and data to characterize risk as outlined in the OMB Bulletin.

•   Negotiate with regulatory authorities about the scope of the risk assessment. When deciding specific inputs, there will now be a wider range of choices, rather than one or two choices.

•   Communicate the results to people unfamiliar with the risk assessment process, due to the increased complexity of the risk characterization portion and the increase in the amount of material requiring explanation.

•   Increase the level of expertise needed to perform quantitative uncertainty analysis for completing a risk assessment. Finding the expertise in a timely fashion may present challenges.

•   Review products due to increased time associated with more complex risk assessments.

c.   If your agency followed the procedures described in the Bulletin, would it affect the time course for production of the risk assessment (that is, the time required from initiation of the risk assessment to delivery to the regulatory decision maker)? If so, please explain why?

The time required will vary depending on the organization and type of risk assessment being conducted. No expected change is anticipated for some risk assessments while a significant increase in time may be required for others. Some organizations within DoD believe that adherence to the provisions listed in Section V: Special Standards for Influential Risk Assessments and in Section IV: General Risk Assessment and Reporting Standards may impact the ability to meet critical and/or regulatory prescribed deadlines unless the allowable timeframes are extended to accommodate the expanded assessments.

d. One of the Bulletin's reporting standards states the need to be scientifically objective by "giving weight to both positive and negative studies in light of each study's technical quality." Please give an example of how this would be implemented by your agency or department.

A requirement to give weight to both positive and negative studies in light of each study's technical quality would generally be a beneficial change. The key point in the question is "in light of each study's technical quality." DoD upholds the principles of scientific objectivity and consideration of all peer-reviewed literature, with an emphasis on appropriate and technically relevant study design for the research.

The ability to be able to select site-specific exposure assumptions and toxicity parameters based upon the latest science, vice the default values required by some regulatory agencies, would be very beneficial. Risk assessors should have the option to evaluate the various studies and discuss in the risk assessment the justification for deviating from the standard default value(s). Currently, some agencies are reluctant to allow the use of site specific exposure assumptions.

The EPA's Final Cancer Guidelines state that well-conducted human studies that fail to detect a statistically significant positive association may have value and should be judged on their own merit. However, it may be difficult to have EPA consider negative studies of "equal weight" with positive studies, particular since the Cancer Guidelines also have a default assumption that states when cancer effects are not found in an exposed human population, this information, by itself, is not generally sufficient to conclude that the chemical poses no carcinogenic hazard to potentially exposed human populations.

Deciding whether to give weight to both positive and negative studies in site-specific risk assessments could be determined by the complexity of the risk assessment necessary for a scientifically sound decision and the benefits, if any, of conducting such an evaluation, since this may significantly increase the time and resources needed to conduct the assessment. If the requirements of the risk assessment include the development of parameters for use in the risk assessment, both positive and negative studies are likely to be used. If parameter development is not required, one may choose to use default parameters.

e. Does your agency use risk assessments conducted by external groups? Would it be helpful to you if risk assessments submitted to your agency by external groups, such as consultants and private industry, met the requirements proposed in the OMB Bulletin?

Products produced by external groups are occasionally used and frequently reviewed by DoD. Risk assessments from external groups are often used when there is a lack of existing regulatory guidance. Contractors frequently conduct human health and ecological risk assessments as part of the DoD Installation Restoration Program. DoD also considers risk assessments published in open scientific literature when examining chemicals for which no regulatory standards exist. Although it would result in an increased contract requirement, it would be beneficial if contractors and private industry met the OMB Proposed Bulletin requirements. Potential benefits include:

- More consistent DoD risk assessments,

- More rapid quality analysis/quality control (QA/QC) review(s),
- Increased transparency when using products prepared by others, and
- Better information on which a risk manager can base a decision.

The use by federal agencies of risk assessments submitted by external organizations, such as consultants and private industry, may increase the pace of such risk assessments and increase the number of toxicity benchmarks available by removing the burden for all toxicity benchmark development from EPA. The use of credible and scientifically defensible risk assessment by external groups would allow EPA to focus on those chemicals of national importance.

Assuming a "zero-sum" game in most programs, the aforementioned requirements may result in additional costs per assessment and thus fewer assessments may be conducted. The value of additional information and analysis would have to be considered along with the importance and impact of the assessment and the effects on overall programs.

DEPARTMENT OF ENERGY

Response to Questions
By the National Research Council Regarding
OMB's Proposed Risk Assessment Bulletin

July 26, 2006

National Research Council's general questions about current risk assessment practices:

- Please provide a brief overview of your current risk assessment practices. Specifically, do you conduct probabilistic risk assessment? Is there a common approach to both risk assessments and uncertainty analysis? How do you currently address uncertainty and variability in your agency's risk assessments?
- Please identify any substantial scientific or technical challenges that you may encounter when conducting risk assessments for your agency.
- What is your current definition of risk assessment, and what types of products are covered by that definition?
- About how long (that is, from initiation of the risk assessment to delivery to the regulatory decision maker) does it take to produce the various types of risk assessments?

DOE Response:

We will address the third bullet first -- What is your current definition of risk assessment, and what types of products are covered by that definition?

In addressing these questions, we do not make a distinction between risk assessments performed by management and operating (M&O) contractors and the Department of Energy (Department or DOE) itself. There is no single definition for "risk assessment;" the term has numerous meanings and uses throughout DOE operations. There are project and budget risk assessments the purpose of which is to assess the risk of specific engineering options and funding risks associated with proceeding with a project. There are accident-related risk assessments the goal of which is to assess the probability of a given event and its consequences to determine risks to assist in planning mitigating actions or design requirements. There are health and environmental risk assessments the goal of which is to assess the potential risk to the public, environment or work force from various DOE actions or alternative actions to support decision-making. There are risk assessments that relate to regulatory decisions. These can overlap; for example, a health risk assessment may be part of a project risk assessment. Common environment, health and safety related risk assessments conducted by DOE include:

- Risk/dose[1] assessments used in optimization analyses (As Low As is Reasonably Achievable, ALARA) studies to support radiation control decisions which can include:
  - o Selection of control equipment to minimize releases to the environment
  - o Selection of operating procedures that protect workers and the public
  - o Development of authorized limits for control and release of property
- Risk/dose assessments in National Environmental Policy Act (NEPA) documents such as Environmental Impact Statements to support DOE programmatic or project decisions
- Risk/dose assessments that support safety analysis reports (SARs) to support nuclear safety and facility safety planning
- Risk/dose assessments in the form of performance assessments and composite analyses to support waste management authorizations.

In responding to these questions, we are assuming that the National Research Council's primary interest, and the focus of the Office of Management and Budget's (OMB) risk guidelines, is health and environmental related risk assessment consistent with the OMB definition in its proposed Risk Assessment Bulletin. We note that most of the risk assessments conducted by DOE would likely not be "influential risk assessments" as defined in OMB's proposed Bulletin.

Regarding the first bullet -- Please provide a brief overview of your current risk assessment practices. Specifically, do you conduct probabilistic risk assessment? Is there a common approach to both risk assessments and uncertainty analysis? How do you currently address uncertainty and variability in your agency's risk assessments?

Probabilistic risk assessment is sometimes employed by DOE in areas such as performance assessments for waste management facilities, safety analyses, and analyses to support real property release limits (*e.g.*, cleanup standards). However, historically, deterministic assessments have been more frequently used. Except where required by regulation or statute (*e.g.*, 40 CFR Part 191 requires certain probabilistic assessments to demonstrate compliance of high-level waste disposal repositories with the standard), the Department allows the analyst (risk assessor) the flexibility of using either deterministic or probabilistic approaches. In either case, analyses most times include an evaluation of uncertainty and variability (or parameter and assumption sensitivity) of the analytical results of the risk assessment. In some cases, these may be addressed through qualitative evaluations or estimates of doses or risks under bounding conditions.

DOE provides guidance and tools to support such assessments and, to the extent possible, to standardize them for the specific type of assessment. For example, DOE

---

[1] It is noted that because one of the major regulatory functions of the Department is radiological protection and nuclear safety, in its assessments, radiation dose is frequently used instead of "health risk." We consider dose to be a surrogate for risk and hence, in responding to the questions, we use risk assessment and dose assessment interchangeably.

developed and maintains the RESRAD family of codes for conducting dose and risk assessments to support radiological decontamination and cleanup decisions for lands, structures and other property (http://web.ead.anl.gov/resrad/home2/). These codes and models provide the ability to conduct either deterministic assessments, with sensitivity and uncertainty assessment capability, or probabilistic assessments.

There also may be specific requirements for assessing bounding risk where for example, in the development of authorized limits for release of property, DOE requires the doses to be assessed for likely and expected uses and then contingency analyses for the worst plausible use (i.e., the use causing the highest potential human exposure given a plausible use) of the property to be released. In the case of low-level waste (LLW) disposal site performance assessments, the primary performance standard assumes undisturbed performance of the closed site. However, additional assessments are required to determine risks caused by intrusion into the site. DOE provides guidance for most areas to help standardize the risk assessments; however, given their varied purposes, a risk assessment for one activity will not necessarily be the same as for another. In addition, consistent with the proposed OMB Bulletin, DOE recommends that the resources expended for a risk or dose assessment be commensurate with the importance of the risk assessment, taking into consideration the nature of the potential hazard, the available data, and the decision's needs. DOE is currently drafting a policy and guidance on risk methodology consistent with OMB Information Quality Guidelines in response to a request from the Defense Nuclear Facilities Safety Board.

Regarding the second bullet -- Please identify any substantial scientific or technical challenges that you may encounter when conducting risk assessments for your agency.

The primary challenge for DOE when conducting risk assessments usually relates to maintaining consistency between various risk assessments and explaining differences when they are warranted. In trying to make assessments be representative of real risks, it is frequently difficult to not assess worst case conditions, particularly where these have been used by others in the past. There is always one more scenario, or one more approach that someone feels deserves assessment. It is frequently a challenge to balance the desire to evaluate some new option with the need to make a timely decision and complete the action. Integrating or taking into consideration the newest science is also a challenge. It generally is difficult to move away from a particular practice or data that has been used in the past, particularly when the new approach may be less conservative (*e.g.*, a situation where the linear-no threshold model of risk may be in question). However, as noted in the questions on "risk assessment practices" below, for the most part, DOE does not deal with such issues because we base our risk assessments on risk and dose factors developed by other agencies and organizations.

One of the technical difficulties is the paucity of data. For example, DOE facilities have very low accident rates, which create large uncertainties in the determination of accident likelihood, especially for high-consequence events. Unlike the commercial nuclear industry, most DOE facilities vary significantly in design and hazard; developing models for the behavior of systems and predicting outcomes is challenging.

Regarding the fourth bullet -- About how long (that is, from initiation of the risk assessment to delivery to the regulatory decision maker) does it take to produce the various types of risk assessments?

The time it takes DOE to complete a "risk assessment" varies greatly and is typically commensurate with the scope, complexity and controversy associated with a project. The range may be from a few months to several years for extremely complex or controversial projects.

National Research Council questions about OMB's definition of risk assessment and applicability:

> • Using the definition of risk assessment described in the OMB Bulletin, are there work products that would now be considered risk assessments that were not previously considered risk assessments? If so, what are they?

> **DOE Response:** No. As noted above, the term has been used more broadly at DOE than in the definition of "risk assessment" in the proposed OMB Bulletin, but all products that meet the OMB definition of risk assessments have always been considered risk assessments by DOE.

National Research Council questions about type of risk assessment (tiered structure):

• In your agency, is there currently a clear demarcation between risk assessments used for regulatory analysis and those not used for regulatory analysis? Is this clear at the outset of the risk assessment?

> **DOE Response:** Yes, the analyst and reviewers know if the risk assessment being developed is to comply with a specific regulation, to support development of a regulation or just to support decision-making with regard to design development, alternative selection or impact assessment.

• In your agency, is there currently a clear demarcation between "influential risk assessment" used for regulatory purposes and other risk assessments used for regulatory purposes? Is this clear at the outset of the risk assessment?

> **DOE Response:** Yes, the proposed OMB definition seems clear, and the proposed Bulletin contains adequate discussion to use as a basis for such

determinations. More specifically, the proposed Bulletin states that the term "influential" should be interpreted consistently with OMB's government-wide Information Quality Guidelines and the agencies' guidelines. DOE has found the term "influential scientific information," which establishes the same standard, to be clear and workable in practice. The term "influential risk assessment" in the proposed OMB Bulletin has not been used by DOE in the past, but in the future, it will be clear to DOE program offices when an assessment is an influential risk assessment.

National Research Council questions about impact of the Bulletin on agency risk assessment practices:

• If applicable, please specify provisions in the Bulletin that can be expected to have a <u>substantial positive effect</u> on the quality, conduct, and use of risk assessments undertaken by your agency.

• If applicable, please specify provisions in the Bulletin that can be expected to have a <u>substantial negative effect</u> on the quality, conduct, and use of risk assessments undertaken by your agency.

DOE Response: We anticipate no substantial effects on agency risk assessments. DOE requirements and guidance for risk assessments are generally consistent with the OMB proposed guidance and hence, risk assessments should not be greatly influenced. As previously noted, most DOE risk assessments would not be classified as "influential risk assessments" under the OMB definition.

• If your agency followed the procedures described in the Bulletin, would it affect the time course for production of the risk assessment (that is, the time required from initiation of the risk assessment to delivery to the regulatory decision maker)? If so, please explain why?

DOE Response: The only issue identified by DOE relates to the peer review process, which Section III of the proposed Risk Assessment Bulletin includes as one of the goals of risk assessment. Although DOE risk assessments undergo peer review, the explicit requirements for peer review in OMB's Bulletin for Peer Review under some circumstances could reduce flexibility and add cost and time to a project if additional mechanisms for peer review need to be employed.

• One of the Bulletin's reporting standards states the need to be scientifically objective by "giving weight to both positive and negative studies in light of each study's technical quality." Please give an example of how this would be implemented by your agency or department.

DOE Response: For the most part, this is not relevant to DOE risk assessments. Risk factors and dose factors, which typically are the most controversial element of a risk assessment and for which there are differing scientific views and studies, are not generated by the Department but rather by other organizations or agencies. For example, for radiation dose and risk assessment DOE uses the recommendations of the Environmental Protection Agency (EPA) (*e.g.*, Federal guidance reports #11, #12 and #13), the National Academies (*e.g.*, BEIR reports), the International Commission on Radiological Protection (ICRP), and the National Council on Radiation Protection and Measurements (NCRP).

Similarly for toxic chemicals, DOE uses risk estimates from EPA (*e.g.*, IRIS database, HEAST Tables). DOE does conduct research as input to its "influential risk assessments" such as DOE epidemiological studies (*e.g.*, atomic bomb survivors, DOE workers) and DOE Office of Science low dose radiation research program (Link to Low-dose Radiation Research Program homepage). However, DOE has not historically conducted the independent studies to consolidate these assessments, but rather has depended on others such as EPA and the National Academies to use the data and studies developed by DOE. DOE does encourage the development of mechanisms to rapidly and routinely update the science such as that described above which underlies the risk assessment process.

• Does your agency use risk assessments conducted by external groups? Would it be helpful to you if risk assessments submitted to your agency by external groups, such as consultants and private industry, met the requirements proposed in the OMB Bulletin?

DOE Response: As noted in the responses to other questions, DOE depends almost exclusively on the risk assessments prepared by others (primarily other Federal agencies or national and international standards organizations) for the toxicity estimates, carcinogenicity estimates and other risk and dose factor information. These values are used in DOE assessments of risk from its operations such as its NEPA documents, performance assessments and so forth. For risk assessments that we conduct such as those supporting the development of cleanup decisions, we frequently support and as appropriate use independent reviews. Therefore, it would be useful if these outside groups followed the OMB Bulletin.

ADDITIONAL QUESTIONS
BY THE NATIONAL RESEARCH COUNCIL
FOR DOE

• What are DOE's current overall challenges regarding risk assessment? Specifically, please address DOE sites that have to be remediated (*e.g.*, Hanford); DOE facilities (*e.g.*, research and test reactors and processing plants); special projects (*e.g.*, Yucca Mountain); and other sites (*e.g.*, Pantex). How will the OMB Bulletin impact the quality, conduct, and use of risk assessments in these cases?

DOE Response: DOE's overall challenges regarding risk assessments conducted for activities such as site remediation are related to the need to obtain from the regulatory agencies, such as EPA, the best and most up to date scientific data for input into the risk assessment models (*e.g.*, carcinogenicity data for specific chemicals of concern) and the best data for the default assumptions.

Unless the Bulletin results in changes to other agencies' regulations or guidance, it is not likely that the Bulletin will significantly affect the quality, conduct or use of risk assessments for these cases. If there is a significant impact on agencies, such as EPA -- which requires the risk assessments for regulatory compliance, issues the guidance on how to prepare the risk assessments, maintains many of the databases with the "approved" data for input into the models such as the carcinogenicity, and provides many of the default assumptions -- then DOE in turn will be affected. In addition, the reporting requirements could prove to be onerous, without improving the overall quality of the risk assessments.

DOE encourages the development of mechanisms to rapidly and routinely update the science underlying the risk assessment process. This is of particular importance to DOE in the context of risk assessment for potential radiation exposure. The Office of Science supports a research program specifically directed at low-dose radiation effects. Integration of scientific advances such as those resulting from the low-dose program into the risk assessment process is necessary to insure that decisions incorporate the latest science.

The statement on page 10 of the proposed Bulletin regarding exemption is very important, but, as we explain below, should be revised: "This Bulletin does not apply to risk assessments that arise in the course of individual agency adjudications or permit proceedings, unless the agency determines that: (1) compliance with the Bulletin is practical and appropriate and (2) the risk assessment is scientifically or technically novel or likely to have precedent-setting influence on future adjudications and/or permit proceedings. This exclusion is intended to cover, among other things, licensing, approval and registration processes for specific product development activities. This Bulletin also shall not apply to risk assessments performed with respect to inspections relating to health, safety, or environment."

The qualifications in (1) and (2) in that paragraph should be removed: if the purpose of a risk assessment is to seek a permit or a license, such as from the Nuclear Regulatory Commission (NRC) or EPA, then those agencies ought to specify the scope and content of the assessment, not DOE. To suggest otherwise (as these two points do by giving DOE managers a chance to make that judgment) sets up a potential for dual, and potentially contradictory, guidance.

The paragraph also needs to exempt, explicitly, all risk and safety assessments being performed preparatory to the safety assessment that is to become part of a permitting or licensing process. Preparatory assessments ought to address the requirements of the regulator(s), not DOE requirements.

A case in point, regarding this potential for dual or contradictory guidance, is with respect to population dose/risk calculations: The proposed Bulletin mentions population dose and risk in many places. Particularly troublesome from a DOE Yucca Mountain project perspective, with calculations for up to a million years, are Section IV, item 4, on page 16 (as also reflected on page 24, item 6 d).

> "4) When estimates of individual risk are developed, estimates of population risk should also be developed. Estimates of population risk are necessary to compare the overall costs and benefits of regulatory alternatives."

For long-term potential dose/risk calculations, the international consensus is shifting away from population doses. The International Commission on Radiological Protection (hence also the NRC and EPA, and even the National Academy of Sciences in their 1995 report on the bases for Yucca Mountain repository standards) acknowledge that for long-term performance or risk assessments future population estimates are highly speculative, making the usefulness of population dose estimates for far future safety evaluations questionable. They are not required for Yucca Mountain repository performance assessments by either EPA or NRC.

In a case where it is appropriate for DOE to assess a population risk, that risk should not be estimated beyond a few hundred years in the future. Similarly, exposures of only the most exposed groups should be assessed (*e.g.*, for emissions or releases from a facility). Exposures beyond a few tens of miles (DOE uses 50 miles as a guideline) from the release point add little to the comparison of alternatives but greatly increase uncertainty and complexity of the analyses.

A Yucca Mountain total system performance assessment is part of an important decision process, so would qualify as an "influential risk assessment," but given the explicit exemption suggested above, the "special standards" for influential risk assessments would not apply to either its pre-licensing or licensing assessments.

APPENDIX
Sources of Guidance Related to DOE Dose or Risk Assessment

- See http://www.directives.doe.gov/directives/current.html#number for
    o   DOE O 435.1 and associated guidance
    o   DOE P 441.1
- DOE 5400.5 and associated guidance (http://www.eh.doe.gov/oepa)
- 10 CFR Part 1021 and related NEPA guidance (http://www.eh.doe.gov/nepa/index.html)
- Office of Science Low Dose Research Program (http://www.sc.doe.gov/ober/LSD/lowdose.html)
- Office of Environment, Safety and Health, epidemiological studies (http://www.eh.doe.gov/health/index.html)
- Assessments related to the performance of high-level radioactive waste repository and management of HLW (http://www.ocrwm.doe.gov/index.shtml)
- Assessments related to performance of the Waste Isolation Pilot Plant for transuranic waste (http://www.wipp.energy.gov/)
- Information on DOE cleanup programs (http://www.em.doe.gov/)

DEPARTMENT OF HEALTH & HUMAN SERVICES   Office of the Secretary

_____

Washington, D.C. 20201

Ellen Mantus, Ph.D.   JUL 28 2006
Study Director
Committee to Review the OMB Risk Assessment Bulletin
Board on Environmental Studies and Toxicology
The National Academies
500 F Street N.W.
Washington, D.C. 20001

Dear Dr. Mantus:

We are pleased to forward HHS responses to the questions posed to federal agencies by the National Academy of Sciences Committee to Review the OMB Risk Assessment Bulletin. HHS is one of the federal agency sponsors of the Committee, and our responses are intended to assist the Committee in its deliberations.

As we indicated during the Committee's recent workshop and public meeting, and expand upon in our enclosed responses, HHS supports the goals of the draft Bulletin, to improve scientific information and encourage the application of sound methodological practices and standards to relevant and appropriate scientific products and situations. The ability of the draft Bulletin to support accomplishment of those goals in a manner that is commensurate with scientific objectives and available science while not overburdening agencies will depend upon a number of factors, including its scope, definition, applicability and requirements for federal agencies, as well as its implementation and interpretation.

Our attached responses to NAS questions reflect potential concerns in several areas. For example, concerns exist that the scope and definition of risk assessment proposed in the draft Bulletin is broad, and could encompass agency scientific, safety and health information products and activities that were not previously considered formal risk assessments in the sense of the National Academy of Sciences' earlier definition, and that do not fit such a model. Second, the draft Bulletin includes technical choices and decisions that one could make in developing a risk assessment, but these practices appear to be expressed as uniform requirements that could inadvertently preclude other appropriate scientific choices and approaches more commensurate with intended scientific and health objectives and the available science. Third, depending on scope and applicability, it will be important to ensure that the Bulletin's requirements do not impede our ability to develop and communicate urgent and time sensitive health and safety information.

We hope that the attached responses will assist the Committee in its deliberations and we would be happy to provide additional information.

                                         Sincerely,

                                         Ann C. Agnew
                                         Executive Secretary to the Department

Enclosure: HHS Responses

HHS-A

U.S. DEPARTMENT OF HEALTH AND HUMAN SERVICES
BACKGROUND INFORMATION ON THE NATIONAL RESEARCH
COUNCIL'S REVIEW OF THE OMB RISK ASSESSMENT BULLETIN[1]

I. QUESTIONS FOR ALL AGENCIES POTENTIALLY AFFECTED BY THE
OMB BULLETIN

A. General questions about current risk assessment practices

1. QUESTION: Please provide a brief overview of your current risk
assessment practices. Specifically, do you conduct probabilistic risk
assessment? Is there a common approach to both risk assessments and
uncertainty analysis? How do you currently address uncertainty and
variability in your agency's risk assessments?

Of the thirteen Department of Health and Human Services (HHS) agencies and
offices, only two, the Food and Drug Administration (FDA) and the Centers for
Disease Control and Prevention (CDC) conduct risk assessments as the term
generally is defined and understood by the NAS in its 1983 report, *Risk Assessment
in the Federal Government: Managing the Process*. Based on the NAS definition, a
risk assessment is a formal and quantitative assessment that includes: (1) hazard
identification, (2) hazard characterization or dose-response assessment, (3)
exposure assessment, and (4) risk characterization.

As noted below, both FDA and CDC use very similar conceptual approaches to risk
assessment although the different contexts (e.g., food, environmental, and
occupation) necessitate differences in these agencies approaches. The National
Institutes of Health (NIH) does not conduct risk assessments as the term is defined
by the 1983 NAS report. Although NIH carries out components of risk
assessments, none of the component products involve quantitative risk assessments
(as discussed, in Section 1.c.).

Scientific assessments are designed and scaled to fit the public health problem at
hand. The type of complex risk assessments contemplated in the Bulletin are not
always appropriate given the magnitude and type of problem, affected population
characteristics, available data, time constraints or resources. As described more
fully in our responses, HHS agencies and offices produce, evaluate and synthesize a
great deal of scientific information, including a number of types of health and safety
assessments that do not follow the NAS paradigm and are not intended to result in
the formal development of a risk estimate—in other words, unlike risk assessments,
they do not develop a statement about the probability that populations or individuals
with the exposure of concern will be harmed and to what degree.

---

[1] The page numbers cited in our answers refer to the pages of the draft Bulletin as released by OMB
for peer review and public comment.

a. FDA

FDA's approach to the conduct of scientific assessments is specific to and dependent upon the scope and purpose of the particular need. FDA's efforts include probabilistic quantitative risk assessments, safety assessments and qualitative risk assessments.

Probabilistic risk assessment. FDA conducts quantitative, probabilistic risk assessments, such as the one on *Listeria monocytogenes* in ready-to-eat foods, available at http://www.foodsafety.gov/~dms/lmr2-toc.html. Factors considered in determining whether a probabilistic quantitative risk assessment is appropriate include: complexity, availability of data, time frame, staff resources, data availability, and the level of certainty needed. With respect to the work of one FDA center, the Center for Food Safety and Applied Nutrition, the procedures used in the selection, commissioning, and conduct of "major" risk assessments (which would generally cover most probabilistic risk assessment of significant complexity) are available at http://www.cfsan.fda.gov/~dms/rafw-toc.html.

Uncertainty and variability. It may be helpful to clarify how FDA uses these terms. *Uncertainty* is typically thought to arise from a lack of data or information. Multiple sources of uncertainty are often considered to be relevant to scientific evaluations and techniques are available to account for or measure some of these uncertainties. *Variability* reflects the fact that all systems or populations have inherent, biological heterogeneity that is not reducible through further measurement or study. Sufficient knowledge is needed to account for both variability and uncertainty, but a key difference between them is that uncertainty reflects incomplete knowledge about a system or population that can be reduced with additional study.

State-of-the art food safety risk assessment models, such as the *Listeria monocytogenes* risk assessment for ready-to-eat foods, use techniques that separately address uncertainty and biological variability. In other risk assessments, FDA identifies sources of uncertainty without clearly distinguishing between variability and uncertainty, because the level of precision needed from the risk assessment does not warrant this separation.

b. CDC

Formal, quantitative risk assessments that are consistent with the NAS 1983 definition are mainly conducted by the CDC's National Institute for Occupational Safety and Health (NIOSH) and the National Center for Environmental Health/Agency for Toxic Substances and Disease Registry (NCEH/ATSDR) in the areas of occupational and environmental health, and conducted by NIOSH and NCEH/ATSDR. CDC's current risk assessment practices are congruent with the practices defined by the NAS. The methods used are data-driven and tailored to the research question under investigation. Typically, workplace exposures of concern are evaluated for potential to cause harm to exposed individuals. Exposures could include chemicals, physical agents, energy, or other hazards in the workplace.

Either human or animal data, or both, are used for quantitative risk assessment, though the preference is to use human data whenever possible. The data are evaluated for applicability to dose-response analysis, availability of human studies, mechanistic information, etc. Dose-response analyses are conducted. Particular emphasis is given to evaluation of alternative models and sensitivity analyses, in order to assess the potential impact of varying data sets or modeling assumptions on the estimated risks.

Probabilistic risk assessment. CDC typically does not conduct probabilistic risk assessments by assigning probability distributions to inputs of a risk equation to generate probability distributions of risk. However, probabilistic methods are used when appropriate and useful, for example, when attempting to characterize uncertainty in exposure or in methodological studies assessing the statistical properties of proposed risk assessment methods. Full probabilistic risk assessments could potentially be developed in the future, given sufficient information on the distributions of exposures, metabolic enzymes, genetic susceptibilities, etc., in the population. However, these data are typically not available for occupational exposures. To date, CDC risk assessment practice has emphasized evaluation of alternative models and assumptions and sensitivity analyses of those models as methods for describing uncertainty, rather than probabilistic modeling.

Uncertainty and variability.
Uncertainty analysis is an essential component of every formal, quantitative risk assessment conducted by CDC. Uncertainty may be evaluated through analysis of different data sets, different endpoints in animal studies, and different hypotheses about the precise mechanism of action, differing assumptions for extrapolation from animals to humans, lack of knowledge of current and historical exposures in human studies and/or differing assumptions regarding statistical models for dose-response or metabolism. CDC risk assessment practice is to explore and describe these uncertainties, to the extent possible, and to evaluate the influence of these various factors on the risk estimates. Current risk assessment research at CDC also assesses the utility of model averaging techniques as a method for addressing model uncertainty in a meaningful and quantitative fashion.

CDC evaluates and describes uncertainty by analysis of alternative models and assumptions, via sensitivity analyses to describe the quantitative impact of alternative assumptions on estimates of risk, and by methods that consider variability and uncertainty of the models in an integrated framework (e.g., meta-analyses, Bayesian approaches). The end result is generally to report a range of plausible risk estimates, which encompass both uncertainty and variability.

c. NIH
NIH does not conduct risk assessments as the term is defined in the 1983 NAS report. However, NIH does carry out components of risk assessments. Since none of the component products involve quantitative risk assessments, NIH does not conduct formal probabilistic analyses, uncertainty analyses or calculations of

variance per se. The National Toxicology Program (NTP) Report on Carcinogens (RoC) provides some indication of the strength of the evidence in its use of two categories of carcinogenic hazards ("known" or "reasonably anticipated to be") and a category of "not listed" when an agent does not meet the criteria for the other two categories. Other NIH products may address uncertainty in the recommendations. Peer-reviewed publications for discovery research typically include a discussion of uncertainty and formal statistical analyses to support a particular conclusion.

2. QUESTION: Please identify any substantial scientific or technical challenges that you may encounter when conducting risk assessments for your agency.

a. FDA
Most challenges that FDA faces in conducting risk assessments are related to funding or resource scarcity rather than substantial scientific or technical issues. Part of FDA's approach to commissioning risk assessments is to consider fully the specific scientific, technical, and informational challenges that are likely to be encountered and the feasibility of overcoming those challenges. The logistics of supporting risk assessment activities remain difficult and involve issues such as availability of staff expertise and availability of funding. Technical challenges include data gaps, lack of access to proprietary information, and the need to develop experimental protocols or models to generate needed data.

b. CDC
Historically at CDC, emphasis has been placed on the use of human data in formal, quantitative risk assessment; however, it is frequently difficult to obtain characterizations of exposures suitable for dose-response analysis. This problem is particularly acute in the case of carcinogens where, because of long disease latencies, the exposures of greatest concern may be decades prior to the conduct of the study, and records of exposure may be sparse to non-existent. In the case of animal studies, data is generally available on both exposure and response, but uncertainty exists as to how to model responses in the low-dose region and how to extrapolate the results from animals to humans.

c. NIH
The NIH does not currently conduct risk assessments as the term is set forth in the 1983 NAS report. However, if the OMB Bulletin definition were to be implemented as currently drafted and strictly applied across government, there may be many additional activities that will need to adhere to the procedures set forth in the Bulletin. Applying those procedures to activities that are not risk assessments now will pose significant challenges. For example, there may be challenges related to understanding active ingredients (e.g., herbal supplements) and providing clear descriptions of key concepts for emerging fields (e.g., gene therapy).

3. QUESTION: What is your current definition of risk assessment, and what types of products are covered by that definition?

Currently, HHS does not have a written definition of "risk assessment" that applies throughout the agency but like most other government agencies worldwide, we rely on the definition of risk assessment put forth by the NAS in its 1983 report, *Risk Assessment in the Federal Government: Managing the Process.* Based on this definition, FDA and CDC are the only agencies within HHS that currently conduct risk assessments.

a. FDA

FDA believes that "risk assessment" refers to a scientific or technical document that assembles and synthesizes scientific information and arrives at a qualitative or quantitative estimation of the extent to which a potential hazard exists and/or the extent of possible risk to human health, safety, or the environment. A complete risk assessment includes the examination of known or potential adverse health effects resulting from human exposure to a hazard. The generally accepted four-part risk assessment paradigm includes: (1) hazard identification; (2) hazard characterization or dose-response assessment; (3) exposure assessment; and (4) risk characterization. Under this definition, we would include only those FDA activities in which there is a formal development of a risk estimate expressed in a scientific or technical document.

b. CDC

CDC distinguishes between scientific assessments, for the purpose of hazard identification, and formal, quantitative risk assessments, for the purpose of characterizing risks numerically. Hazard identification studies often are focused narrowly on whether exposure to a given hazard is associated with significant injury or disease. That is, the response may be measured quantitatively, while the exposure is not. Such studies are valuable in identifying hazards, but do not lend themselves to quantitative exposure-response analysis and full risk characterization. Formal, quantitative risk assessments generally follow the NAS definition of exposure assessment, hazard identification, exposure-response analysis, and risk characterization. CDC has reserved the term "risk assessment" for quantitative analyses which follow the NAS paradigm; i.e., to full quantitative risk assessments, rather than applying the term to the sub-components of a full risk assessment.

CDC formal, quantitative risk assessments range from relatively brief documents – i.e., when only a very limited amount of data are available and only a simplistic analysis can be performed – to extensive analyses, when large amounts of data are available and extensive sensitivity analyses are conducted. For example, an epidemiological study may report only an average exposure and a summary measure of excess risk in an occupational cohort. Without access to the individual data from the study, only a simple linear analysis can be performed. A toxicologically-based risk assessment might also be very simplistic, if there is only one data set available and little controversy on how to extrapolate it to humans, e.g., for a site of contact irritant effect. In every case, an effort is made to develop both a central estimate of risk and statistical confidence limits, and to explore alternative models if the data are adequate to do so. On the other hand, an epidemiologically-based risk assessment using individual data from a large cohort, or a toxicologically-based risk assessment with multiple studies and/or multiple endpoints, could involve numerous models and an extensive exploration of the sensitivity of the final risk estimate to the various modeling assumptions. CDC formal, quantitative risk assessments are peer-reviewed and published in the scientific literature.

c. NIH

The NIH has no formal definition for risk assessment but regards the definition of risk assessment in the 1983 NAS report *Risk Assessment in the Federal Government: Managing the Process* as the authoritative source for the definition of risk assessment. Under this definition, none of the analytical reports and other products prepared by the NIH is considered a risk assessment.

4. QUESTION: About how long (that is, from initiation of the risk assessment to delivery to the regulatory decision maker) does it take to produce the various types of risk assessments?

a. FDA

It depends upon the complexity and nature of the risk assessment (and on how that term is defined). Factors that affect time to completion include scope of data and analysis, extent of public participation, and nature of peer review.

b. CDC

Formal, quantitative risk assessments at CDC range from several months for very simple analyses to a year or more for very complex and extensive analyses. Additional time is required for publication of the analyses in official CDC publications or peer reviewed journals. However, there are activities conducted on very short timelines that would be considered risk assessments under the Bulletin's proposed definition, for example, hazard assessments involving infectious exposures that are conducted under emergency situations.

c. NIH

The NIH does not currently conduct risk assessments as the term is defined in the 1983 NAS report. However, if the OMB Bulletin definition of risk assessment were to be implemented, it would take NIH longer to develop its products. The procedures of the Bulletin would add a number of steps but the specific length of time needed for each product would also depend on the complexity of the science and the complexity of the product's message. In general, most guidance documents and information bulletins can be prepared in less than 18 months. The RoC takes approximately 2.5 years for each agent under review.

II. Questions about OMB's definition of risk assessment and applicability

5. QUESTION: Using the definition of risk assessment described in the OMB Bulletin, are there work products that would now be considered risk assessments that were not previously considered risk assessments? If so, what are they?

The Bulletin (page 9) states that " Documents that address some but not all aspects of risk assessment are covered by this Bulletin" as is information that could be used for risk assessment purposes. Among the Bulletin's specific examples of products that fall under the Bulletin are NTP substance profiles, ATSDR toxicological profiles, FDA tolerance values, and NIOSH current intelligence bulletins and criteria documents, and risk assessments. The Bulletin also refers to the "Surgeon General's Report on Smoking and Health" and [NIH] "alerts to the public about the risks of taking long-term estrogen therapy" as risk assessments (page 5). However, under HHS's current understanding of risk assessment, only a minority of ATSDR toxicological profiles and NIOSH current intelligence bulletins and criteria documents are considered risk assessments. All the other HHS information products that are cited are not considered to be risk assessments. For example, FDA tolerance values are considered to be determinations of an acceptable level of hazard associated with a particular exposure.

Under the Bulletin's proposed definition of risk assessment, several HHS agencies including NIH, CDC and FDA would be most significantly impacted. However, other HHS agencies and offices (e.g. the Agency for Healthcare Research and Quality (AHRQ), the Substance Abuse and Mental Health Administration (SAMHSA) and the Office of Public Health and Science (OPHS)) would be affected as well. Since almost any health information product contains some discussion of safety or risk, it could be interpreted to fall under the Bulletin's definition of risk assessment.

For example, a major program area for AHRQ is the development of information on effectiveness and comparative effectiveness of health care interventions. To the extent that the effectiveness of an intervention is the demonstration that the benefits outweigh the risks, and that patient safety involves risks associated with the intervention, the Bulletin's broad definition of risk assessment could be construed to apply. Thus, the Bulletin could impose major new requirements on AHRQ and other HHS agency information products.

a. FDA

The definition of risk assessment currently in the draft Bulletin could effectively include almost any scientific analysis or review conducted by FDA. Second, the current definition may be broad enough to encompass peer-reviewed scientific journal articles cited in support of a regulation or a public health advisory. FDA does not currently consider these types of documents to be risk assessments.

Third, some exposure or hazard assessments might be interpreted under the Bulletin to be "risk assessments" because of uncertainties created by the definition of "risk assessment" when read in conjunction with Section II.1, "applicability," which states that the Bulletin's standards apply to "all agency risk assessments available to the public." The Bulletin (at page 8) states that the definition of risk assessment applies to documents that *"could be used* for risk assessment purposes, such as an exposure or hazard assessment *that might not constitute a complete risk assessment"* (emphases added). The same difficulty reappears on page 9 which states that "Documents that address some but not all aspects of risk assessment are covered by this Bulletin."

Fourth, the definition of "risk assessment" arguably applies to a wide array of documents or presentations. For example, a "PowerPoint" presentation could become a "risk assessment" if the printed slides are construed to be a "scientific or technical document." A speech discussing risk assessment on a specific matter could similarly be argued to be a "risk assessment" if the speech is printed or reduced to a transcript, thereby creating a "scientific or technical document."

Finally, while many FDA product approval activities may be excluded because they are "individual agency adjudications or permit proceedings," the draft Risk Assessment Bulletin would, under a broad interpretation of the Bulletin, continue to apply to other comparable FDA activities which, either by law or regulation, pertain to a class of products (as in the case of some risk classifications for devices). The draft Bulletin, at page 10, 2nd paragraph, expressly states that it *does* cover "risk assessments performed with respect to classes of products." To make clear that this broader interpretation is not correct, and to avoid costly disruptions to FDA activities relating to classes of products and to avoid dissimilar treatment for agency adjudications that pertain to a class of products, the Bulletin should explicitly exclude agency adjudications or permit proceedings even where a class of products is involved. This approach is sensible, where similar products raise the same issue of risk and where that issue related to an agency adjudication or permit proceeding.

b. CDC

Risk assessment activities as defined by the NAS definition constitute a moderate portion of CDC's overall activities and are largely conducted by NIOSH and NCEH/ATSDR. Under the definition of risk assessment proposed in the OMB Bulletin, much of the scientific work conducted by CDC could be subject to this Bulletin. This broader definition of risk assessment would now include epidemiologic or correlational studies, hazard reviews, site-specific studies, risk assessments reported in journal articles, and summaries of the scientific literature. The purpose of most of CDC's scientific work is to describe patterns of disease, illness, and health behaviors. Although the intent and methodologies are not congruent with the NAS definition of risk assessments such products could be interpreted to be covered by the Bulletin. This expansion of the NAS definition of risk assessment to include component parts of a risk assessment substantially broadens the scope of CDC work products covered by the provisions of this draft Bulletin.

Under the NAS definition, few CDC documents focus exclusively on risk assessment. In many cases, CDC risk assessors collect the relevant exposure and hazard data, conduct the appropriate quantitative exposure-response and uncertainty analyses and provide the risk assessment as one component of a broader health or safety document. Much of the core work of NIOSH and NCEH/ATSDR involves exposure and hazard assessments in large epidemiologic and toxicologic studies and smaller health hazard evaluations. The purpose of most of this work is to assemble and synthesize scientific information to determine whether a potential to human health hazard exists. In addition, CDC formal, quantitative risk assessments are sometimes conducted in response to requests from other agencies, such as OSHA, MSHA or EPA. The risk assessment product, in that case, may be a published journal article, technical report, testimony or comments to the requesting agency.

The draft Bulletin defines risk assessment as "a scientific and/or technical document that assembles and synthesizes scientific information to determine whether a potential hazard exists and/or the extent of possible risk to human health, safety or the environment." The preamble specifies that "for the purposes of this Bulletin, this definition applies to documents that could be used for risk assessment purposes, such as exposure or hazard assessment that might not constitute a complete risk assessment as defined by the National Research Council." CDC publishes Alerts, Hazard Reviews, Fact sheets, Information Circulars, Workplace Solutions, and other informational documents, many of which contain hazard identification, exposure assessment and occasionally quantitative risk assessment. These documents are not currently considered to be risk assessments, using the NAS definition, unless they contain full quantitative risk assessments. For example, NIOSH Criteria Documents frequently contain risk assessment information used to develop Recommended Exposure Limits (RELs) or other recommended standard provisions to protect worker health and safety. Although CDC has not considered all Criteria Documents to be risk assessments as defined by NAS, many do contain quantitative risk assessments. Current Intelligence Bulletins (CIBs), on the other hand, are more variable. Some CIBs contain quantitative risk assessments, but many offer only hazard assessment or exposure assessment information. Therefore, calling all CIBs and Criteria Documents risk assessments would be a new requirement for CDC.

Other examples of the CDC activities that would now be covered under the Bulletin's proposed definition are the epidemiologic investigations that involve the analysis of available scientific information to determine the extent of risk to human health:

1) Investigation into anthrax deaths and illnesses resulting from intentionally contaminated mail. Waiting for literature reviews of all available papers and peer reviewed studies and development of the range of all scientific opinions and the

likelihood of all plausible alternative assumption would have delayed recommendations for addressing the threat.

2) Investigation into recent outbreak of mumps illness and the development of new policies on vaccination of healthcare workers. In this outbreak, emergency input from the Advisory Committee on Immunization Practices (ACIP) and the Healthcare Infection Control Practice Advisory Committee (HICPAC) were obtained to assist in the development of new policy based on preliminary epidemiologic information obtained during the investigation of cases of disease. The changes in policy were then quickly published in the MMWR as real time recommendations to control an ongoing outbreak.

3) Investigation of the agent, risk factors and epidemiology of SARS. This was a previously unrecognized disease so there was no literature specific for this agent. However, as with Anthrax investigations, to wait for the development of all scientific opinions and to address the range of all scientific opinions and plausible explanations would have delayed publications of interim analyses and the establishment of control measures.

Another example of work products that comprise a significant portion of CDC scientific activities are "syntheses of scientific evidence" that might now be included under the OMB definition of risk assessment, but not under the NAS definition. Surgeon General Reports (SGR) are an example of such activities where the purpose is to provide clear and definitive conclusions about the strength of science on the relationships between exposure to potential hazards such as tobacco smoke and health effects. SGRs have not been characterized as risk assessments. An SGR on tobacco use is cited in the Bulletin as a type of risk assessment that would be included under the OMB definition and the Bulletin characterizes the widely adopted model of evidence review as "an actuarial analysis of real-world human data" which does not reflect the methodology used for SGRs. The evidence review methods were established for the 1964 report, and refined over the past twenty-nine reports. The evidence review methodology used by the SGRs has been widely cited as the gold standard for considerations of potential causality based primarily upon epidemiological data. This approach does not use a probabilistic risk assessment, but applies the well-defined rules of causality first listed in the 1964 report and more fully re-defined in the 2004 SGR, Chapter 1. Expert judgment regarding the consistency, strength, specificity, coherence, biological plausibility, and dose-response gradient of the evidence are obtained in a structured and systematic peer-review and senior scientific review process. As stated in many past SGRs and as explicitly stated in Chapter 1 of the 2004 report, the SGR evidence review process separates the evidence review and determinations of causality from implications or policy recommendations. Chapter 1 of the 2004 report reviewed this methodology and the criteria for causality conclusions.

c. NIH

If the definition of risk assessment described in the OMB Bulletin were implemented as written and applied, the following reports and other products developed by the NIH could be considered risk assessments:

NTP Report on Carcinogens. The Report on Carcinogens (RoC) is an informational scientific and public health document first ordered by Congress in 1978 that identifies and discusses agents, substances, mixtures, or exposure circumstances that may pose a hazard to human health by virtue of their carcinogenicity. The RoC is published biennially and has a formal process for preparation that includes scientific peer review and multiple opportunities for public comment. This document is intended for hazard identification only (as clearly noted in its Introduction). However, under OMB's proposed definition of risk assessment, the Bulletin specifically identifies this report as an "influential risk assessment" because it addresses "some but not all aspects of risk assessment" (page 9).

Guidance to Medical Professionals. NIH routinely develops and disseminates guidance documents intended to aid medical professionals in providing health care in the United States. These guidance documents address critical issues associated with patient care and professional safety such as the proper methods for handling potentially hazardous biological material (e.g. human blood) and methods for reducing nosocomial infections. NIH staff generally prepares these documents after consultation with a broad array of medical professionals. The documents possibly fall under the Bulletin's definition of risk assessment due to their implication of a hazard or risk if the guidance, which they provide, is not followed.

- Guidance to the Research Community. In a similar manner, the NIH also develops and disseminates guidance documents for laboratory researchers regarding the safe conduct of basic and clinical research. These guidance documents usually apply to emerging therapies (e.g. gene-based therapies), new technologies (e.g. use of recombinant DNA products) or the management of clinical trials. As with guidance to medical professionals, NIH staff generally prepares these documents after broad consultation. They may be subject to the Bulletin under its current definition of risk assessment because their guidance could imply/identify a hazard or risk.

- Discovery Research with Direct Potential Impact on Risk Assessments. The Intramural Research Programs of the various NIH Institutes all conduct discovery research that may, on a case-by-case basis, have direct bearing on a risk assessment being considered by another federal agency. Of special note in this category would be clinical trials, epidemiology studies and toxicology studies that are large and generally carry considerable weight in agency's risk assessments. Even though these studies are intended for peer-reviewed journal articles or the NTP Technical Report series, the Bulletin's new definition of risk assessments could include studies of this type.

Health Information Documents. These are documents, generally prepared by NIH staff after outside consultation, and are intended as guidance to the general public on health related information. Most likely to fall under the broad definition of risk assessment in the Bulletin would be health alerts (e.g. on the safety of commonly used herbal supplements or on the safety of long-term estrogen) or information on personal choices to lead a healthier lifestyle (e.g. modifying diet to control diabetes). Because these imply potential hazards or risks, they are included in the definition in the Bulletin.

III. Questions about type of risk assessment (tiered structure)

6. QUESTION: In your agency, is there currently a clear demarcation between risk assessments used for regulatory analysis and those not used for regulatory analysis? Is this clear at the outset of the risk assessment?

a. FDA

FDA understands the term "regulatory analysis" as OMB does—i.e., as meaning an assessment of the potential costs and benefits of a regulatory action pursuant to E.O. 12866 and OMB Circular A-4. For risk assessments as FDA currently uses the term (i.e., those that result in a formal development of a risk estimate), there is no clear demarcation between risk assessments done to support economic analyses and those done for other Agency purposes. In general, any economic analysis is done after the risk assessment is completed, and does not influence the risk assessment, except to the extent there are specific variables that economists need to include to perform a sound economic analysis.

b. CDC

Formal risk assessments conducted by NIOSH and NCEH/ATSDR are not specifically developed to support regulatory analysis (cost-benefit or cost effectiveness analyses), nor is any distinction made in conducting risk assessments that may end up as part of another agency's regulatory analysis. There are units within the agency with delegated regulatory authority such as the Division of Global Migration and Quarantine (DGMQ), which has regulatory authority around migrating populations (immigrants, refugees, travelers, cargo and animals). Specifically, DGMQ has regulatory authority (through delegation from the Secretary of HHS) to prevent the introduction, transmission, and spread of communicable diseases in the US, under 42 C.F.R. Part 70. Because of this DGMQ regularly assesses findings for regulatory analysis and needs to conduct risk assessments to determine the best way to meet legal and regulatory responsibilities. Sometimes DGMQ needs to quickly execute an action, sometimes within minutes (i.e., a quarantine order, if a plane load of passengers is sitting at an airport with an ill passenger on board), and there would not be time to comply with the proposed Bulletin. Even embargos usually need to be enacted rather quickly; within hours to days. Findings and assessments performed by DGMQ can lead to regulatory changes, in essence making DGMQ part of the regulatory decision-making process.

c. NIH

The NIH does not currently conduct risk assessments as the term is defined in the 1983 NAS report. In addition, the NIH is not a regulatory agency. Although some of the NIH scientific products previously discussed might be used by regulatory agencies for regulatory analysis, the NIH has no control over their use, and it is not evident at the outset of any of NIH research whether a product will be used for regulatory analysis.

7. QUESTION: In your agency, is there currently a clear demarcation between "influential risk assessment" used for regulatory purposes and other risk assessments used for regulatory purposes? Is this clear at the outset of the risk assessment?

a. FDA

It is not always clear at the outset of a risk assessment that it will be influential. At the outset, FDA conducts and reviews risk assessments depending on the nature of the risk assessment, FDA's estimate of its significance (influential or "highly influential" as those terms are defined by OMB), and on the risk management decisions the risk assessment will support.

The distinction between "influential risk assessment" and other risk assessments derives from the Information Quality Act and OMB and OMB and agency guidelines pursuant to it. FDA's guidelines are posted as part of the HHS Information Quality website at http://aspe.hhs.gov/infoquality/Guidelines/fda.shtml#viic. Under FDA's guidelines, scientific information is considered "influential" if it is:

> disseminated information that results from or is used in support of agency actions that are expected to have an annual effect on the economy of $100 million or more or will adversely affect in a material way the economy, a sector of the economy, productivity, competition, jobs, the environment, public health or safety, or State, local or tribal governments or communities.

As FDA's Guidelines note, "the definition applies to 'information' itself, not to decisions that the information may support."

b. CDC

NIOSH quantitative risk assessments are sometimes used by OSHA and MSHA to support rulemaking. NIOSH makes no methodological or scientific distinctions between "influential risk assessments" and other risk assessments. NIOSH risk assessments are grounded in the best available science and rely on the most robust methods available. NIOSH uses the same approach whether or not they are used for, or are intended to inform, regulatory action. All NIOSH risk assessments are conducted with the goal of evaluating the potential hazards or risks in order to protect workers' health and safety.

IV. Questions about impact of the Bulletin on agency risk assessment practices

8. QUESTION: If applicable, please specify provisions in the Bulletin that can be expected to have a <u>substantial positive effect</u> on the quality, conduct, and use of risk assessments undertaken by your agency.

> **a. FDA**
> FDA has been a leader in conducting risk assessments that meet high standards for accuracy, transparency, and stakeholder involvement. Thus, the draft Bulletin will reinforce FDA's commitment to high quality risk assessments.

> **b. CDC**
> The Bulletin provides many standards which most agencies already adhere to as good practice, at least where it specifies criteria to be applied to quantitative risk assessments. CDC's formal, quantitative risk assessments reflect a philosophy and commitment to the same tenets described in the draft Bulletin, but these measures already represent CDC current practices. Specifically, CDC occupational risk assessments clearly state the informational needs driving the risk assessment and the objectives of the assessment. They also summarize the scope of the risk assessment, delineating the population of concern and, when appropriate and necessary for the purpose of the risk assessment, they consider confounding factors. CDC typically reports multiple risk estimates, including central estimates and appropriate upper or lower bounds. Great effort is made to produce objective, scientifically defensible, accurate, reproducible and transparent risk assessments.

Since CDC formal, quantitative risk assessments are frequently used by other agencies (OSHA and MSHA) to support regulatory actions, the risk assessments must not only meet the standards of scientific peer review, but also must be defensible in rulemaking hearings. Transparency and reproducibility helps ensure that other scientists can determine the objectivity, scientific soundness and accuracy of CDC risk assessments and enhance the credibility of CDC formal, quantitative risk assessments. CDC also strives to clearly explain the basis for all critical assumptions in its quantitative risk assessments, in particular when alternative assumptions might be used. When appropriate, comparisons are made to other published risk assessments in the scientific literature, characterizing uncertainty and variability, and explain how choices of studies or effects influence the formal, quantitative risk assessment

9. QUESTION: If applicable, please specify provisions in the Bulletin that can be expected to have a <u>substantial negative effect</u> on the quality, conduct, and use of risk assessments undertaken by your agency.

As drafted, the Bulletin's definition of risk assessment could be interpreted to cover a wide range of health information disseminated by HHS. Most importantly, this may result in delays in the release of critical scientific data such as public alerts about serious risks to public health and patient safety. Further, the Bulletin's proposed scope and requirements will involve substantial time, effort, and costs.

Given the Bulletin's proposed definition of risk assessment, specific examples where provisions of the Bulletin may have substantial negative effects across HHS include:

* Because most documents are presumed to be available to the public under the Freedom of Information Act (FOIA) (unless an exemption applies), making the Bulletin applicable to risk assessments that are available to the public (discussed on page 9, last paragraph, and also in Section II.1 on page 23) may result in agency resources being spent on satisfying the Bulletin even for analyses that are preliminary or are either not relied on or rejected by the agency.

* The Bulletin (on pages 13-14) appears to conflict with previous OMB Bulletins as to whether risk assessments *must* meet the provisions of the Safe Drinking Water Act (SDWA) or whether agencies can *adapt* SDWA provisions as appropriate and as OMB currently allows under the Information Quality Guidelines.

  Detailed requirements concerning statements about assumptions and placing risks in context and perspective with other risks would create additional requirements on risk assessors and may require judgment outside of their area of expertise.

  The requirement (at Section V.2 (pages 17 and 25)) directing agencies to find and examine previously conducted risk assessments "from qualified scientific organizations" and to "compare these risk assessments to the agency's risk assessment" will impose additional requirements to evaluate the scientific rigor and aims of the comparison studies and the expertise and objectivity of their contributors.

* The requirement at pages 20 and 25 that influential risk assessments identify the nature, difficulty, feasibility, cost, and time associated with undertaking research to close data gaps and remedy limitations goes well beyond the likely expertise of the risk assessors themselves will require additional resources and will not improve the quality of the risk assessment itself.

a. FDA

If a broad definition of risk assessment is used, application of the Bulletin may result in substantial increases in the time and resources needed to do scientific analyses that are not currently considered to be risk assessments. Considering the limited resources currently available, this would decrease resources for groups performing non-risk assessment scientific reviews and create a disincentive for conducting thorough scientific analyses of a non-risk assessment nature. Since many scientific reviews we conduct are not developing formal risk estimates, the reviews cannot specify:

> Multiple estimates of risk;
> Appropriate upper-bound or lower-bound estimates of risk;
> * Each significant uncertainty in the risk assessment process and studies that would assist in resolving the uncertainty; and
> Peer-reviewed studies which support or fail to support the risk estimates.

The issue of scope is also of concern if, as some have suggested to the NAS, the Bulletin expands to include the activities or "individual agency adjudications or permit proceedings." For example, FDA conducts approximately 100 food contact substance notification reviews annually. If these reviews fell within the definition of "risk assessment" and had to comply with the standards of the Bulletin, it would be very difficult for us to meet statutory timelines for response.

More specific examples where the Bulletin may have substantial negative effect include:

- The definition of "risk assessment" (Section I.3), when read in conjunction with Section II.1 ("Applicability"), could transform documents into "risk assessments" under the Bulletin when neither the agency nor the document's authors intended the document to be a true risk assessment.

- The section on updating risk assessments (Section VI on pages 21 and 25) may impose an additional burden on agencies where risk assessments are used to support regulations. Outside parties may attempt to use the update provision as a mechanism to challenge existing rules – not the underlying risk assessment. However, regulations that impose a significant economic impact on a substantial number of small entities are already subject to periodic review under the Regulatory Flexibility Act, and FDA believes that mechanism, which provides for a more comprehensive review at ten year intervals, is more appropriate and better satisfies the need for periodic review.

b. CDC

The largest and most direct negative impact of the draft Bulletin is the proposed broad definition of risk assessment. By utilizing a definition of risk assessment that includes not only quantitative risk assessment, but also all the individual studies that may eventually lead to a risk assessment (e.g., exposure assessment, epidemiology studies, toxicology studies, hazard identification and evaluation), the Bulletin creates confusion in the scientific community by holding a broad array of supporting science to the same standards and requirements as a full quantitative risk assessment. Such standards cannot be applied practically to studies that identify hazards or provide the groundwork for more formal quantitative risk assessment. The Bulletin's definition of risk assessment dilutes the effectiveness of such standards and could severely limit the number supporting studies available for quantitative risk assessment by directing them to conduct repetitive and unnecessary analyses. These additional activities would slow the pace of research and require extra resources. Unlike formal, quantitative risk assessments, public health assessments and health consultations incorporate subjective evaluation and best professional judgment. Many of the requirements outlined in the OMB Bulletin are not applicable to this qualitative decision making process.

Particular examples where this provision may not be appropriate include occupational and environmental health hazard evaluations, public health emergency outbreak investigations (e.g. Epi Aids) and epidemiologic studies. Health hazard evaluations are a public health practice activity designed to solve problems at worksites and prevent occupational disease among workers at that site. Specifically, they are investigations to learn whether workers are experiencing work-related health effects or exposed to hazardous materials or harmful conditions. CDC scientists conducting health hazard evaluations conduct exposure and health assessments, often making judgments based on professional expertise and expert knowledge of industry practices. Occupational health hazard evaluations are designed to be rapid evaluations providing employers, employees, and employee representative's relevant information related to the prevention of occupational exposures and work-related health effects. Applying the standards in this draft Bulletin would be unworkable for health hazard evaluations because of the need to provide results and recommendations in a timely manner.

Another core function of CDC that does not meet the NAS definition, but would be subject and likely impacted by the standards of this draft Bulletin is industry-wide exposure assessment and epidemiologic studies. CDC scientists conduct industry-wide field studies to determine the incidence and prevalence of acute and chronic disease in a working population or their offspring and to determine the nature and extent of exposure to potentially hazardous agents in the work environment. The epidemiologic studies conducted by CDC do not establish definitive risk levels, but provide supporting evidence for the presence or lack of an association between exposure and adverse outcome. The broad application of this draft Bulletin to such epidemiological industry-wide field studies would be problematic because collecting data for formal risk characterizations in these would studies would be impractical and resource prohibitive.

CDC already operates by many of the "standards" as best practices for formal, risk assessments and best practices appropriate to other scientific activities, thereby making it difficult to assess the impact of other provisions of the Bulletin particularly for formal, quantitative risk assessments. However, characterization of every possible uncertainty and extensive evaluation of each assumption and derived parameter on the final risk estimate could result in a confusing, less straight-forward document that is entirely consistent with the language in this draft Bulletin, but would not serve the public or the risk assessment community well.

The Bulletin seems to equate all types of epidemiologic studies with risk assessments regardless of whether numerical estimates or a quantitative model is included in the epidemiological evaluation. The broad application of the Bulletin to epidemiologic studies would be problematic and impractical. Epidemiologic studies do not establish risk levels. For example, from page 6, in "Actuarial analysis of real-world human data" the relevance of etiologic epidemiologic methods is mischaracterized as "such assessments by combining actuarial analyses with biologic theory and medical expertise." The activities of defining cohorts, conducting exposure assessment, ascertaining outcomes and properly analyzing the association of exposure and outcome while controlling for confounding and evaluating effect modification in epidemiologic studies provide supporting evidence for the presence of or lack of an association between exposure and illness.

This issue is especially of concern for emerging hazards, where a complete package of toxicologic and epidemiologic data may not yet exist. The draft Bulletin notes that "risk assessments of infectious agents pose special challenges since the rate of diffusion of an infectious agent may play a critical role in determining the occurrence and severity of an epidemic" and that "Scientific understanding of both biology and human behavior are critical to performing accurate risk assessments for infectious agents." However, in addition to the fact that the source of an infectious agent is not static and instead increases and spreads as time lapses (especially for diseases with very short incubation periods (hours to days), there are several other important factors that the Bulletin does not take into consideration:

1) Federal investigations into risks of infectious diseases often involve those diseases with high or undefined morbidity and/or mortality.

2) The risk of developing signs and symptoms of disease can occur after even one exposure to undetectable 'levels" of the infectious agent.

3) The need to stop exposures from occurring, and thus limit illness and death, requires rapid analyses of the source of the infectious agents and the risk factors for exposure and development of disease and rapid responding public health action taken on a basis of incomplete and evolving data.

4) The public expects and demands that provisional recommendations on means to stop or mitigate the spread of infectious disease be made available as quickly as possible. The goal of scientific completeness must be balanced with the cost of inaction.

5) Recommendations may evolve over time as more information is obtained, but control efforts cannot wait for completion and certification of each step required by this Bulletin.

6) Infectious disease risk assessments typically are published later as scientific articles in peer reviewed journals and/or are presented at scientific forum. It is in

these venues that scientists present background data from literature reviews, their methodology, the range of their results and discuss in detail any uncertainties and comparisons with the results of others.

7) Surveillance for infectious diseases and the publication of surveillance data, while used to understand "risk," are conducted/collected using established case definitions, which serve to enhance objectivity. Interrupting this process for certification would jeopardize timely data collection, and potentially undermine a critical public health activity.

8) Immediate data collection on adverse events must occur during an "event."

An important part of the health assessment process is our ability to communicate the findings of our activities to the public. We have learned that the public is often confused by the complexities of health science and wants clear, understandable and accurate answers. The Bulletin directs all risk assessments to include an evaluation of alternative models, provide a range of risk estimates using different exposure assumptions, discuss sources of uncertainty, conduct a sensitivity analysis, etc. The inclusion of such information would make it more difficult to develop a clear, user-friendly, unambiguous message for the public.

The Bulletin fails to allow for additional emerging statistical methodologies beyond the expert panel method. Additionally, the requirement to address only clearly adverse human health effects may have unintended public health consequences because of the increasing importance of biomarkers.

It is unclear whether this draft Bulletin is intended to apply to journal articles. If so, the requirements would be impractical. It would be helpful if the final Bulletin include a specific exclusion for journal articles similar to the language in the Peer Review Bulletin.

c. NIH

Given the Bulletin's proposed definition of risk assessment, some activities carried out by the NIH will be significantly impacted. Risk assessments should be considered special documents since their entire focus pertains to the overall integration of materials into a common document that predicts uncertain risks. In some cases, it is possible to provide sufficient information to judge the uncertainty of the eventual predictions, in others it is not. This is not an issue for each single piece of evidence entering a risk assessment and these individual parts should not be subject to guidelines solely intended for risk assessment documents. Of special concern to the NIH are guidelines developed by Institutes within the NIH to inform the public and studies conducted by NIH researchers to identify factors affecting human health that play a pivotal role in risk assessments (such as epidemiology and toxicology studies). In the opinion of the NIH, these do not, on their own, constitute risk assessments and should be explicitly excluded from the Bulletin.

If these types of activities are considered risk assessments and subject to the requirements of the Bulletin, it will have serious ramifications on the ability of the NIH to provide the basic scientific evidence needed by other agencies to develop scientifically sound risk assessments. More importantly, if the research and scientific activities supported by the NIH are required to undergo the full process suggested by the Bulletin for risk assessments – even though they are not risk assessments – the NIH would face serious challenges in providing the public with timely scientific research to inform public health decisions.

10. **QUESTION: If your agency followed the procedures described in the Bulletin, would it affect the time course for production of the risk assessment (that is, the time required from initiation of the risk assessment to delivery to the regulatory decision maker)? If so, please explain why?**

   a. FDA

It is difficult to answer this question given the uncertainty surrounding the draft's current definition of "risk assessment." Following the Bulletin's procedures will likely not affect the time required for many complex probabilistic risk assessments because, for those assessments, we currently follow practices that are consistent with the Bulletin. However, the Bulletin could affect the time course for production of other types of scientific review that, although we do not consider them to be "risk assessments," might nonetheless be considered as falling under the proposed Bulletin.

Additionally, particularly for agencies that sometimes deal in controversial issues, the draft Bulletin may result in challenges as to whether an agency interpreted the Bulletin correctly. For example, for influential risk assessments, the draft Bulletin would compel an agency to respond to "significant" comments and would presume that "scientific" comments are "significant" (see Section V.9). It also expects agencies to prepare a "response-to-comment" document that "should provide an explicit rationale for why the agency has not adopted the position suggested by the commenter" and "why the agency position is preferable." Section V.9 may adversely affect risk assessment practices at FDA by diverting resources to respond to "significant" comments or to resolving disputes as to whether a comment was "scientific" or "significant." There may be instances where parties (particularly competitors) may disagree over the "science" to be applied, whether a comment is "significant," or even whether conventional scientific concepts are applicable or recognizable. In the latter case, individuals or firms advocating the use of "unconventional" or "alternative" therapies may have their products fall within the broad, statutory definitions of "drug" or "device" in the Federal Food, Drug, and Cosmetic Act and would argue that individuals trained in "conventional" science or medicine are either biased or not qualified to evaluate the merits of their products. In such situations, the "science" to be used or considered could become an issue under the Bulletin. One way to avoid such disputes would be to respond to _all_ comments, but this would place even more demands on limited agency resources for little or no apparent benefit.

As another example, the draft Bulletin, at Section VIII (pages 22 and 26), "Deferral and Waiver," allows an agency head to waive or defer "some or all of the requirements...where warranted by compelling rationale." If an agency defers meeting a requirement, the draft Bulletin states that the agency shall comply with the risk assessment requirements "as soon as practicable." However, the Bulletin provides little or no insight as to how an agency would justify a deferral or waiver, and it is unclear who decides whether an agency's rationale is "compelling" or whether agencies may be challenged on this issue.

b. CDC

If the Bulletin were to apply to only formal, quantitative risk assessments as defined by NAS and the goals and "standards" in the draft Bulletin are treated as "best practices," implementation would not substantially slow the pace of producing risk assessments. However, if a more prescriptive implementation was followed and separate peer reviews required for the risk assessment outside the context of the document it was intended for, the result could be a substantial slowing in the risk assessment process.

One recurring message from the public and other agencies is the importance of releasing information a timely manner. This is especially important for public health assessments and health consultations. If the public's health is at risk, messages must be disseminated as quickly as possible, so that appropriate corrective actions can be implemented. Current CDC scientific activities that would now be considered risk assessment under the proposed OMB definition would be subject to the extensive set of requirements for formal, quantitative risk assessments and pose challenges to the timeliness of information release. It would take considerable time and effort for health assessors to address all of the requirements of this Bulletin and thereby compliance could significantly delay the release of our documents, with potential adverse consequences for public health.

Additionally, the Bulletin implies that in certain circumstances, agencies shall await further research to attain "scientific completeness" before conducting a risk assessment. The goal of scientific completeness must be balanced with the cost of inaction. There must be the ability to conduct the best risk assessment with the "best" available data and inclusion of uncertainty caveats to address urgent public health needs.

For those supporting studies not previously considered risk assessment, there could be a substantial slowing of delivery and use when formal, quantitative risk assessments are conducted having a substantial impact on the quantitative risk assessor and then to the decision maker because of new and time-consuming requirements.

If public health assessments and health consultations were included in the scope of the Bulletin, application of all aspects of the Bulletin under site specific activities would be challenging and resource intensive and potentially, have a deleterious impact on public health because they are often performed under circumstances requiring rapid communication of results to affected parties.

Implementation of the proposed Bulletin also could result in substantial delay in SGR releases. In the history of the twenty-nine SGRs on Smoking and Health for example, the typical time required to complete the reports has varied from less than a year to over 5 years. Rapid expansion of scientific peer-reviewed literature in recent years has added to the technical and scientific challenge in completing the SGRs in a timely fashion. The time from completion of the review volume to publication of the final SGR now takes from 12-18 months. If SGRs were subject to the requirements described in the Bulletin, then the current challenge for timely dissemination would be exacerbated. The language in the Bulletin implies that the review process of such work products should be subject to public comment from all parties. Adding the requirement for public participation and comment to this process likely would add a large volume of comments, which would affect the timeliness of the reports without adding improvements in the scientific quality to the report.

c. NIH

The NIH does not currently conduct or use risk assessments according to the definition set forth in the 1983 NAS report. However, the NIH is concerned that, if strictly applied in its current form, the Bulletin may have a negative impact on the conduct of NIH research programs. The products outlined previously (in Answer 5c) that might be subject to the procedures of the Bulletin have historically been developed as independent, science-driven, public health documents or as research activities. If these activities are required to undergo the full process outlined in the Bulletin for risk assessments, the NIH will face serious challenges in providing the public with timely scientific research to inform public health decisions. The provisions in the Bulletin are likely to blur the distinction between the independent scientific review and research funded by the NIH and the use of that information in making public health policy decisions.

11. **QUESTION: One of the Bulletins's reporting standards states the need to be scientifically objective by "giving weight to both positive and negative studies in light of each study's technical quality." Please give an example of how this would be implemented by your agency or department.**

HHS scientific products are currently based upon a complete and thorough review of the science giving weight to both positive and negative studies.

a. FDA

FDA already considers both positive and negative studies, as well as their quality, when it reviews the full range of scientific research. Before beginning a risk assessment, it is appropriate to establish criteria for including or excluding studies from the assessment. If needed, weighting factors based on the quality of the study data can also be established or determined before the risk assessment is conducted.

Consequently, FDA does not believe the draft Bulletin's reporting standards on scientific objectivity will necessitate any significant changes to existing FDA practices.

b. CDC

CDC typically evaluates all relevant studies of acceptable quality in its quantitative risk assessment. Negative studies are evaluated along with positive studies in forming a risk assessment strategy. Specifically, negative studies are assessed in light of the quantitative risk assessment to determine if they are consistent and to suggest any inconsistencies in the database that might warrant explanation. The SGRs have always considered all available peer-reviewed literature, considering all positive and negative studies. This consideration of the consistency of the data always has been central to the SGR evidence review process. Another example is when a positive rat cancer bioassay is compared with one or two negative epidemiology studies. When quantitative information on dose is available, it is possible to compare the animal and human studies and determine if the epidemiology studies had sufficient power to detect the observed dose response. If they do, and the results are incompatible, it might suggest looking closer at mechanistic information or species susceptibility. If the epidemiology studies did not have sufficient power or the statistical analyses suggests no inconsistency, greater confidence can be derived in using the animal data to predict human response, even in light of the nominally "opposite" human results.

However, if the Bulletin is interpreted to mean that an agency should give some sort of quantitative weight to each study based on an evaluation of the technical quality of the study, this is not currently done at CDC, nor is it clear how this could be objectively implemented. Weighting based on perceived technical quality would require substantial professional judgment and carrying that quantification into some sort of adjustment of the final risk numbers is not technically feasible at this time.

12. QUESTION: Does your agency use risk assessments conducted by external groups? Would it be helpful to you if risk assessments submitted to your agency by external groups, such as consultants and private industry, met the requirements proposed in the OMB Bulletin?

a. FDA

FDA, on occasion, does rely on risk assessments conducted by external groups, including contractors. We also may receive documents or submissions during notice-and-comment rulemaking or in adversarial proceedings that could be considered "risk assessments" as defined by the draft Bulletin. As the FDA does with any scientific information, we would evaluate any such risk assessments to determine whether they may appropriately be considered in our decisionmaking pursuant to the Information Quality Act and other legal authorities.

b. CDC

Although CDC does not typically contract its quantitative risk assessments, it does evaluate others' risk assessments of the same hazard and compare them to CDC assessments. If the draft Bulletin were to be applied to government agency risk assessments, it would be helpful if quantitative risk assessments conducted by external groups also met the same requirements when those assessments are used by a government agency.

ADDITIONAL NAS QUESTION FOR FDA

12. QUESTION: Dr. Galson indicated at the public meeting that there were problems with the application of OMB requirements to certain types of assessments. Can FDA suggest specific language to exclude those problematic assessments from OMB requirements, rather than just offering examples of those assessments? In other words, how would FDA describe in general terms the types of assessments it would like to see excluded?

Risk assessment is a tool for addressing public health problems and should be scaled to fit the public health problem at hand. The risk assessments according to the proposed Bulletin definition and requirements may not always be appropriate depending on the magnitude of the problem, time constraints, resources, affected population characteristics or available data. Rather than describing in general terms the types of assessments we would like to see excluded, we suggest three significant revisions to the text of the draft bulletin to clarify and better define what should be included.

First, we propose that the Bulletin's definition of "risk assessment" be revised so that it is consistent with the definition of that term in domestic and international risk assessment communities. OMB's draft definition is broad because it defines "risk assessment" as "a scientific and/or technical document that assembles and synthesizes scientific information to determine whether a potential hazard exists and/or the extent of possible risk to human health, safety or the environment" (page 8). We suggest that "risk assessment" should refer to a "scientific and/or technical document that assembles and synthesizes scientific information *and arrives at a qualitative or quantitative estimation of the extent to which* a potential hazard exists and/or the extent of possible risk to human health, safety, or the environment." A risk assessment does not, itself, determine the presence of a hazard (as the Bulletin's proposed definition implies). Furthermore, not all syntheses of scientific information are risk assessments. This change would be effective in removing from the purview of the Bulletin several of the types of activities that we do not feel are appropriately brought under the bulletin.

Second, we recommend that the Bulletin define or interpret "scientific information" as it relates to the definition of "risk assessment." The definition of "scientific information" should be relatively narrow and encompass "factual inputs, data, and models." While ordinarily there may be a common understanding of the meaning of "scientific information," our recommendation results from the existence of a broad definition of the term in the OMB Peer Review Bulletin (70 FR 2664 (January 14, 2005)). There, "scientific information" is defined as "factual inputs, data, models, analyses, technical information, or scientific assessments based on the behavioral and social sciences, public health and medical sciences, life and earth sciences, engineering, or physical sciences" and includes _any_ communication or representation of "knowledge, such as facts or data...." Clarifying the definition of "scientific information" in this particular context would help avoid the application of the OMB risk assessment bulletin to FDA documents and other federal documents that are not appropriately considered "risk assessments" either by their authors or by the scientific community.

Third, we recommend that OMB revise the Bulletin to be more consistent with the OMB Peer Review Bulletin in terms of scope and exemptions. The Peer Review Bulletin, for example, applied to "influential scientific information" and imposed additional requirements to "highly influential scientific assessments," and the requirements applied to information that an agency disseminated to the public. In contrast, the draft risk assessment bulletin would apply to _all_ risk assessments regardless of whether they are disseminated[2] or influential. In terms of exemptions, the Peer Review Bulletin contained an express exemption for "[a] health or safety dissemination where the agency determines that the dissemination is time-sensitive...." The Draft Risk Assessment Bulletin, however, omits a "time-sensitive" health or safety exception and provides only a weak agency deferral and waiver authority that requires the agency to comply with Bulletin requirements as soon as practicable. The Draft Risk Assessment Bulletin also omits exceptions for regulatory impact analyses, and negotiations involving international trade or treaties where compliance with the Bulletin "would interfere with the need for secrecy or promptness;" such express exemptions existed in the Peer Review Bulletin. As with the suggestions noted above, this clarification would help protect against unintended application of the Bulletin to less relevant activities.

---

[2] The reason why the draft risk assessment bulletin reaches more documents is because Section II.1 uses the phrase "all agency risk assessments *available to the public*..." (emphasis added) and because the bulletin explains that "available to the public" includes documents that are made available to the public or required to be disclosed under the Freedom of Information Act (FOIA). Note, however, that the OMB Peer Review Bulletin and the Information Quality Act use a different construct; the information must be "disseminated" to the public. It would be easier for agencies, OMB, and interested parties to use the same construct as the OMB Peer Review Bulletin and the Information Quality Act so that peer review and risk assessment standards apply to information "disseminated" to the public. A single interpretation would be easier to implement, easier to understand, and avoid disputes as to whether one or both bulletins applied to an agency document. We also believe that the draft risk assessment bulletin's "available to the public...under the Freedom of Information Act" construct is impractical because, in general, the presumption is that *everything* is available under FOIA *unless* an exemption applies. Consequently, even a preliminary risk assessment that an agency does *not* rely upon and *rejected* by the agency would be subject to the risk assessment bulletin because the preliminary risk assessment could be "available to the public" under FOIA.

DEPARTMENT OF HOUSING AND URBAN DEVELOPMENT RESPONSE

TO THE

BACKGROUND INFORMATION ON NRC REVIEW OF THE OFFICE OF MANAGEMENT AND BUDGET RISK ASSESSMENT BULLETIN

QUESTIONS FOR ALL AGENCIES POTENTIALLY AFFECTED BY THE OMB BULLETIN

July 26, 2006

General questions about current risk assessment practices

- **Current risk assessment practices.**
  - HUD does not conduct probabilistic risk assessments, but rather uses data to focus on the central tendency of the data, or the central estimate, typically means or medians. This is largely due to the fact that the data are not amenable to aggressive statistical data manipulation
  - HUD addresses uncertainty analysis where the data are amenable to the required statistical analysis.
  - HUD currently addresses uncertainty and variability in risk assessments by describing the confidence level of the mean (either arithmetic or geometric).

- **Substantial scientific or technical challenges of risk assessments.**

  - There is substantial variability in housing stock. These variables include: construction methods and materials; age; maintenance, repair, and renovations; climate and meteorological impact; design and operation of plumbing, electrical, heating, ventilation, and air conditioning systems; ownership, occupancy and uses; socio-economic factors; state and local building codes and enforcement;
  - Most existing housing risk-related research not sponsored by HUD or other Federal agencies is limited in scope and is not amenable to application to national impacts.
  - Congressional authority and appropriations may limit the scope of research to support the risk assessment.
  - Privacy concerns and the general information collection requirements associated with gathering the necessary data are often restrictive and/or cumbersome.
  - Because HUD does not conduct many risk assessments, it cannot support full time equivalent staff for the analyses. Therefore it is necessary to seek outside support to complete the requisite research and analysis for the risk assessment, and there are a limited number of qualified contractors who are available.

- **HUD's current definition of risk assessment, and associated products.**

HUD Response to National Research Council Questions
Review of the OMB Risk Assessment Bulletin

- ○ HUD relies on OMB Circular A-4 for its risk assessments.
- ○ HUD also addresses Congressional and Executive requirements, such as:
  - the Small Business Regulatory Enforcement Fairness Act (SBREFA);
  - the Regulatory Flexibility Act;
  - Unfunded Mandates Reform Act (UMRA);
  - Executive Order 13132, entitled Federalism (64 FR 43255, August 10, 1999);
  - Executive Order 13175, entitled Consultation and Coordination with Indian Tribal Governments (59 FR 22951, November 6, 2000);
  - Executive Order 13045, entitled Protection of Children from Environmental Health Risks and Safety Risks (62 FR 19885, April 23, 1997);
  - National Technology Transfer and Advancement Act of 1995 ("NTTAA"); and
  - Executive Order 12898, entitled Federal Actions to Address Environmental Justice in Minority Populations and Low-Income Populations (59 FR 7629, February 16, 1994).

- **Risk assessments time frames.**

  - ○ The period to complete an original risk assessment is usually two years from the time the need for the assessment is identified until a final work product is available for public comment. In some cases, this can be shortened to about six months where an original risk assessment can be adapted for amendments to existing regulations.

Questions about OMB's definition of risk assessment and applicability

- New risk assessment not previously considered if HUD uses the proposed OMB Bulletin definition.
  - ○ Because inspections and adjudications are explicitly not covered by the proposed bulletin, HUD believes that no additional programs will require risk assessments.
  - ○ HUD supports these exclusions, although additional clarification of the definitions may be helpful.

Questions about type of risk assessment (tiered structure)

- Demarcation between HUD risk assessments used for regulatory analysis and other analyses.
  - ○ Environmental and health issues which may warrant risk assessments for regulatory analysis are limited to a few programs. Analysis for most programs is limited to risks associated with significant economic impact.

HUD Response to National Research Council Questions
Review of the OMB Risk Assessment Bulletin

- **HUD current demarcation between "influential risk assessment" used for regulatory purposes and other risk assessments used for regulatory purposes.**
    - As for the case discussed in the previous answer, environmental and health issues which may warrant risk assessments for regulatory analysis are limited to a few programs. Analysis for most programs is limited to risks associated with significant economic impact.

Questions about impact of the Bulletin on agency risk assessment practices

- **Provisions in the Bulletin that can be expected to have a <u>substantial positive effect</u> on the quality, conduct, and use of risk assessments undertaken by HUD.**
    - HUD anticipates that meeting the additional cost and time requirements when using risk assessments will improve the quality, conduct and use of risk assessments.

- **Provisions in the Bulletin that can be expected to have a <u>substantial negative effect</u> on the quality, conduct, and use of risk assessments undertaken HUD.**
    - HUD believes the cost and time effects will not have substantial negative effects.

- **Effect on the time course for production of the risk assessment (that is, the time required from initiation of the risk assessment to delivery to the regulatory decision maker) if HUD followed the procedures described in the Bulletin.**
    - HUD believes that the time course will have to be extended to ensure the procedures are properly followed.

- **Please give an example of how HUD would implement the Bulletin's requirement for scientific objectivity by "giving weight to both positive and negative studies in light of each study's technical quality."**
    - HUD has always considered positive, negative, and inclusive studies in its regulatory risk analysis.
    - In order to enhance transparency, HUD would ask the author to identify the sources of funding for all research studies. This will aid in evaluating what weight to give to all studies, whether positive or negative.

- **HUD's use of risk assessments conducted by external groups.**
    - HUD welcomes the submission of risk assessments submitted by external groups, and meeting the requirements proposed in the OMB Bulletin will provide added weight to their consideration. HUD will still look for peer review to ensure that the study did not introduce bias due to financial support by a stakeholder with a strong position before the study was initiated, among other considerations.

HUD Response to National Research Council Questions
Review of the OMB Risk Assessment Bulletin

ADDITIONAL ISSUES FOR HUD

- Consideration of baseline conditions when evaluating alternative mitigation options for regulatory analysis may be inappropriate where there is a statutory requirement.
- The definition or guidelines for the determination of what constitutes a significant comment would be useful for consistency.
- Organizational structure, administrative procedures and statutory authority may affect the deferral and waiver process.

U.S. DEPARTMENT OF THE INTERIOR
COORDINATED AGENCY RESPONSE ON OMB'S PROPOSED RISK ASSESSMENT BULLETIN

Prepared by:
Office of Policy Analysis (PPA)

Introduction

The Department of Interior (DOI) has reviewed the Office of Management and Budget's (OMB) Office of Information and Regulatory Affairs (OIRA) proposed risk assessment bulletin, along with the accompanying set of questions developed by the National Research Council (NRC) of the National Academy of Sciences.

The DOI's comments are provided below. The attached comments represents DOI's best effort to compile information from all Interior agencies and is not necessarily comprehensive, given the short time-frame required for a response. Comments on the proposed Bulletin, and answers to the questions posed by the NRC could be developed in greater detail given additional time.

Many DOI activities appear to be outside the scope of the proposed Bulletin, given the exemptions described in the section titled "Requirements of This Bulletin."

July 31, 2006
Draft DOI Response to OMB Risk Assessment Bulletin

AGENCY RESPONSES TO THE PROPOSED BULLETIN

Bureau of Reclamation (BOR)

General Comments:

The Bulletin is focused on risk assessment with regard to human health, safety and the environment. The failure analysis of physical structures is addressed to a limited extent. Consider expanding discussion of aspects of risk assessments for physical structures to include the integration of scientific data, simulations and analysis data, failure analysis, and expert elicitation (where expert elicitation provides probabilistic valuation integrating data, analysis, experience, and professional judgment when statistical data is not readily available).

Consider a Department of Homeland Security Module for the bulletin to address security risk assessments, the implications of transparency and communications given the sensitive nature of security risk dissemination.

Specific Comments:

Page 10, Section III: Goals, 3. Goals Related to Effort Expended. Add: The level of effort to be expended should also consider the likelihood that an additional increment of data/analysis would alter the conclusion or decision to be made.

Page 12, Section IV: General Risk Assessment and Reporting Standards, 2. Standards Relating to Scope, third paragraph, modify first sentence as shown in italics: The third step in framing the scope of the risk assessment entails identifying the affected entities, the population to which the hazard applies, and those impacted economically by decision making.

Fish and Wildlife Service (FWS)

General Comments:

The Service is concerned that the Bulletin appears to favor "central tendencies" or expected outcomes as the best approach or the best science. It is the view of the Service that the best science is that which is objective, explicit and complete and the ends or parts of a distribution that we focus on is guided by policy and social values. However, we do agree with the Bulletin that risk assessment cannot be designed independently of context and thus, other norms besides "central tendencies" or middle/most likely risk values could be just as important. As a result, the Service believes there is no absolute standard for treating uncertainty. We agree that there is a need to avoid being selective when gathering or processing information but it is equally important to report results in the same context.

July 31, 2006
Draft DOI Response to OMB Risk Assessment Bulletin

The Bulletin contains exemptions for single product toxics labeling and the Service is concerned that this might lead to human health and environmental risks that could be foreseen if the exemption was not in place.

There are a number of places in the Bulletin where terms or phrases are not clearly defined. For example, in Section II, 2b, ii, the phrase "scientifically or technically novel or likely to have precedent-setting influence on future adjudications and/or permit proceedings" could use more explanation.

Specific Comments:

Page 1, Summary – OMB and the Office of Science and Technology Policy (OSTP) describe this bulletin as "technical guidance" yet some sections of the Bulletin, including the critical implementation section at the end (the formally titled "Risk Assessment Bulletin" section) create an impression that these are *requirements*.

Page 3 – The statement is made that "Federal agencies *should* implement the technical guidance provided in this Bulletin, recognizing that the purposes and types of risk assessments vary." (Italics added. See comment on page 1 above, and pages 23-24, below). Similarly, the statement "The technical guidance provided here addresses the development of the underlying documents that may help inform risk management and communication, but the scope of this document does not encompass how federal agencies should manage or communicate risk" highlights the fact that the Bulletin is advisory and does not constitute a set of absolute requirements. The Service recommends that the Bulletin be edited to clearly indicate that it is guidance to Federal agencies.

Page 4, paragraph 2 – The use of a "screening level assessment" to determine that a potential risk does not exist, and therefore is not of concern, appears to allow agencies to not fully assess potential risks and will likely result in incomplete or erroneous assumptions about the actual risks to human health or the environment.

Page 5, paragraph 4 – The comments in this paragraph of the Bulletin regarding the "high doses used in experiments" versus "the [presumed] low doses typically found in the environment" reveal that potentially the Bulletin assumes that toxic elements and compounds are always in low amounts in the environment. A single example (*e.g.*, mercury and its prevalence in the human environment and accumulation in a variety of seafood "doses") reveals that such an assumption is potentially incorrect.

Page 8, Title – The title of the section "The Requirements of This Bulletin" is inconsistent with other sections indicating that the Bulletin is technical guidance.

Page 9, Section II: Applicability. The paragraph states that "a rule of reason should prevail in the appropriate application of the standards in this Bulletin." The example given is a screening-level risk assessment, which would be exempt from the standard of "neither minimizing nor exaggerating the nature and magnitude of risk." The paragraph goes on to say that quantitative risk assessments should provide a range of risk estimates.

July 31, 2006
Draft DOI Response to OMB Risk Assessment Bulletin

Many screening-level risk assessments are quantitative, in that numbers for both exposure and thresholds of harm are compared, typically by taking ratios. The Service believes that calculating a range of risk estimates defeats the purpose of a screening-level assessment. This apparent contradiction should be resolved.

Page 11, Section IV: General Risk Assessment and Reporting Standards. The section begins by stating that risk assessments must "meet the three key attributes of utility, objectivity, and integrity in IQA guidelines. Objectivity is defined in IQA guidelines in terms of accuracy, clarity, completeness, and lack of bias. While all of the attributes are desirable and positive, lack of bias has special considerations in risk assessments. Bias may be relatively easy to overcome in a scientific exercise of measurement, data analysis and presentation. In this scientific process, risk assessment is what is done after the raw data are condensed; it is essentially speculation. Bias is difficult to control in this situation, requiring those who will use the risk assessment to agree beforehand on how it will be done.

Page 14, "Standards Related to Objectivity", paragraph 2. The statements referring to "...the best available, peer reviewed science and supporting studies conducted in accordance with sound and objective scientific practices" modifies the definition and concept of "best available scientific and commercial information" per the Endangered Species Act. Is that what the Bulletin intended to do?

Page 14, section IV. 4. This section implies that risk is directly measured as part of a risk assessment, making the application of objectivity standards straightforward. This is clear in the first paragraph: "When determining whether a potential hazard exists, weight should be given to both positive and negative studies." In the second paragraph, there are references to peer-reviewed science and data collected by accepted or best available methods. In reality, risk is seldom directly measured and objectivity standards are difficult to apply to the risk characterization. The objectivity standards may be applied to the data that are used as input to risk assessments. However, the risk assessments themselves typically require assumptions about input data, modeling of these data, or comparisons among input data to estimate risk. These activities are arbitrary or speculative in nature rather than strictly scientific. This distinction needs to be made in the guidelines. Otherwise, most risk assessments may be held to objectivity standards that can only be reasonably applied to input data.

Page 16, item 5. re: central estimates and expected risks – The Service believes that reliance on a central estimate alone in determining expected risks, is problematic, even in "non-influential" (per definition of the Bulletin) risk assessments because short-term, high-range values can have devastating effects even when an average does not. We recommend that this section of the guidance receive further, scientifically-focused, attention to make sure it provides a more accurate discussion of "expected risk."

Page 16, section 7 1). The use of the term "baseline risk" is confusing and should be clarified. Typically, baseline is used for conditions as they currently exist. The reason "anticipated countermeasures" should be understood to "capture the baseline risk" needs to be explained.

July 31, 2006
Draft DOI Response to OMB Risk Assessment Bulletin

Page 18, last paragraph – The statement that "When model uncertainty is substantial, the central or expected estimate may be a weighted average of the results from alternative models" appears to be sound guidance as long as agencies have latitude to take other approaches if circumstances demand.

Page 23. The actual bulletin begins here, while the bulk of the preceding material was "supplementary information." In Section II, Applicability, the "rule of reason" described in the supplementary information is missing. Although the phrase "to the extent appropriate" precedes the phrase "all agency risk assessments...shall comply...," it is overshadowed by all the requirements listed in the remaining pages of the bulletin. While requirements for transparency and similar attributes have obvious utility, requirements for procedures like population risk estimates and the use of probability distributions do not. Because some agencies have a long history of performing risk assessments with stakeholders, OMB should consult with them on the likely consequences of an overly prescriptive approach to risk assessment. For example, the need to reach consensus on the conduct of the assessment among risk assessors, risk managers, and other stakeholders may need to take precedence over some procedures required by the guidelines. Otherwise, arriving at meaningful decisions may be much more difficult. Such advice should at least be as prominent in the bulletin as the prescriptive measures.

Minerals Management Service (MMS)

For the purposes of this Bulletin, the term "risk assessment" refers to a document that assembles and synthesizes scientific information to determine whether a potential hazard exists and/or the extent of possible risk to human health, safety or the environment. The purpose of this Bulletin is to enhance the technical quality and objectivity of risk assessments prepared by federal agencies by establishing uniform, minimum standards.

MMS' two largest programs are Minerals Revenue Management (MRM) and Offshore Mineral Management (OMM). MMS' mission includes 1) the protection of lives, resources and property while managing offshore mineral resources and 2) ensuring industry compliance with revenue mandates, receipt of fair market value on the oil and gas produced, and the timely disbursement of revenues to localities, tribes and the Treasury. The "royalty side" of the MMS operations has more difficulty incorporating the details from the Bulletin, and therefore looks to additional sources for guidance in this area.

MRM does face various risks, and attempts to prepare risk assessments. A working definition of risk is "future events or conditions that may or may not occur that will positively or negatively affect agency objectives." A risk assessment is the identification of these future events or conditions along with an estimate of their impacts and the likelihood of occurrence. MMS appreciates the need for an integrated approach such as this, and continues to incorporate best practices across government and industry. However, since the Bulletin focuses on health, safety, and the environment, its impact on risk assessment practices is minimal (or none) for MRM, and unclear for OMM. For

July 31, 2006
Draft DOI Response to OMB Risk Assessment Bulletin

OMM, the procedures in the Bulletin may affect the time course for risk assessments conducted internally, but should not affect those risk assessments that are contracted out, since the procedures described in the Bulletin could be included in the contract.

Note: The administrative areas within MMS incorporate the risk-based principles of OMB Circular A-123 in conducting internal control assessments.

Agency Responses to the NRC Questions—Questions and Agency Responses

General questions about current risk assessment practices

- **Please provide a brief overview of your current risk assessment practices. Specifically, do you conduct probabilistic risk assessment? Is there a common approach to both risk assessments and uncertainty analysis? How do you currently address uncertainty and variability in your agency's risk assessments?**

BOR: Reclamation conducts probabilistic risk assessments to evaluate dam safety issues at approximately 250 Reclamation owned dams. These risk assessments are used for prioritization of workload, evaluation of the need for risk reduction measures, selection of preferred alternatives, and verification that completed risk reduction measures were effective in reducing risk. Reclamation uses event tree-based models to evaluate risk, and integrates uncertainty and variability in the analyses by having technical staff estimate probability distributions for each event in the tree. Distributions of risk are then computed through Monte Carlo simulation of the event trees.

FWS: Risk assessment practices are used by several different Service programs. The Fire Coordination staff use risk assessment practices to make predictions about equipment and staffing needs for both wildland fire suppression and for controlled burns. Safety and Health staff use risk assessment practices to evaluate certain work activities to determine the potential risks these activities pose to human health. The Aquatic Nuisance Species (ANS) program uses risk assessment practices to evaluate the potential for ANS to invade a specific water body. The Endangered Species Program is engaged in assessing risks to Federal listed threatened and endangered species. These analyses are more along the lines of classical strategic decision-making as opposed to classical risk assessment analyses. Classical risk assessment analyses are principally conducted by the Environmental Contaminants (EC) and Natural Resource Damage Assessment and Restoration (NRDAR) Programs. These programs frequently rely on agencies like the Environmental Protection Agency (EPA) and the Department of Defense to conduct a significant portion of the assessments needed.

Many of the risk assessments performed by the Service are qualitative or deterministic. Probabilistic risk assessments are sometimes a component of risk assessment as related to the Comprehensive Environmental Restoration, Compensation, and Liability Act of 1980 (CERCLA) and as guided by the EPA. In general, the Service does not conduct probabilistic risk assessments very frequently.

July 31, 2006
Draft DOI Response to OMB Risk Assessment Bulletin

Generally, for contaminant-related issues, the Service uses EPA-recommended approaches.

At this point, the Service cannot provide a complete listing of all approaches used in each program or region, however, the two excerpts provided below provide some insight into approaches used by Service personnel:

[excerpt from the regional response of one Service region reflecting the approach taken by staff from the Contaminants Program]

> Our uncertainty/variability analyses summarize the assumptions made for each element of the assessment and evaluate the validity of those assumptions, the strengths and weaknesses of the analyses, and attempts to quantify – to the greatest practicable extent – the uncertainties associated with each risk we identify. In our deterministic environmental risk assessments, we discuss uncertainty related to selection and quantification of constituents of potential ecological concern (CPECs), receptor selection, exposure estimation, effects estimation, and risk characterization. We also identify and thoroughly discuss in our uncertainty analyses significant data gaps that may have hindered or prevented the full determination of potential risk.

[excerpt from the regional response of one Service region reflecting the approach taken by staff from the Contaminants Program]

> Uncertainty is addressed primarily through the use of standard uncertainty factors; variability is addressed through the use of ranges and measures of central tendency

MMS: MMS, in some cases, relies on the regulatory review process and participation of the scientific community to identify the need for risk assessments. Reviews and analyses of offshore operational data are also done in-house to support reviews of Outer Continental Shelf operations. MMS also conducts probabilistic risk assessment for meeting or failing to meet the fair market value requirement for Royalty-in-Kind.

- **Please identify any substantial scientific or technical challenges that you may encounter when conducting risk assessments for your agency.**

BOR: The most significant challenge for Reclamation is the treatment of low-probability, but high-consequence events. Ensuring the safety of dams through probabilistic risk assessment requires assurance that the dams will safely perform their intended purpose even under extreme events not likely to have been experienced in recent history. While available data are insufficient for a statistically-based estimate of event probabilities, Reclamation has conducted significant investigations to develop tools for inferring estimates of hydrologic and seismic event probabilities through a variety of scientific and engineering processes.

July 31, 2006
Draft DOI Response to OMB Risk Assessment Bulletin

FWS: One of the most substantial scientific/technical challenges the Service faces is related to the complexity of the systems that are the focus of risk assessments and the limited data that are available to evaluate risk. When conducting risk assessments the Service is usually interested in evaluating risk to a variety of species as a result of exposure to one or more chemicals or trace elements. In most cases, toxicity data for the species of interest does not exist and this challenge is compounded when data does not exist for the most sensitive life stage. Similarly, the Service is challenged by the extrapolation of laboratory studies to wild populations and extrapolation of studies of one species to another. In general, a lack of data on wild populations and species in decline poses difficulties in risk assessment.

MMS: MMS may contract out a risk assessment on new and/or emerging technologies. Another challenge is to anticipate future events, such as hurricanes and their severity, and evaluate their likelihood.

- **What is your current definition of risk assessment, and what types of products are covered by that definition?**

BOR: For Reclamation, risk assessment activities include identification of potential risks, data collection and information analysis for computing risks, assembling a team of technical experts to develop risk models and report estimated risks, and decision-making regarding Reclamation actions to be taken to address the risk. Reclamation work products include risk analysis reports, decision documents, and workload priorities.

FWS: A process to provide a qualitative and/or quantitative appraisal of the likelihood that adverse effects are occurring or may occur in plants and animals (other than humans) as a result of exposure to one or more stressors, which are defined as any physical, chemical, or biological entity that can induce an adverse ecological response. Stressors can be biological (*e.g.* invasive exotic species) and physical (*e.g.* mechanical destruction of habitat), as well as chemical (i.e. hazardous substances).

MMS: A risk assessment is the identification of future events or conditions along with an estimate of their impacts and the likelihood of occurrence in program operations. Risk management is the creation and implementation of strategies to minimize the impacts or likelihood.

- **About how long (that is, from initiation of the risk assessment to delivery to the regulatory decision maker) does it take to produce the various types of risk assessments?**

BOR: Assuming the preliminary technical analysis has been performed, the time to prepare a risk analysis report varies from a couple of weeks to several months. The shorter time frame is associated with screening-type studies performed to determine the value of conducting further detailed studies to estimate risk. The longer time frame is associated with assembling technical experts in a team to conduct risk analysis and

July 31, 2006
Draft DOI Response to OMB Risk Assessment Bulletin

compile recommendations for decision makers, regarding the need for and selection of actions to reduce risk.

FWS: Risk assessments are intended to be time-efficient, cost-effective, analyses that facilitate defensible appraisals of the significant effects of stressors on natural resources at spatial and temporal scales relative to the Federal statutes, regulations, and policies which the Service is charged to uphold. The scale, complexity, protocols, data needs, and investigational methods used in a given assessment are determined by circumstances at or associated with the site being investigated, in conjunction with the fiscal and staffing constraints. Thus, the timelines vary considerably.

MMS: Varies, contracted risk assessments may take up to 2 years from problem identification to delivery.

Time to produce internal risk assessments depends on the complexity of the subject.

Questions about OMB's definition of risk assessment and applicability

*   **Using the definition of risk assessment described in the OMB Bulletin, are there work products that would now be considered risk assessments that were not previously considered risk assessments? If so, what are they?**

BOR: Based on the OMB Bulletin, there are no work products in the Dam Safety Program that would now be considered a risk assessment that were not previously considered risk assessments.

FWS: OMB's definition appears to more broadly define risk assessment, or risk assessment-like processes, than what the Service has historically called risk assessment. For example, some of the processes and procedures within the Endangered Species Program most likely will fall under OMB's definitions.

MMS: No, regarding human health, safety, and environment issues as addressed in the Bulletin.

Questions about type of risk assessment (tiered structure)

*   **In your agency, is there currently a clear demarcation between risk assessments used for regulatory analysis and those not used for regulatory analysis? Is this clear at the outset of the risk assessment?**

BOR: Reclamation is not a regulatory agency, therefore none of its risk assessments have a regulatory purpose. However, Reclamation clearly understands the importance of defining the purpose and scope of a risk assessment prior initiating work on the risk model. This is addressed in Reclamation's methodology for dam safety risk assessment.

FWS: While some work may be more directly linked to policy, most of the ecological risk assessments the Service undertakes—including most other risk assessments or risk

July 31, 2006
Draft DOI Response to OMB Risk Assessment Bulletin

assessment-type work (following the definition of risk assessment in the policy bulletin) —have a link to statutes and/or regulations.

MMS: It varies. In general, MMS does not make a distinction. However, initiated risk assessments and analysis will likely relate in one manner or another to our regulatory authority granted in the Outer Continental Shelf Lands Act.

•   **In your agency, is there currently a clear demarcation between "influential risk assessment" used for regulatory purposes and other risk assessments used for regulatory purposes? Is this clear at the outset of the risk assessment?**

BOR: Since Reclamation is not a regulatory agency, and the risk assessments conducted by Reclamation are used for decisions at specific facilities, there is no need for the Bureau to distinguish between "influential" and other types of risk assessment.

FWS: The Service believes the necessary guidance from the OMB Peer Review Bulletin and the Service's own Information Quality Act guidelines provide the necessary framework to make the demarcation clear.

MMS: No.

Questions about impact of the Bulletin on agency risk assessment practices

•   **If applicable, please specify provisions in the Bulletin that can be expected to have a substantial positive effect on the quality, conduct, and use of risk assessments undertaken by your agency.**

BOR: Reclamation believes that government-wide guidance regarding risk assessment offers the opportunity for greater consistency among a variety of technical applications where risk assessment can assist in decision making, provided that some of the key challenges facing the technical staff implementing these methods are addressed.

FWS: The Service believes that the presence of a risk assessment bulletin will stimulate discussion within the agency at all levels, and will increase awareness of appropriate guiding principles when risk assessments are produced.

MMS: Since the Bulletin deals with health, safety, and the environment, it would not affect how certain risk assessments are done. It is unclear if the provisions in the Bulletin would have a substantial positive or negative effect on future risk assessments. A Risk Management instruction guide will help answer this question.

•   **If applicable, please specify provisions in the Bulletin that can be expected to have a substantial negative effect on the quality, conduct, and use of risk assessments undertaken by your agency.**

BOR: Given Reclamation's current commitment to probabilistic risk analysis for Dam Safety decision making, Reclamation sees no negative impacts in that area. It is less clear whether or not there would be an expectation to extend the application of probabilistic risk assessment to other areas of Reclamations programs.

FWS: If it is the intent of the Bulletin to drive more risk assessment work to be probabilistic, the Service anticipates that it would negatively affect the Service as a result of anticipated increased costs and time required to complete probabilistic risk assessments. If influential risk assessments carry with them more requirements, then costs will rise, as more staff time is required to complete them.

MMS: Since the Bulletin deals with health, safety, and the environment, it would not affect how certain risk assessments are done. It is unclear if the provisions in the Bulletin would have a substantial positive or negative effect on future risk assessments. A Risk Management instruction guide will help answer this question.

- **If your agency followed the procedures described in the Bulletin, would it affect the time course for production of the risk assessment (that is, the time required from initiation of the risk assessment to delivery to the regulatory decision maker)? If so, please explain why?**

BOR: Reclamation foresees no substantial affects in the area of Dam Safety.

FWS: It might increase the time and cost depending on the application of the "influential risk assessment" concept, and if the Bulletin's guidance is in reality a set of "requirements."

MMS: In certain areas of MMS, it could affect the risk assessments being contracted out since the procedures described in the Bulletin could be included in the contracted assessments. In other MMS areas, the Bulletin's procedures may extend the timeline for the risk assessments conducted by MMS staff.

- **One of the Bulletin's reporting standards states the need to be scientifically objective by "giving weight to both positive and negative studies in light of each study's technical quality." Please give an example of how this would be implemented by your agency or department.**

BOR: Reclamation's methodology specifically calls for teams conducting risk assessments to evaluate information both in support of and contrary to a given premise in estimating the likelihood of an event. This information can include scientific data, theoretical analysis, and engineering judgment. This methodology acknowledges that there may be multiple sources of data, and that some sources of data may provide conflicting interpretations of the likelihood of an event.

FWS: The Service currently does not have formal direction on such a technique. However, a useful approach might include the following: 1) identify applicable studies, primarily from peer-reviewed scientific journals; 2) evaluate the applicability and technical quality of the study in relation to the objectives of the risk assessment; 3) rank

July 31, 2006
Draft DOI Response to OMB Risk Assessment Bulletin

each study based on its quality and how well it supports the objectives of the assessment; 4) use the most highly ranked studies to develop values such as toxicity reference values, home ranges, assimilation efficiencies etc.

MMS: MMS cannot provide examples at this time.

- **Does your agency use risk assessments conducted by external groups? Would it be helpful to you if risk assessments submitted to your agency by external groups, such as consultants and private industry, met the requirements proposed in the OMB Bulletin?**

BOR: Reclamation only uses risk assessments conducted by external groups to the extent that they are contracted to expand program accomplishment. Reclamation requires these risk assessments to meet the same standards as risk assessments performed internally by Reclamation staff. Therefore the benefits of an OMB risk assessment bulletin would be only those addressed by previous questions.

FWS: The Service, at times, uses risk assessments developed by external groups but not without evaluating them carefully first. Improving risk assessments is a laudable goal, whether for Federal agencies or the private sector. The Service suggests that consultants and industry be urged to follow the same guidelines as those provided by OMB.

MMS: MMS contracts for specific risk assessments. It is undeterminable if this Bulletin would be helpful.

U.S. DEPARTMENT OF LABOR

Responses to Questions from the National Research Council's Committee to Review the Proposed OMB Risk Assessment Bulletin

The Department of Labor (DOL) appreciates the opportunity to respond to questions from the National Research Council's Committee to review the proposed OMB Risk Assessment Bulletin. Within DOL, analyses of safety and health risks are performed by both the Occupational Safety and Health Administration (OSHA) and the Mine Safety and Health Administration (MSHA). Both agencies use similar approaches and must meet similar statutory and other legal obligations in conducting such assessments. For clarity, our responses to these questions primarily reference OSHA but generally apply in an analogous manner to MSHA.

General questions about current risk assessment practices

- Please provide a brief overview of your current risk assessment practices. Specifically, do you conduct probabilistic risk assessment? Is there a common approach to both risk assessments and uncertainty analysis? How do you currently address uncertainty and variability in your agency's risk assessments?

Risk assessments are generally performed in connection with promulgating safety and health rules; as such, risk analyses disseminated by these agencies are subject to statutory requirements governing regulatory decision making as well as the public rulemaking process, during which the risk analyses undergo rigorous scientific and technical review by scientific experts and the interested public. OSHA's analyses of workplace risks are disseminated to the public as a component of Federal Register notices of proposed and final rules.

In promulgating safety and health standards, OSHA uses the best available information to evaluate the risk associated with exposures to workplace hazards, to determine whether this risk is severe enough to warrant regulatory action, and to determine whether a new or revised rule will substantially reduce this risk. OSHA makes these findings, referred to as the "significant risk determination", based on the requirements of the Occupational Safety and Health Act, the Supreme Court's interpretation of the Act in the "benzene" decision of 1980 (Industrial Union Department, AFL-CIO v. American Petroleum Institute, 448 U.S. 607), and other court decisions. To make its determinations of the significance of the risk, OSHA relies on analyses of scientific and statistical information and data that describe the nature of the hazard associated with employee exposures in the workplace, and derive estimates of lifetime risk assuming that employees are exposed to the hazard over their working life (usually taken to be 45 years). This corresponds to the first two components of the risk assessment paradigm described by the National Research Council (NRC) in 1983, i.e., hazard identification and exposure-response analysis.

OSHA generally relies on the risk approaches, practices, policies, and assumptions used by the agency in previous regulatory actions unless there is convincing scientific rationale to adopt an alternative. OSHA does not have formal risk assessment guidelines like the EPA.

For health risks, OSHA most often has relied on epidemiological data, but will estimate risk from animal data where adequate human data are not available or where it is useful to compare risk estimates derived from both human and animal data. OSHA generally uses widely accepted approaches to estimate risk in the range of exposures of interest to the agency (*e.g.*, at the current exposure limit and at exposure levels being considered to set new or revised limits). Because risk assessment is used to support findings of the significance of risk, OSHA finds it most useful to quantitatively estimate risk by extrapolating from the observed range of exposure to the range of interest; as such, approaches such as the use of uncertainty factors or EPA's margin-of-exposure approach is less useful for OSHA's regulatory purposes.

OSHA will typically address model uncertainty by comparing results from alternate models that are compatible with scientific evidence on mode of action. OSHA will usually conduct sensitivity analysis where there is reasonable data to support it and when it is useful to facilitate regulatory decision making. Most often, OSHA bases its regulatory decisions on a range of central estimates of risk derived from the best supported models. The key assumptions and uncertainties in the assessment are identified and their impact discussed. OSHA has not generally derived quantitative uncertainty distributions for its risk estimates.

OSHA addresses risks to vulnerable and/or susceptible employee populations in its quantitative risk assessments when there is scientific evidence to support potential differences in risk. Quantitative variability in risk is characterized when the appropriate data and models are available; for example, OSHA accounted for biological variability in using a physiologically-based pharmacokinetic model to estimate cancer risk in its methylene chloride rulemaking. Variability in employee exposures is usually addressed as part of the OSHA feasibility analysis and not in the assessment of risk.

Analyses of safety risks conducted by OSHA to support safety standards are quite different from health risk analyses in terms of the kinds of data and information available to the Agency. The goal of a safety risk analysis is to describe the numbers, rates and causal nature of injuries related to the safety risks being addressed. OSHA has historically relied on injury and illness statistics from the Bureau of Labor Statistics (BLS), combined with incident or accident reports from OSHA's enforcement activities, incident or accident reports submitted to the record from the private or public sectors, testimony of experts who have experience dealing with the safety risks being addressed, and information and data supplied by organizations that develop consensus safety standards, such as the American National Standards Institute or ASTM International (formerly known as the American Society for Testing and Materials).

Part of what can be considered the risk analysis also appears in OSHA's Economic Analysis for proposed and final rules. The Economic Analysis includes an analysis of employee exposures to the hazard of interest, estimates of the sizes of the exposed employee populations in affected industry sectors, and an analysis of the numbers of exposure-related illnesses that occur in those populations and the numbers of illnesses potentially avoided by the new standard. Thus, the remaining two components of the NRC risk assessment paradigm, exposure assessment and risk characterization, are conducted by OSHA to fulfill Executive Order requirements to evaluate the benefits of regulation. Information and data typically relied upon by the Agency to conduct these analyses include exposure data generated by OSHA's enforcement activity, exposure data submitted to the record by industry or labor organizations, industry studies conducted by the National Institute for Occupational Safety and Health (NIOSH), and data obtained by OSHA or its contractors during the conduct of site visits to industrial facilities. In addition, OSHA has usually relied on statistics published by the BLS or the U.S. Census to develop estimates of the size of the population at risk. OSHA does not typically conduct probabilistic uncertainty analysis as part of its exposure assessment and risk characterization, but does conduct sensitivity analysis to describe the effect of uncertainties in estimates of exposure or population-at-risk on benefits estimates.

- Please identify any substantial scientific or technical challenges that you may encounter when conducting risk assessments for your agency.

One of the biggest challenges in chemical risk assessment at OSHA is determining quantitative risk estimates for non-cancer endpoints, especially if it involves extrapolation from experimental animals to humans and extrapolation outside the observable range. As mentioned above, OSHA statutes and policies required to support regulatory action are not readily compatible with the uncertainty factor/margin of exposure approaches favored by EPA and other agencies to evaluate non-cancer risks.

Analysis of safety risks present unique challenges to OSHA. While OSHA can sometimes be quite confident of the number of injuries or fatalities caused by a hazard (due to the availability of fatality and injury statistics from the Bureau of Labor Statistics), there is sometimes uncertainty about the population-at-risk and extent of employee exposure to safety hazards. In large part, this is due to the difficulty of ascertaining certain exposure metrics for safety hazards, unlike the situation that exists for chemical exposures. In addition, it is difficult to quantify precisely the effect of preventive measures on safety risks since quantitative exposure-response relationships are difficult to construct. Instead, the effects of preventive measures on risk are often a matter of expert judgment and practical experience in implementing safety programs.

BLS routinely groups the mining industry with the oil and gas sectors when reporting national statistics, because the mining industry is small in size compared to other industries. Therefore, sufficient data are not readily available to MSHA to make meaningful statistical inferences.

For both safety and health regulatory projects, OSHA faces a challenge in estimating the effect on risk of certain mitigation measures such as employee training, competency certification, exposure assessment, and certain procedural requirements. There is a general lack of quantitative data on the beneficial effects of such practices and OSHA generally describes their effects in qualitative terms.

- What is your current definition of risk assessment, and what types of products are covered by that definition?

As described in response to the first question above, OSHA typically considers risk assessment to mean hazard identification and estimation of lifetime risk associated with exposure to a hazard over a working lifetime. OSHA has not, in the past, treated exposure assessment or risk characterization as part of its "risk assessment," although OSHA does conduct these analyses as part of its estimation of the benefits of regulatory alternatives.

- About how long (that is, from initiation of the risk assessment to delivery to the regulatory decision maker) does it take to produce the various types of risk assessments?

This obviously depends on the scope and complexity of the assessment, the availability of existing analyses, and the priority given the regulatory project within the agency. For its most recently completed risk assessment, OSHA required about 2.5 years to develop an assessment of health risks associated with exposure to hexavalent chromium. This included work to produce and review the risk analyses, evaluate key studies, develop and review the written health effects and dose-response documents, and conduct and respond to an outside peer review of the dose-response analysis before the assessment was ready to pass on to decision makers.

Analysis of safety risks generally take less time, ranging from weeks for an assessment of risks that are already characterized by BLS, to a year or more for risks that have not been so classified.

Questions about OMB's definition of risk assessment and applicability

- Using the definition of risk assessment described in the OMB Bulletin, are there work products that would now be considered risk assessments that were not previously considered risk assessments? If so, what are they?

As mentioned above, the exposure assessment and risk characterization analyses conducted by OSHA as part of the agency's benefits assessment have not been considered to be part of what OSHA disseminates as a risk assessment.

It is possible that some non-regulatory informational products developed by OSHA can fall into the Bulletin's definition of risk assessment where the information contains hazard statements or hazard information. For example, OSHA recently published guidance documents to assist employers and employees in reducing exposures to perchloroethylene in dry cleaning establishments and glutaraldehyde in health care facilities. Both of these documents contain information on potential adverse health consequences of exposure (cancer in the case of perchloroethylene and asthma for glutaraldehyde) as well as exposure control recommendations believed by OSHA to be effective in reducing these risks. Such documents might be regarded under the Bulletin as "a synthesis of scientific information to determine whether a potential hazard exists."

Questions about type of risk assessment (tiered structure)

- In your agency, is there currently a clear demarcation between risk assessments used for regulatory analysis and those not used for regulatory analysis? Is this clear at the outset of the risk assessment?

As described above, to date OSHA has conducted what the agency regards as risk assessments only as part of regulatory analyses.

- In your agency, is there currently a clear demarcation between "influential risk assessment" used for regulatory purposes and other risk assessments used for regulatory purposes? Is this clear at the outset of the risk assessment?

The Department of Labor Information Quality Guidelines defines "influential" information as that having a "clear and substantial impact on important public policies and private-sector decision making." Generally, this is interpreted to mean information having an annual impact of $100 million or more. In most cases, it will be evident to OSHA at the outset of a risk assessment whether the assessment is or is not likely to be influential under this definition. However, since the impact of a regulation depends on the scope of the regulation as well as the nature of the individual provisions in the regulation, it is not always clear at the outset that the regulation can reasonably be expected to have an impact of $100 million annually. The actual impact of a regulation is usually determined well after a risk assessment has been initiated since the results of the assessment in part are necessary to make regulatory decisions that can affect the size of the impacts.

Questions about impact of the Bulletin on agency risk assessment practices

- If applicable, please specify provisions in the Bulletin that can be expected to have a substantial positive effect on the quality, conduct, and use of risk assessments undertaken by your agency.

Most of the Bulletin's provisions should have a positive effect on the transparency, objectivity, and technical completeness of agency risk assessments. OSHA believes that its risk assessments have typically complied with these quality standards and, since the agency's risk assessments are conducted as part of notice and comment rulemaking, they have always achieved a high degree of transparency and have typically been subject to rigorous scientific scrutiny and debate.

- If applicable, please specify provisions in the Bulletin that can be expected to have a substantial negative effect on the quality, conduct, and use of risk assessments undertaken by your agency.

The Bulletin's provisions for deriving quantitative distributions of model uncertainty and variability, wherever feasible, could add significant time to some risk assessments where such analyses are not critical to fully inform regulatory decision makers. In particular, such analyses have not been necessary to adequately characterize safety risks. These provisions may also require conducting formal uncertainty analysis of OSHA's exposure assessments and benefits analyses performed as part of the agency's economic impact assessments. As explained above, these assessments have not been generally regarded by OSHA as part of its risk assessment.

One possible negative impact relates to provisions IV.3 and IV.5, which specify that, wherever possible, risk estimates based on all plausible assumptions and models be quantitatively evaluated. OSHA believes the wording of the requirement could provide credibility to some risk analyses that may not be supported by scientific evidence and, thus, could undermine the technical rigor of the assessment. OSHA would prefer that the Bulletin make clear that quantitative evaluation of risk be based on those assumptions and models that are clearly consistent with supporting scientific evidence, for example regarding a chemical agent's mode of action.

Provision IV.6 of the proposed Bulletin would require that an executive summary of the risk assessment include information that would place the risk estimates in context with other risks that might be familiar to the target audience. OSHA does not generally engage in such comparative risk analyses for decision making purposes since OSHA's regulatory decisions must be based on consideration of the significance of risk and the extent to which those risks would be reduced by the regulatory action (as well as other factors such as technologic and economic feasibility). OSHA has had a long history of considering risks to be clearly significant if employees are exposed to a lifetime risk of 1 death or case of serious harm per 1,000 employees; thus, evaluating the significance of the risk does not involve making comparisons of that risk to other risks.

Provision IV.7 of the proposed Bulletin would require that agencies provide information on the onset of adverse effects and on the timing of corrective measures and associated reduction in risk. For chronic health effects, information that describes the relationships between reduction in exposure and reduction in risk (for example, cessation lag models) is not generally available. OSHA's benefits analyses clearly identify assumptions made by the Agency to describe how benefits are believed to accrue following regulatory action, and such assumptions are usually based on what is known about the latency of the disease(s) of interest. For example, for chemically related lung cancer, OSHA has often assumed a latency of 20 years from first exposure for purposes of describing how benefits can be expected to accrue after exposures are reduced in response to a new regulation. However, until specific information on the actual relationships between cessation of exposure and reduction in chronic disease risk becomes available, OSHA does not anticipate that it will be possible to construct alternative assumptions for evaluating the benefits.

- If your agency followed the procedures described in the Bulletin, would it affect the time course for production of the risk assessment (that is, the time required from initiation of the risk assessment to delivery to the regulatory decision maker)? If so, please explain why?

OSHA believes that the Bulletin's provisions to develop quantitative distributions of model uncertainty and variability, wherever feasible, could add significant time to some risk assessments without necessarily increasing the utility of the risk assessment for Agency decision makers.

- One of the Bulletin's reporting standards states the need to be scientifically objective by "giving weight to both positive and negative studies in light of each study's technical quality." Please give an example of how this would be implemented by your agency or department.

OSHA usually considers both positive and negative studies in its risk assessments and makes hazard determinations based on evaluating the quality of each study included. The agency will often look to reconcile positive and negative data, using additional scientific information if necessary. OSHA's recently published evaluation of the scientific evidence for an increased cancer risk among employees exposed to hexavalent chromium is an example of how OSHA considers positive and negative studies on technical merit based on a weight of evidence scheme.

- Does your agency use risk assessments conducted by external groups? Would it be helpful to you if risk assessments submitted to your agency by external groups, such as consultants and private industry, met the requirements proposed in the OMB Bulletin?

OSHA always considers risk assessments submitted by outside groups during its rulemakings, whether or not they meet the OMB Bulletin's standards or DOL's Information Quality Guidelines. Clearly, higher quality risk assessments that comply with these guidelines are more likely to be helpful to OSHA.

THE DEPARTMENT OF TRANSPORTATION'S RESPONSES TO QUESTIONS POSED BY THE NATIONAL RESEARCH COUNCIL'S COMMITTEE TO REVIEW THE OMB RISK ASSESSMENT BULLETIN

QUESTIONS FOR ALL AGENCIES POTENTIALLY
AFFECTED BY THE OMB BULLETIN

The Department of Transportation (DOT) is pleased to submit to the Office of Management and Budget (OMB) responses to the questions posed by the National Research Council's Committee to Review the OMB Risk Assessment Bulletin that relate to the substance of OMB's proposed draft Risk Assessment Bulletin (the Bulletin).

By way of background, the DOT is a diverse department that consists of ten operating administrations, and the Office of the Secretary, each of which has statutory responsibility for a wide range of regulations. For example, the DOT regulates safety in the aviation, motor carrier, railroad, mass transit, motor vehicle, commercial space, and pipeline transportation areas. The DOT also regulates aviation consumer and economic issues and provides financial assistance and writes the necessary implementing rules for programs involving highways, airports, mass transit, the maritime industry, railroads, motor vehicle safety, and natural gas and hazardous liquid pipeline transportation. It writes regulations carrying out such disparate statutes as the Americans with Disabilities Act and the Uniform Time Act. Finally, the DOT has responsibility for developing policies that implement a wide range of regulations that govern internal programs such as acquisition and grants, safety statistics, access for the disabled, environmental protection, energy conservation, information technology, occupational safety and health, property asset management, seismic safety, and the use of aircraft and vehicles.

General Questions about Current Risk Assessment Practices

Question 1:

Please provide a brief overview of your current risk assessment practices. Specifically, do you conduct probabilistic risk assessment? Is there a common approach to both risk assessments and uncertainty analysis? How do you currently address uncertainty and variability in your agency's risk assessments?

Response:

The DOT does not provide written guidance as to how the DOT operating administrations should conduct risk assessments[1] so there is no common approach to risk assessments and uncertainty analyses within the DOT operating administrations. As a result, the operating administrations employ varied risk assessment practices that range from informed judgment to probabilistic risk assessments.

For example, one operating administration, the National Highway Traffic Safety Administration (NHTSA), researches the incidence, severity and causes of injury relating to motor vehicle crashes when it assesses risk. NHTSA does not, however, typically

---

[1] OMB's Bulletin defines the term "risk assessment" as "a document that assembles and synthesizes scientific information to determine whether a potential hazard exists and/or the extent of possible risk to human health, safety or the environment." Bulletin at 2.

conduct formal probabilistic risk assessments. Rather, it addresses risk by defining the target populations for specific safety-related countermeasures by maintaining several databases that measure the annual incidence of crashes, as well as the characteristics of those crashes. These databases provide a sample-based annual estimate of all crash types, but also provide a complete annual census of fatal crashes. The databases are occasionally supplemented by special studies that address specific injury or safety problems and by research that employs biomechanical test devices and crash tests of motor vehicles. NHTSA synthesizes all of these data sources to estimate the target population that is at risk due to specific vehicular or behavioral characteristics.

Another operating administration, the Pipeline and Hazardous Materials Safety Administration (PHMSA), conducts both probabilistic risk assessments and qualitative risk assessments to support its regulatory functions. PHMSA also employs risk assessments to allocate resources, measure performance, prioritize workload, develop strategies, and refine PHMSA's overall mission. The scope and comprehensiveness of the risk assessments that PHMSA conducts vary with the nature and impact of the issues being addressed and the potential value of the risk assessments in its risk management decisions.

A third DOT operating administration, the Federal Aviation Administration (FAA), typically conducts risk assessments, including probabilistic risk analyses, for regulatory analysis, investment analysis and procurement. The FAA conducts risk assessments to evaluate the effects of proposed industry-wide mitigations against broad categories of aviation accidents. The FAA maintains guidance documents that promote the use of risk assessments by providing information on topics such as: (i) risk and uncertainty, (ii) risk assessment of benefit-cost results, (iii) sensitivity analyses, (iv) monte carlo analyses,[2] and (v) decision analyses.

Question 2:

Please identify any substantial scientific or technical challenges that you may encounter when conducting risk assessments for your agency.

Response:

To the extent that the DOT operating administrations conduct risk assessments, the challenges that they have typically encountered involve a lack of data relating to the nature of the risks at issue.

---

[2]A monte carlo study acknowledges the fact that raw data are often uncertain; instead of knowing exactly what the "cost" of something is, we may have a probability distribution of the cost. A monte carlo study combines the uncertainties and determines, given the uncertainties, the probability distribution for the outcome at issue -- for example, in a cost-benefit analysis, what the probability is that the benefits will exceed the costs.

For example, NHTSA maintains databases that contain comprehensive information regarding the circumstances, causes, and impacts of motor vehicle crashes. However, NHTSA must frequently assess the impacts of countermeasures that target specific injury groups or crash circumstances that are not found in its databases. Additionally, at times, NHTSA must estimate impacts due to specific causal factors that are not well documented in police reports, which are the basis for most of the information in its databases, or in NHTSA's investigative reports. If supplemental studies are unavailable to address these issues, NHTSA may have to rely on imperfect proxy measures to develop its risk assessments.

PHMSA similarly relies on databases and incident reporting systems to estimate the probability of accidents involving pipelines and hazardous materials. Although PHMSA utilizes commodity flow surveys[3] jointly prepared by the Departments of Commerce and Transportation, its ability to achieve a high degree of confidence in its estimates is hampered by the limited availability of data.

In addition, it should be noted that agencies' ability to collect data is restricted by the Paperwork Reduction Act.

Question 3:

What is your current definition of risk assessment, and what types of products are covered by that definition?

Response:

The DOT does not have a standard definition of risk assessment, and within the DOT, the definition varies based upon the operating administration that is defining the term. Similarly, the types of products that are included in the definition of risk assessment vary depending on which operating administration is conducting the risk assessment.

For example, the FAA defines risk assessment as an assessment, either qualitatively or quantitatively, of the probability of some hazard occurring and the potential impact(s) or consequence(s) of that occurrence. According to the FAA, a risk assessment addresses the questions of what can happen, how likely it is that the event will occur, and what the consequences of the event will be. The FAA applies the risk assessment process to products including regulatory analyses and investment analyses of air traffic control services and airport infrastructure to support procurement decision-making.

PHMSA defines risk assessment as a determination of risk context and acceptability, often relative to similar risks. PHMSA's definition encompasses risk analysis, which

---

[3]The Commodity Flow Survey captures data on shipments originating from selected types of business establishments located in the 50 states and the District of Columbia. Respondents provide the following information about their establishment's shipments: domestic destination or port of exit, commodity, value, weight, mode(s) of transportation, the date on which the shipment was made, and an indication of whether the shipment was an export, hazardous material, or containerized.

PHMSA defines as the study of risk in order to understand and quantify risk so that it can be managed. PHMSA employs risk assessments as a tool to better understand the risks associated with the transport of hazardous materials by all of the DOT operating administrations and energy transportation by pipelines.

In contrast to the FAA and PHMSA, NHTSA does not have a current definition of risk assessment. It does, however, interpret the Bulletin's definition of risk assessment to apply primarily to an agency's estimates of fatalities and injuries that result from specific vehicular or behavioral characteristics. NHTSA believes that according to the Bulletin's definition of risk assessment, risk assessments are used in regulatory analyses or evaluations, and special studies, and they define the target population that is addressed by regulatory or behavioral programs.

Question 4:

About how long (that is, from initiation of the risk assessment to delivery to the regulatory decision maker) does it take to produce the various types of risk assessments?

Response:

The DOT does not have a standard time frame for producing risk assessments; the time required to produce risk assessments varies widely from days to years, depending on the complexity of the issue. Factors that influence the time parameters include: the importance and complexity of the project, the level of the estimated risk, the number of the alternatives being considered, the availability of information, the sensitivity of results to changing assumptions, and the consequences of an incorrect decision.

For example, when the FAA evaluates the urgency of a risk, it may conduct a preliminary risk analysis based on the limited data that is immediately available to it. If the urgency indicates higher than acceptable short-term risk, interim actions may be put in place or quick attempts to refine the analysis are pursued. In rare instances of very high risk, future flight may be restricted until interim mitigations (*e.g.* inspections or operational restrictions) can be put in place. For the typical unsafe condition on a particular product, a more in-depth risk analysis takes approximately several weeks or months. This is to account for collecting available data, coordinating meetings with manufacturers and/or airlines, and evaluating possible mitigations.

Questions about OMB's Definition of Risk Assessment and Applicability

Question 5:

Using the definition of risk assessment described in the OMB Bulletin, are there work products that would now be considered risk assessments that were not previously considered risk assessments? If so, what are they?

<u>Response:</u>

As discussed above, the regulatory analyses that are conducted by the DOT operating administrations incorporate elements of risk assessment, even though the operating administrations may not have typically considered them to be risk assessments. Nonetheless, the Bulletin's expansive definition of risk assessment includes some risk assessment activities that the DOT's operating administrations presently undertake.

For example, NHTSA does not typically conduct formal risk assessments, and in the past, it has not considered its target population estimates to be risk assessments. However, NHTSA interprets the Bulletin's risk assessment definition to include estimates of populations at risk due to specific vehicular or behavioral characteristics. Similarly, the Research and Innovative Technology Administration (RITA) believes that some of its activities would come within the Bulletin's definition of a risk assessment. As an example, RITA points to its Travel Statistics Program, which requires independent data collection and analysis that involves aspects of motor vehicle occupant fatalities.

Questions about Type of Risk Assessment (Tiered Structure)

<u>Question 6:</u>

In your agency, is there currently a clear demarcation between risk assessments used for regulatory analysis and those not used for regulatory analysis? Is this clear at the outset of the risk assessment?

<u>Response:</u>

There is generally not a clear line of demarcation between DOT risk assessments that are generated for regulatory analysis and DOT risk assessments that are generated for other purposes. However, as a practical matter, analysts are typically aware at the outset of a risk assessment whether the assessment is for regulatory or non-regulatory purposes.

The FAA explains that as the scope of a risk assessment does not necessarily vary based on whether or not the assessment is for regulatory or non-regulatory analysis, a clear demarcation would serve no practical purpose. Another operating administration, NHTSA, gave a similar explanation, noting that its analysts are well aware of when risk assessments are used for regulatory purposes because the assessments are developed in the context of, and included within, the regulatory document.

<u>Question 7:</u>

In your agency, is there currently a clear demarcation between "influential risk assessment" used for regulatory purposes and other risk assessments used for regulatory purposes? Is this clear at the outset of the risk assessment?

Response:

The DOT does not currently have a clear line of demarcation between "influential risk assessments" used for regulatory purposes and other risk assessments used for regulatory purposes. One operating administration, NHTSA, notes that the only practical demarcation for "influential risk assessments" occurs when an estimate of a population at risk is associated with a regulation of sufficient scope that it requires probabilistic uncertainty analysis. In such cases, NHTSA will include in its analysis a variation in estimates of the population at risk.

Questions about Impact of the Bulletin on Agency Risk Assessment Practices

Question 8:

If applicable, please specify provisions in the Bulletin that can be expected to have a substantial positive effect on the quality, conduct, and use of risk assessments undertaken by your agency.

Response:

The DOT believes that it already complies with many of the substantive guidelines in the Bulletin. Nonetheless, the DOT believes that the overall effect of the Bulletin on the quality, conduct, and use of the DOT's risk assessments will be positive. Indeed, the DOT supports the stated purpose of the Bulletin to enhance the quality and objectivity of risk assessments that are performed by Federal agencies.

Additionally, the DOT agrees with Section III of the Bulletin, which provides that agency efforts should be commensurate with the importance of the risk assessment. See Bulletin at 11. The DOT believes that this guideline will help prevent unnecessary expenditures of agency resources when preparing risk assessments. At a time of significantly reduced budgetary resources, the DOT maintains that it is critical that the benefits from the Bulletin's requirements justify the costs of complying with those requirements.

Question 9:

If applicable, please specify provisions in the Bulletin that can be expected to have a substantial negative effect on the quality, conduct, and use of risk assessments undertaken by your agency.

Response:

The DOT has several concerns that some of the guidelines in the Bulletin, if rigidly interpreted, may result in a substantial negative effect on its preparation of risk assessments.

First, several provisions of the Bulletin may discourage the use of risk assessments in the future. For example, the DOT is concerned that Standard 3 in the Bulletin (standards related to characterization of risk) may introduce unnecessary complexities into the risk assessment process by requiring the risk assessment to contain a range of risk estimates so that the public is aware of whether the nature of the risk is conservative. Such a requirement, however, is time consuming, not always necessary, and could deter the DOT's operating administrations from employing such assessments. Standard 3 requires, in relevant part, that "[w]hen a quantitative characterization of risk is provided, a range of plausible risk estimates should be provided." Bulletin at 13. An alternative approach might be to state: "Uncertainty in the data and assumptions should be evaluated to the degree necessary to demonstrate that the analysis conclusions are relatively insensitive to that uncertainty or to provide risk bounds that encompass the range of uncertainty."

Second, the DOT believes that the Bulletin may considerably prolong the preparation of risk assessments. For example, if Standard 3 in the Bulletin were applied to risk assessments that were conducted by agencies through advisory committees, it might be much more difficult for the agencies to perform risk analyses and respond in a timely manner to unsafe conditions. When working outside the agency structure, for example, agencies face the burden of trying to (i) evaluate and document bounds and uncertainties and (ii) perform a complete review of prior studies. Additionally, Section III.5 of the Bulletin requires agencies to "follow appropriate procedures for peer review and public participation in the process of preparing the risk assessment." Bulletin at 11. The DOT understands that this would require its operating administrations to respond to public comments. An exception should be added to the guidelines for agencies that plan on proceeding under a notice-and-comment rulemaking, in order to avoid unnecessary delay.

Third, some of the guidelines in the Bulletin could be exploited against the DOT by regulated entities in order to frustrate the DOT's regulatory powers or evade regulation. For example, a requirement that analysis from influential risk assessments be "capable of being substantially reproduced" could be employed by regulated parties to purposely delay rulemakings. Even studies detecting low probability risks sometimes involve a great deal of technical judgment, and the same expert judgment process can produce different results over time. Especially in health and safety areas, there has to be an appropriate balance between expert judgment and scientific certainty before action is taken.

Finally, many of the risk assessment guidelines that are set forth in the Bulletin are more appropriate for health risk assessments than for the types of transportation safety risk assessments common at the DOT. Thus, this could cause an unnecessary negative effect; a remedy would be to make many of the requirements discretionary for safety decisions, depending on the particular circumstances of each assessment.

Despite the above-referenced concerns, the DOT understands that many of the negative effects of the Bulletin could be minimized through the application of the Bulletin's "rule of reason," which could provide the DOT operating administrations with sufficient discretion and flexibility to apply the guidelines when they are appropriate. However, further clarification could lessen the possibility of future disputes over what is reasonable.

Question 10:

If your agency followed the procedures described in the Bulletin, would it affect the time course for production of the risk assessment (that is, the time required from initiation of the risk assessment to delivery to the regulatory decision maker)? If so, please explain why?

Response:

The DOT's adherence to the guidelines in the Bulletin would entail a more formalized risk assessment process that would affect the time and resources that are necessary to complete risk analyses.

For example, one standard under Section IV is that agencies shall place the risk in perspective/context with other risks familiar to the target audience. This standard may make sense if the risk being evaluated is expressed in an obscure metric or involves odds that are difficult for readers to fathom. However, NHTSA's risk measures are typically expressed in very straightforward terms—deaths and injuries from traffic crashes. These are easily understood concepts and token comparisons to other types of injury statistics would be superfluous to the point of the analysis. Further, there is no reason to include information on the timing of exposure and the onset of adverse effects, or to develop estimates of individual risk.

By way of another example, if the peer review component in the Bulletin is interpreted as requiring "formal peer review," then significant delay—as much as six months—would likely occur. Other requirements, such as those for characterization of risk, could also cause delay.

Question 11:

One of the Bulletin's reporting standards states the need to be scientifically objective by "giving weight to both positive and negative studies in light of each study's technical quality." Please give an example of how this would be implemented by your agency or department.

Response:

Currently, the DOT operating administrations are generally scientifically objective when evaluating studies, even though the method by which the studies are evaluated may vary.

Some operating administrations already review and analyze pertinent literature as a routine part of their analytical tasks, and will continue notwithstanding the outcome of the Bulletin. Indeed, there are DOT operating administrations that presently evaluate both positive and negative studies in light of each study's technical quality. For example, NHTSA already considers both positive and negative studies when preparing risk assessments. If NHTSA is unable to establish a clear quality-based preference for conflicting studies, the results of both studies may be presented either as a range or through a sensitivity analysis.

However, other modal administrations make wide use of advisory committees that have broad representation, including individuals with significant technical expertise. In those situations, it is not clear whether there would be any additional benefit to literature searches that could be time consuming.

Question 12:

Does your agency use risk assessments conducted by external groups? Would it be helpful to you if risk assessments submitted to your agency by external groups, such as consultants and private industry, met the requirements proposed in the OMB Bulletin?

Response:

If risk assessments are conducted by external groups, it would be helpful if those risk assessments generally met the requirements proposed in OMB's Bulletin. However, the DOT does not believe that such risk assessments should be required to follow the Bulletin's guidelines. Rather, the guidelines should act as a "best practices" for external assessments. One DOT operating administration, NHTSA, notes that when it employs contractors for research and development, the requirements to which its contractors are subject are substantially similar to the Bulletin's requirements. A requirement mandating complete adherence to the Bulletin's guidelines by contractors that conduct risk assessments could discourage the submission of useful and relevant information by external groups. They could, however, be advised that any variations from the "best practices" in the OMB Bulletin would need appropriate justification.

EPA Answers to Questions posed by NRC in its review of the Proposed OMB Risk Assessment Bulletin – August 3, 2006

I. Introduction

Below please find EPA's answers to the questions posed by NRC to EPA (and other federal agencies) about the Proposed OMB Risk Assessment Bulletin. We have numbered the questions for readability. (In some cases, the order of the questions has been rearranged, *e.g.* question 1).

Answers were prepared in the Office of the Science Advisor with input from other Offices. Many answers were based on the general comments presented by EPA to NRC at its public meeting in June. Others were written specifically in response to this request or were drawn from existing EPA publications, primarily:

US EPA 2004; An Examination of EPA Risk Assessment Principles and Practices. EPA/100/b-04/001; www.epa.gov/osa/ratf.htm

US EPA 2002; Guidelines for Ensuring and Maximizing the Quality, Objectivity, Utility, and Integrity, of Information Disseminated by the Environmental Protection Agency. EPA/260R-02-008; www.epa.gov/oei/quality/informationguidelines
US EPA 2006; EPA's Peer Review Handbook, 3rd Edition; EPA/100/B06/002; http://www.epa.gov/peerreview

II. NRC Questions and EPA Responses

QUESTIONS FOR ALL AGENCIES POTENTIALLY AFFECTED BY THE OMB BULLETIN

General questions about current risk assessment practices

NRC Question 1. A. Please provide a brief overview of your current risk assessment practices.

In 2004, EPA published a staff paper entitled "An Examination of EPA Risk Assessment Principles and Practices" (*Staff Paper*) that described its risk assessment practices at that time. This paper was developed in large part in response to public comments[1] requested by OMB on EPA's risk assessment practices. While it does not represent official EPA policy, it was reviewed and approved for publication and presents an analysis of EPA's general risk assessment practices at that time. Chapter 1, pages 1-6, and Chapter 2, pages 11-16 provide a good overview of our current practices.

---

[1] On February 3, 2003 (68 FR 22, pp. 5492-5527) OMB requested public comment on "ways in which 'precaution' is embedded in current risk assessment procedures through 'conservative' assumptions in the estimation of risk" and "Examples of approaches in human and ecological risk assessment...which appear unbalanced."

NRC Question 1 B. Specifically, do you conduct probabilistic risk assessment?

EPA typically uses deterministic approaches to characterize risk, although, increasingly often, in the Office of Pesticide Programs (OPP), in the Office of Solid Waste and Emergency Response (OSWER), and for criteria pollutants in the Office of Air Quality Planning and Standards (OAQPS), EPA applies probabilistic techniques for characterization of exposure or risk.

EPA has published a number of documents related to probabilistic assessments: these include the March 1997 *Guiding Principles for Monte Carlo Analysis* (USEPA, 1997b), the May 1997 Policy Statement (USEPA, 1997c), and the December 2001 Superfund document *Risk Assessment Guidance for Superfund: Volume III — Part A, Process for Conducting Probabilistic Risk Assessment* (USEPA, 2001a)"
Section 3.4.3 of Chapter 3 of the Staff Paper described generally how EPA uses probabilistic analyses with respect to hazard assessment.

" EPA cancer and other risk assessments have not included full probabilistic uncertainty analyses to date, primarily due to the need to develop relevant probability distributions in the toxicity part of risk assessment. However, quantitative statistical uncertainty methods are routinely applied in evaluation of fitting of dose-response models to tumor data, and quantitative uncertainty methods have been used to characterize uncertainty in pharmacokinetic and pharmacodynamic modeling."

OPP increasingly is using probabilistic techniques for characterization of exposure.

OSWER routinely uses probabilistic techniques for evaluating risks from wastes, specifically in the fate, transport and exposure components of assessments used for a variety of management decisions and rules. OSWER has also used PRA to characterize variability and uncertainty in exposure assessments on a site-specific basis. Superfund has a guidance document (US EPA 2001).

For criteria air pollutants, OAQPS has conducted probabilistic exposure analyses and for some air pollutants (*e.g.*, particulate matter, ozone) and health endpoints it has conducted probabilistic risk assessments incorporating statistical uncertainty in exposure-response and concentration-response relationships.

In addition, in July of 2005, EPA was a co-sponsor of a Contemporary Concepts in Toxicology Workshop on Probabilistic Risk Assessment (www.toxicology.org/AI/MEET/PRA_meeting.asp) and has a workgroup within the Risk Assessment Forum that is considering ways to promote probabilistic analyses, including a risk assessor—risk manager dialogue, and a clearinghouse for EPA probabilistic assessments.

U.S. Environmental Protection Agency (USEPA). (1997). Guiding principles for Monte Carlo analysis. EPA/630/R-97/001. Risk Assessment Forum, Office of Research and Development, Washington, DC.

U.S. Environmental Protection Agency (USEPA). (1997). Policy for use of probabilistic analysis in risk assessment at the U.S. Environmental Protection Agency. Fred Hansen, Deputy Administrator. Science Policy Council, Washington, DC. (http://www.epa.gov/osa/spc/2polprog.htm)

U.S. Environmental Protection Agency (USEPA). (2001). Risk assessment guidance for Superfund: Volume III - Part A, Process for conducting probabilistic risk assessment. EPA 540-R-02-002. Office of Emergency and Remedial Response, Washington, DC. http://www.epa.gov/oswer/riskassessment/rags3a/.

NRC Question 1 C. How do you currently address uncertainty and variability in your agency's risk assessments?

EPA has been increasingly making efforts to more completely characterize uncertainty in its risk estimates. EPA's 1986 set of Risk Assessment Guidelines explicitly stated the importance of characterizing uncertainty. EPA's Exposure Assessment Guidelines developed this theme further for the exposure assessment part of risk assessment. EPA's Risk Characterization Policy provided even more direction for describing uncertainty in risk estimates.

Chapter 3 of the Staff Paper discusses EPA's practices in the areas of uncertainty and variability. Below is an excerpt from the overview of the chapter.

"Uncertainty and variability exist in all risk assessments. Even at its best, risk assessment does not estimate risk with absolute certainty. Thus, it is important that the risk assessment process handle uncertainties in a predictable way that is scientifically defensible, consistent with the Agency's statutory mission, and responsive to the needs of decision makers (NRC, 1994). Instead of explicitly quantifying how much confidence there is in a risk estimate, EPA attempts to increase the confidence that risk is not underestimated by using several options to deal with uncertainty and variability when data are missing. For example, in exposure assessment, the practice at EPA is to collect new data, narrow the scope of the assessment, use default assumptions, use models to estimate missing values, use surrogate data (*e.g.*, data on a parameter that come from a different region of the country than the region being assessed), and/or use professional judgment. The use of individual assumptions can range from qualitative (*e.g.*, assuming one is tied to the residence location and does not move through time or space) to more quantitative (*e.g.*, using the 95th percentile of a sample distribution for an ingestion rate). This approach can also fit the practice of hazard assessment when data are missing. Confidence in ensuring that risk is not underestimated has often been qualitatively ensured through the use of default assumptions."

Most recently, EPA has begun to place increased emphasis on use of quantitative uncertainty analyses in its risk assessments, and, in its IRIS assessments, will be moving away from promoting a single value for both non-cancer and cancer effects and will instead recognize and quantify the range of uncertainty in estimates of potential hazard and risk.

NRC Question 1 D. Is there a common approach to both risk assessments and uncertainty analysis?

EPA has a long history of the development of risk assessment guidance to foster consistent practices between and within different effect areas, *e.g.* carcinogenicity, neurotoxicity, or for different categories of assessments, *e.g.* cumulative risk assessment, benchmark dose analysis. Approaches to uncertainty analysis are less well developed at this point, but are a goal for the Agency. Section 3.3.3 of the *Staff Paper* on uncertainty analysis describes a general EPA tiered approach.

"Over the years, improved computer capabilities have created more opportunities to characterize uncertainty. As a result, advocates promote such characterization in all cases. We need to be judicious in which methods we apply, such as Monte Carlo analysis. Uncertainty analysis is not a panacea, and full formal assessments can still be time- and resource-intensive. Further, the time and resources needed to collect an adequate database for such analyses can be a problem. While uncertainty analysis arguably provides significant information to aid in decision making, its relative value is case-specific and depends on the characteristics of the assessment and the decision being made. In some cases, a full probabilistic assessment may add little value relative to simpler forms. This may occur where more detailed uncertainty analysis (or analysis focused on non-critical uncertainties) does not provide information which has any impact on the overall decision."

"Accordingly, EPA's practice is to use a "tiered approach" to conducting uncertainty analysis; that is, EPA starts as simply as possible (*e.g.*, with qualitative description) and sequentially employs more sophisticated analyses (*e.g.*, sensitivity analysis to full probabilistic), but only as warranted by the value added to the analysis and the decision process. Questions regarding the appropriate way to characterize uncertainty include:

a) Will the quantitative analysis improve the risk assessment?

b) What are the major sources of uncertainty?

c) Are there time and resources for a complex analysis?

d) Does this project warrant this level of effort?

e) Will a quantitative estimate of uncertainty improve the decision? How will the uncertainty analysis affect the regulatory decision?

f) How available are the skills and experience needed to perform the analysis?

g) Have the weaknesses and strengths of the methods involved been evaluated?

h) How will the uncertainty analysis be communicated to the public and decision makers? "

NRC Question 2. Please identify any substantial scientific or technical challenges that you may encounter when conducting risk assessments for your agency.

The principal scientific challenge relates to limited data.

Data limitations relate to reliance on available data and may include qualitative hazard characterization without identification of the full range of potential hazards; quantitative analyses with limited data points; reliance on animal data for estimating risks to humans; an absence of hazard or exposure data on susceptible lifestages at potential risk; and reliance on data on individual chemicals when estimating risks likely to involve exposure to multiple agents.

Specific data limitations may be seen: for evaluation of countervailing risks, *e.g.* for implications of reduced income, as an indirect impact; for defining the timing of exposure and onset of the adverse effects, reduction, or cessation of adverse effects; or for estimating population risk from safety assessments, *e.g.* reference doses.

There are many places within the exposure to outcome continuum where additional data can be quite instrumental either in establishing the adversity of exposure or in reducing the uncertainty in an assessment. EPA encourages, wherever possible, the development of more biological data, or other data for refining risk assessments.

EPA has recently placed increased emphasis on mode of action information in its cancer risk assessments as a way of evaluating alternative (non-linear) dose response models. These data can play an important role in defining the biological plausibility of alternative models.

EPA has also recently emphasized a preference for data-derived uncertainty factors rather than the default assumptions used in safety assessment (Reference Dose) calculations, such as the data-derived factors used in intra-species extrapolation.

Another important consideration is the increasing role of biochemical data or newer types of data, *e.g.*, genomics, in defining events that may be linked with adverse outcomes and become valid endpoints for risk assessment.

Technical challenges may include application of multiple models with limited datasets, estimation of indirect countervailing risks of alternatives, and others.

EPA-5

There are areas of risk assessment for which the application of some probabilistic and statistical methods is not straightforward and additional guidance may need to be developed. For example, quantitative uncertainty analysis (of which 2-dimensional Monte-Carlo assessments is one example) and probabilistic hazard assessment are areas in which techniques are available but for application within the Agency, EPA believes there could be benefit from development and articulation of guidance in their application for some risk assessments. As another important example, consider that much of the historical effort in risk assessment has been devoted to "safety assessment" - development of adequate margins of exposure or safety for key variables to prevent toxicity of products, failure of structures, etc. Such safety analyses may not be quickly replaced with more extensive calculations of statistical bounds and probabilities.

Application of central estimates and confidence bounds in dose response assessments may also require further development prior to routine application. Development of guidance, and in some contexts, derivation of central estimates and statistical bounds may require further methods development. These proposed methods and applications should be subject to peer review prior to application. What is meant by central estimates may need more discussion or guidance. The definition of central estimates may be context specific, i.e. may vary or even not be appropriate, depending on the regulatory and statutory context. There is a need for flexibility to make these determinations.

There are a number of additional areas in risk assessment where there may be technical challenges.

These include:

- the state of development of methodologies, and understanding statutory needs and specific context as issues for *e.g.* reporting results as population risks;
- the need for clear definitions, an understanding of the needs for the decision, the statutory environment, and the specific context, in distinguishing between central estimates and expected risks;
- limited or no data to support a quantitative measure of the relative plausibility of alternative risk estimates; and
- the need for caution (See NRC, 1994) in treating fundamentally different predictions as quantities that should be averaged.

Level of uncertainty in risk estimates is a central issue addressed in EPA risk assessments. This uncertainty is inherent in both exposure estimates and estimates of potential effects (*e.g.*, weight of evidence and dose/response). For our most influential assessments (*e.g.*, National Ambient Air Quality Standards (NAAQS)), EPA conducts quantitative uncertainty analysis for both exposure and effects. However, because of unquantifiable model uncertainty, the large number of input parameters and limited data on their distribution, even the most comprehensive uncertainty analyses do not present the true distribution of uncertainty. EPA has efforts underway to further develop methods to address uncertainty including expert elicitation.

In many assessments (especially for exposure assessments) where distributional information is not available, uncertainty is partially characterized by providing several discrete sets of assumptions that span the range of potential values. In many cases where data are inadequate, default values or high end values (intended to not underestimate risks) are used in the analysis. In such cases their potential impact on the assessment is characterized.

For cancer potency assessments EPA follows the approach in its 2005 Cancer Guidelines (i.e., provide confidence limits, based on the point of departure (POD), and indicate risks may be as low as zero). In some cases a range of potency estimates is presented. In others alternative approaches (which EPA believes are adequately supported) are discussed.

For most non-cancer effects (*e.g.* RfDs in IRIS), EPA typically presents confidence limits where PODs are derived from benchmark dose analyses. However, RfDs are typically presented as point estimates and the uncertainty around those estimates are unknown. As for cancer assessments, the risk often may be as low as zero. Uncertainty factors and a qualitative confidence characterization are also presented.

Alternative models/Model Uncertainty: EPA utilizes expert judgment based on the available data to focus the choice of models to be evaluated. For our most significant assessments (*e.g.*, NAAQS), the quantitative implications of these alternatives are more fully explored. For most Agency exposure assessments programs typically use a single preferred exposure model to develop exposure estimates. Such models have been peer reviewed and their performance and limitations are well documented. Where new models are used, model uncertainties are presented.

As noted in EPA's Cancer Guidelines, many aspects of model uncertainty in risk assessment related to human health hazards (*e.g.*, the use of animals as a surrogate for humans) are difficult to quantify. Further, the bases for analyses of many of these aspects of risk assessment often rest on science policy choices or inference guidelines that have been justified based on the available general evidence and peer reviewed as generic science policy default choices.

Defining adversity is both a challenging and complex issue.

Endpoints chosen as points of departure or as critical effects are not always adverse per se. However, they may well be associated with adverse outcomes, and if the evidence is sufficient, appropriately and often serve as the critical endpoints in risk assessments. Example: The use of blood acetylcholinesterase inhibition as an endpoint, or the use of precursor effects to prevent frank toxicity (as in the recent NRC recommendations regarding perchlorate).

Adversity is not a yes/no phenomenon in many, many situations, so endpoint selection is governed by the considerations in EPA's risk assessment guidelines and professional judgment.

Evidence comes in many levels of quality and detail, and it is the weight of the evidence, or its integrated whole, that will often support a judgment, not simply the "best evidence".

Finally, as another technical challenge facing EPA, there is also our evolving understanding of both the science and engineering processes involved in improving the conceptual model for describing and modeling chemical fate/transport in the environment. A recent example is the consideration of organic chemicals in the generation of gases for waste placed in a landfill.

NRC Question 3. What is your current definition of risk assessment, and what types of products are covered by that definition?

From EPA Staff Paper, section 1.1.1

> "The most common basic definition of risk assessment used within the U.S. Environmental Protection Agency (EPA) is paraphrased from the 1983 report Risk Assessment in the Federal Government: Managing the Process (NRC, 1983), by the National Academy of Sciences' (NAS's) National Research Council (NRC):
>
> Risk assessment is a process in which information is analyzed to determine if an environmental hazard might cause harm to exposed persons and ecosystems."

EPA has long embraced the idea that a risk assessment consists of analyses that embrace the four steps described in NRC 1983: hazard identification, dose response assessment, exposure assessment, and risk characterization. Implicit in the completion of these steps is the notion of the characterization of the magnitude or extent of the potential hazards.

In carrying out its mission, EPA conducts a wide range of analyses that fall within this definition. A series of presentations to the NRC committee examining Toxicity Testing and Assessment of Environmental Agents (1-19-06), made by EPA speakers from programs that regulate air, water, solid waste, toxic substances and pesticides, describes the regulatory environment and the range of EPA products. Many of EPA's programs rely on hazard identification and dose response assessments developed by the Office of Research and Development under its IRIS program.

EPA-8

NRC Question 4. About how long (that is, from initiation of the risk assessment to delivery to the regulatory decision maker) does it take to produce the various types of risk assessments?

Assessments vary widely in their complexity and in the time needed for their production and completion.
For examples:

- review of pre-manufacture notices under the Toxic Substances Control Act to support a concern for significant hazard or exposure must take place within ninety days of submission;
- provisional peer review toxicity values for Superfund sites may be completed in weeks or a few months;
- more complex assessments including Integrated Risk Information System (IRIS) assessments, site-specific assessments, or pesticide registration risk assessments may take one to five years; and
- some of the most complex assessments (*e.g.* dioxin, Libby Montana site-specific risk assessment) in which there is significant controversy and significant new data, the time needed may extend well beyond five years.

It should be noted that much of this time is due in part to requirements not only for rigorous scientific evaluation, but also coordination across the Agency, internal peer review, interagency review, external peer review and final approvals.

Questions about OMB's definition of risk assessment and applicability

NRC Question 5. Using the definition of risk assessment described in the OMB Bulletin, are there work products that would now be considered risk assessments that were not previously considered risk assessments? If so, what are they?

OMB's definition applies the term "risk assessment" to work products that are less than complete risk assessments, *e.g.* hazard characterization and dose response assessments such as IRIS entries. EPA does not see a big change in its practices as a result of this new, more inclusive definition. EPA recognizes, that many of these products, do end up as a major basis of subsequent, fully developed risk assessments.

Questions about type of risk assessment (tiered structure)

NRC Question 6. In your agency, is there currently a clear demarcation between risk assessments used for regulatory analysis and those not used for regulatory analysis? Is this clear at the outset of the risk assessment?

In general, most EPA risk assessment activities are tied to some aspect of a regulatory analysis, even if they do not result in a full (four step) risk assessment.

While the regulatory purpose should generally be apparent at the outset of the assessment in the planning and scoping phase, the ultimate regulatory needs and uses may only evolve over time and may be different for different settings, and different customers.

With respect to actions that may need regulatory impact analyses (RIAs), and that could be subject to OMB Circular A-4, some actions clearly do, some do not, and for some the need may only become apparent as an assessment is developed.

OMB Circular A-4 advocates a flexible approach to these analyses, stating (p. 3):

> *"You will find that you cannot conduct good regulatory analysis according to a formula. Conducting high-quality analysis requires competent professional judgment. Different regulations may call for difference emphases in the analysis, depending on the nature and complexity of the regulatory issues and the sensitivity of the benefit and cost estimates to the key assumptions."*

EPA agrees with this emphasis on professional judgment and consideration of the differences in the nature and purpose of an Agency's assessments related to A-4 and to all risk assessments.

There is a need for flexibility given the variety of statutory mandates and types of assessments to which the section would apply. Differences between RIAs and risk analyses conducted for other purposes mean that not all standards should be applicable to all regulatory risk assessments. They should, of course, where appropriate, maintain consistency with the requirements of Circular A-4.

NRC Question 7. In your agency, is there currently a clear demarcation between "influential risk assessment" used for regulatory purposes and other risk assessments used for regulatory purposes? Is this clear at the outset of the risk assessment?

EPA has set out a number of criteria for determining whether an assessment is an influential risk assessment and considers it a case by case process, with, then, no clear demarcation point. These judgments are made in part to determine what upcoming assessments are subject to peer review, and so are made early in the process.

EPA interprets *influential risk assessment* to mean any risk assessment (or component), as defined above, that meets the OMB Peer Review Bulletin's definition of "influential scientific information," which is, "scientific information the agency reasonably can determine will have or does have a clear and substantial impact on important public policies or private sector decisions," as described in EPA's Peer Review Handbook, 3rd edition. The Handbook states:

"Generally, determinations whether a scientific and/or technical work product is "influential" will occur on a case-by-case basis. The continuum of work products covers the range from the obviously influential, which clearly need peer review, to those products which clearly are not influential and don't need peer review. There is no easy, single "yes/no" test that applies to the whole continuum of work products for determining whether a work product is influential scientific information.

The novelty or controversy associated with the work product may determine whether it is influential scientific information. Influential scientific information may be novel or innovative, precedential, controversial, or emerging ("cutting edge"). An application of an existing, adequately peer-reviewed methodology or model to a situation that <u>departs significantly</u> from the situation it was originally designed to address may make peer review appropriate. Similarly, a modification of an existing, adequately peer-reviewed methodology or model that <u>departs significantly</u> from its original approach may also make peer review appropriate. Determining what constitutes a "significant departure" is the responsibility of the decision maker (SPC Peer Review Handbook, 3rd edition, section 2.2.3)."

The Handbook also provides criteria to evaluate whether products should be considered influential. " Generally, scientific and/or technical work products that are used to support a regulatory program or policy position and that meet one or more of the following factors would be considered to be influential scientific information:

       a) Establishes a significant precedent, model, or methodology;
       b) Likely to have an annual effect on the economy of $100 million or more, or adversely affect in a material way the economy, a sector of the economy, productivity, competition, jobs, the environment, public health or safety, or State, Tribal, or Local governments or communities;
       c) Addresses significant controversial issues;
       d) Focuses on significant emerging issues;
       e) Has significant cross-Agency/interagency implications;
       f) Involves a significant investment of Agency resources;
       g) Considers an innovative approach for a previously defined problem/process/methodology;
       h) Satisfies a statutory or other legal mandate for peer review."

Questions about impact of the Bulletin on agency risk assessment practices

NRC Question 8. If applicable, please specify provisions in the Bulletin that can be expected to have a substantial positive effect on the quality, conduct, and use of risk assessments undertaken by your agency.

EPA supports the broad goal of this OMB Bulletin to improve the quality, objectivity, utility, and integrity of risk assessments. Many of the Bulletin's standards are drawn from National Research Council (NRC) reports that EPA supported and whose recommendations have been endorsed by EPA. Many of the approaches presented in the supplementary information section of the proposed Bulletin ("Preamble") have already been adopted by EPA:

- in our quality system which includes our implementation of the OMB Information Quality Guidelines and OMB Peer Review Bulletin;
- in the EPA Risk Characterization Handbook (www.epa.gov/osa/spc/2polprog.htm)
- in the EPA Staff Paper on Risk Assessment Principles and Practices; and
- in other EPA guidance, guidelines, and policies.

Further, EPA is engaged in a wide variety of activities to advance risk assessment practices:

- agency wide workgroups including a Probabilistic Analysis Workgroup, and a task force on Expert Elicitation;
- in specific activities in different program offices and regions, particularly the National Center for Environmental Assessment (NCEA); and
- in support of intramural research in EPA labs and support of extramural research on risk assessment practices (*e.g.* Resources for the Future report on uncertainty analysis).

EPA supports the general goals described in section III of the Proposed Bulletin. These goals call for dialogue between risk assessors and decision makers in order to define the objectives of the assessment. This dialogue, in turn defines the scope and content of the risk assessment considering professional judgment and the costs and benefits of acquiring additional data before initiating the assessment. The goals provide flexibility in the type of risk assessment based on the hazard, the data, and the decision needs; furthermore the goals indicate that the level of effort be matched to the importance of the assessment. In contrast, sections IV and V describe the twenty standards referred to above as requirements in categorical and mandatory terms; for example, "All influential risk assessments shall…" (Sec V), or "…the agency shall include a certification explaining that the agency has complied with the requirements of this bulletin".

The contrast between the flexibility described in the general goals and the prescriptive nature of the twenty proposed standards makes unclear what will be required in any one of the enormous variety of circumstances under which EPA and other agencies work. This in turn may lead to unrealistic expectations within and outside the Federal government regarding compliance with the proposed Bulletin.

The Bulletin should integrate the flexibility described in the goals in Section III with the standards in Sections IV and V.

Because of the breadth of the areas covered in the standards, and the complexity of their application and implementation, EPA suggests that OMB consider the model used for the Information Quality Guidelines, that is, to issue general guidance, and to ask each Agency to develop guidance appropriate for the scope of its activities, which OMB would review.

EPA believes that it could provide substantial compliance with the standards in the proposed Bulletin through compliance with its Information Quality Guidelines, Peer Review Policy, Risk Characterization Policy, Monte Carlo Policy, its Risk Assessment Guidelines, and other existing, related guidelines, policies, and guidance.
Development of EPA guidance based on compliance with those specific Agency policies, guidelines, and guidance, EPA believes, would provide considerably greater detail and thereby promote greater transparency and clarity in its practices, for those within and outside the government.

EPA believes that this process would ensure greater consistency and integration with current practices, while advancing the practice of risk assessment in the specific areas described in the standards.

NRC Question 9. If applicable, please specify provisions in the Bulletin that can be expected to have a <u>substantial negative effect</u> on the quality, conduct, and use of risk assessments undertaken by your agency.

We see the issues here as essentially related to clarity, transparency, and conduct of risk assessments.

<u>Aspects related to clarity and transparency include:</u>

Sections VIII and IX

While Section IX gives OIRA and OSTP responsibility for overseeing implementation of the Bulletin, it does not outline any roles and responsibilities for decision-making, resolution of disagreements between agencies and OMB, certifications, waivers, exemptions, and other areas. The document should describe how interactions between OMB and the Agencies will work in implementing the Bulletin.

Implementation of the deferral and waiver section VIII is unclear and ambiguous in what is required; that is, when is a standard being "waived" as opposed to just being applied "flexibly?"

While the proposed Bulletin does provide an opportunity to waive or defer some or all of the indicated standards, this opportunity is defined in a very limited way. Under Section VIII, only the agency head may waive or defer the standards, which would likely result in an undue expenditure of great effort and time within the Agency. In addition, deferral only delays the implementation of full compliance with the Bulletin and does not provide any real relief. The proposed Bulletin does not describe any criteria for granting a waiver or for providing for exemptions, but it indicates that even deferral is expected to be a rare event.

Scientific "defaults" or "inference guidelines" play an important role for EPA in providing a consistent and peer reviewed means of addressing recurring, fundamental issues of science policy in its risk assessments. The proposed Bulletin does not address this aspect of risk assessment practice that is discussed in the 1983 NRC "redbook" and specifically described for different areas in the EPA Risk Assessment Guidelines. However, as emphasized in the 2005 Cancer Guidelines, EPA sees that a critical analysis of all the available information relevant to assessing risk is the starting point from which default options may be invoked to address uncertainty or the absence of critical information.

Aspects related to Conduct of Risk Assessments

Those aspects of the Bulletin that could have the greatest negative impact on conduct, in addition to those that may pose technical challenges, are those that have a potentially broad scope, *e.g.*, those that call for multiple analyses. The primary negative effect might be increased need for time and/or resources.

The standards of the proposed Bulletin would come into play for a large class of agency products and, if categorically adopted, would mandate a high level of analysis and development of characterization that goes beyond most current EPA practice in risk assessment.

While EPA appreciates that fact that the Bulletin does not create legal rights (Section XI), challenges that claim that the risk assessment or supporting analyses have not fully carried out the practices established by the Bulletin come in many other fora. Such claims could pose an additional burden.

Several standards discuss multiple analyses, including: IV 5, a quantitative evaluation of reasonable alternative assumptions; and V 5, portrayal of results based on different effects observed and/or different studies; We have some general concerns about these analyses as drafted:

- their scope may be impractical;
- one should consider the value added (benefits) of these analyses versus their costs as a function of the importance of the assessment, and their relative value in comparison to collecting data;
- multiple analyses may pose risk communications challenges;
- and in some cases, the complexity of the analyses may limit their feasibility.

Section V 9. states: Consider all significant comments received on a draft risk assessment report and:

a. issue a "response-to-comment" document that summarizes the significant comments received and the agency's responses to those comments; and
b. provide a rationale for why the agency has not adopted the position suggested by commenters and why the agency position is preferable.

EPA conducts its peer reviews and public involvement in line with its defined policies in these areas and consistent with the OMB Peer Review Bulletin, which provides for different processes for influential scientific information and highly influential scientific assessments. This section goes beyond those guidelines by calling for a response to comment package for all influential risk assessments, and also in its call not only to explain the basis for the agency position, but also to explain why other approaches were not taken, and why. This goes beyond the peer review procedures even for highly influential scientific assessments and most practice we know of in this area.

NRC Question 10. If your agency followed the procedures described in the Bulletin, would it affect the time course for production of the risk assessment (that is, the time required from initiation of the risk assessment to delivery to the regulatory decision maker)? If so, please explain why?

If EPA followed all of the procedures described in the twenty standards, assessments could take considerably longer. If alternatively, scoping and planning lead to an appropriately defined assessment in terms of its scope, as noted in the goals section, then those assessments should be efficient, and there would be a limited impact on current timelines.

NRC Question 11. One of the Bulletin's reporting standards states the need to be scientifically objective by "giving weight to both positive and negative studies in light of each study's technical quality." Please give an example of how this would be implemented by your agency or department.

Weight of Evidence analyses, to which the Agency subscribes, embrace the notion of consideration of all the evidence, consistent with its quality. Thus, any published EPA risk assessment, should satisfy this standard in that sense. The phrase "giving weight to both positive and negative studies" has quantitative connotations and the term "consideration" may be preferable.

See also, section 4.4.2, page 72 of the *Staff Paper* which illustrates how positive evidence has not uncritically been accepted in analysis of carcinogenicity data.

NRC Question 12. Does your agency use risk assessments conducted by external groups? Would it be helpful to you if risk assessments submitted to your agency by

external groups, such as consultants and private industry, met the requirements proposed in the OMB Bulletin?

Yes, in some cases the Agency has relied upon assessments conducted by external groups, including NRC panels, the World Health Organization, the Canadian government, ATSDR, and CAL-EPA. In general, their conformity with the requirements of the Bulletin, as feasible and appropriate, would be a laudable goal both for those whose assessments may be used as well as more broadly for those who might wish to propose alternative analyses for consideration.

ADDITIONAL QUESTIONS FOR SPECIFIC AGENCIES: EPA

NRC Question 13. Regarding pesticides specifically, what risk-assessment activities will be covered by the Bulletin and what risk-assessment activities will be exempted?

The Agency agrees with the OMB bulletin that risk assessments for permitting or licensing programs should be exempt. Thus, pesticide risk assessments or actions under FIFRA would be excluded given that pesticide registration/re-registration program is a licensing program. However, the proposed Bulletin did indicate that actions that involve assessment / reassessment of tolerances for pesticide residues on food would be subject to the Bulletin (page 10, par. 2). EPA's Office of Pesticide Programs conducts risk assessments in support of the establishment of tolerances under Federal Food Drug and Cosmetic Act (FFDCA). Because pesticide risk assessments supporting tolerances are tied to the pesticide registration/re-registration program (i.e., licensing), such risk assessments should also be exempted from the OMB bulletin. Furthermore, all new food tolerances are impacted by the short PRIA (Pesticide Registration Improvement Act) time frames (2 years and less). Although pesticide risk assessment tied to the registration/re-registration program (licensing) should be exempted, we agree with OMB that certain pesticide risk assessments that have significant science issues that are debated by the scientific community and that have intra- and inter-agency impact on regulatory decisions of broad consequences (*e.g.*, arsenicals) should be subject to the Bulletin.

NRC Question 14. Does EPA have any examples of the application of the 1996 requirements of the Safe Drinking Water Act, as described on page 13 of the Bulletin? Can any examples be provided to the committee? If none are available, can EPA provide an explanation?

EPA has *adapted* these requirements in its implementation of the Information Quality Guidelines (US EPA, 2002[2]). Thus, any assessments published subsequent to our completion of that document should be consistent with the elements described therein.

In issuing its IQGs, EPA *adapted* the SDWA principles. As EPA explained in its IQGs, "EPA conducts and disseminates a variety of risk assessments. When evaluating environmental problems or establishing standards, EPA must comply with statutory requirements and mandates set by Congress based on media (air, water, solid, and hazardous waste) or other environmental interests (pesticides and chemicals). Consistent with EPA's current practices, application of these principles involves a "weight-of-evidence" approach that considers all relevant information and its quality, consistent with the level of effort and complexity of detail appropriate to a particular risk assessment." EPA committed to ensure, to the extent practicable and consistent with Agency statutes and existing legislative regulations, the objectivity of our dissemination of influential scientific information regarding human health, safety or environmental risk assessments by applying an adaptation of the SDWA principles.

EPA adapted the SDWA principles in the Agency's IQGs, "in light of our numerous statutes, regulations, guidance and policies that address how to conduct a risk assessment and characterize risk" in order to:

- Implement SDWA principles in conjunction with and in a manner consistent with Agency statutes, existing legislative regulations, and our existing guidelines and policies for conducting risk assessments.
- Accommodate the range of real world situations that EPA confronts in the implementation of our diverse programs. For example, EPA's adaptation covers situations where EPA may be called upon to conduct "influential" scientific risk assessments based on limited information or in novel situations, and recognizes that all "presentation" information called for in the SDWA principles may not be available in every instance. Our adaptation recognizes that the level of effort and complexity of a risk assessment should also balance the information needs for decision making with the effort needed to develop such information.
- Enable EPA to use all relevant information, including peer reviewed studies, studies that have not been peer reviewed, and incident information; evaluate that information based on sound scientific practices as described in our risk assessment guidelines and policies; and reach a position based on careful consideration of all such information (i.e., a process typically referred to as the "weight-of-evidence" approach). As noted in our IQGs, EPA uses a weight of evidence approach, in which a well-developed, peer-reviewed study would generally be accorded greater weight than information from a less well-developed study that had not been peer-reviewed, but both studies would be considered.

---

[2]US EPA (December 2002). Guidelines for Ensuring and Maximizing the Quality, Objectivity, Utility, and Integrity of Information Disseminated by the Environmental Protection Agency (EPA/260R-02-008). Washington, DC, Office of Environmental Information

- Allow EPA to use terms that are most suited for environmental (ecological) risk assessments. EPA assessments of ecological risks address a variety of entities, some of which can be described as populations and others (such as ecosystems) which cannot.

The Bulletin should clarify that it does not modify or supersede OMB-approved agency adaptations of the SDWA risk assessment principles in their Information Quality Guidelines.

NRC Question 15. Does EPA have a working definition of "expected risk" or "central estimate"? The agency indicated in its 1986 cancer guidelines (51FR33992-34003) that central estimates of low-dose risk, based on "best fit" of the observed dose-response relationship, were meaningless—that "fit" in the high-dose region provided no information about "best fit" in the region of extrapolation. The newer cancer guidelines appear to adopt the same thinking. Has the Agency changed its view on this point? If so, why?

EPA finds the terms central estimate and expected risk to be quite different and does not use them interchangeably. EPA documents discuss central estimates from a specific model, for example, with respect to both cancer dose response assessment and for derivation of maximum likelihood estimates for points of departure (PODs). In contrast, discussion of the notion of expected risk, (not a specifically defined term, to our knowledge) in a risk assessment usually involves a particular exposure distribution, and relies on a series of judgments about whom (average consumer, top 5% of those exposed) we expect to be exposed. For safety assessment, an additional complication is a limited ability to describe what effect is expected above a reference dose.

EPA's 2005 cancer guidelines differ significantly from its 1986 guidelines with regard to the treatment of the "central estimate" of cancer risk. In particular, the 2005 guidelines distinguish between the dose-response function within the range of data from that which is used to extrapolate to lower doses. In contrast, the 1986 guidelines use one model (the linearized, multistage model) both to fit the data and to extrapolate to lower doses. The 2005 guidelines discuss the following issues not mentioned in the 1986 guidelines.

1. A preference for biologically-based dose-response models when there is adequate scientific support for them.

2. The potential for biologically based modes of action that are non-linear at low doses (even in the absence of a biologically based dose-response model).

3. The utility of central estimates, and estimates of confidence limits, when practicable, conforming with OMB and EPA guidelines on data quality.

**NASA Responses to National Academy of Sciences
Questions Posed on Office of Management and Budget's Proposed
Risk Assessment Bulletin**

July 25, 2006

**QUESTIONS FOR ALL AGENCIES POTENTIALLY
AFFECTED BY THE OMB BULLETIN**

General questions about current risk assessment practices

Question 1: Please provide a brief overview of your current risk assessment practices. Specifically, do you conduct probabilistic risk assessment? Is there a common approach to both risk assessments and uncertainty analysis? How do you currently address uncertainty and variability in your agency's risk assessments?

NASA Response:

NASA defines risk in a very broad sense.[1] Risk is the expression of likelihood (probability) and severity of scenarios leading to potential undesired consequences with respect to achieving established and stated program objectives which generally fall into two categories: technical and programmatic. Technical objectives are associated with attributes such as safety and performance. Programmatic objectives are associated with attributes such as schedule and cost. When specifically considering technical risk, the undesired consequences of interest to NASA include:
- Death, injury, or illness to a member of the public.
- Loss of crew.
- Mission failure.
- Death, injury, or illness to ground crew and other workforce (occupational).
- Earth contamination.
- Planetary contamination.
- Loss of, or damage to, flight systems.
- Loss of, or damage to, ground assets (program facilities and public properties).

Regardless of the type of risk that may be of interest for specific circumstances, assessments performed at NASA for technical risks typically involve the definition and characterization of three components of risk:
- The sequence of possible events that constitute a risk scenario (events leading to an undesired consequences)
- The probability of the risk scenario occurring(expressed qualitatively or quantitatively),
- The severity of the consequences that constitute the outcome of the risk scenario (expressed qualitatively or quantitatively).[2]

---

[1]NASA Procedural Requirements (NPR) 8000.4 defines risk as "the combination of the probability that a program or project will experience an undesired event (such as a cost overrun, schedule slippage, safety mishap, environmental exposure, or failure to achieve a needed scientific or technological breakthrough or mission success criteria) and the consequences, impact, or severity of the undesired event, were it to occur."

[2]This is done in the form of the numeric magnitude of the parameter, or a set of parameters that best represent the impact of consequences.

In addition to NASA's mission-related risk assessments, external regulatory agencies at the Federal and State levels may require NASA to conduct project-specific (*e.g.*, nuclear missions) or site-specific risk assessments to evaluate the extent of environmental contamination, potential threat to human health (including occupational exposures), and the environment or evaluate remediation response alternatives. In these cases, NASA utilizes the risk assessment technical procedures approved by the regulating agency, in conformance with the requirements of the regulating agency.

Application of Probabilistic Techniques for the Assessment of Technical Risks

NASA uses the scenario-based modeling framework for probabilistic risk assessment (PRA) of space systems. This framework is employed primarily because space-related accidents with adverse safety consequences are too infrequent to assess directly the risk using actuarial assessments. This scenario-based modeling framework involves the following steps:

1. Define a set of undesired consequences (*e.g.*, loss of crew, loss of mission)
2. Develop for each undesired consequence; a set of off-normal trigger conditions or events is which, if uncontained or unmitigated, can lead to the undesired consequences. These disturbances are referred to as initiating events (IEs).
3. Employ various systematic techniques to identify risk scenarios (sequences of events) that start with an IE and end at an undesired consequence (called an "end state" in PRA). These scenarios include hardware failures, human errors, and physical phenomena.
4. Evaluate, using Bayesian approaches, the probabilities of these scenarios based on available evidence, expert judgment, and data from similar systems. Evaluating uncertainties is an important part of this activity. The probabilities are updated as new information is gained.

To date, NASA has performed a number of scenario-based PRA studies, two of them for major programs, namely the Space Shuttle and the International Space Station [1,2]. PRA techniques are now being used in trade studies for the new exploration systems [3 ,4]. In addition, numerous risk assessments have been conducted to support the decision process for the launch of radioactive materials.[3] [5]

To improve the quality of PRAs and to formalize its integration with engineering activities, NASA has developed procedures and requirements for PRA methods and applications. NASA is currently in the process of developing procedures for how to use PRA to support risk-informed decision making. The following is a list of PRA-related documents that NASA has developed:

---

[3]These assessments/evaluations are required under the requirements of Presidential Directive/National Security Council Memorandum Number 25 (PD/NSC-25), "Scientific or Technological Experiments with Possible Large-Scale Adverse Environmental Effects and Launch of Nuclear Systems into Space." NASA missions involving the launch of radioactive materials must also comply with the provisions of the National Environmental Policy Act of 1969 (42 U.S.C. 4321 et seq.).

- NASA Procedural Requirements (NPR) 8705.5: Probabilistic Risk Assessment Procedures for NASA Programs and Projects (http://www.hq.nasa.gov/office/codeq/doctree/87055.htm)
- NASA NPR 8715.3: Chapter 2 (System Safety) of NASA General Safety Program Requirements (updated version pending release)
- Probabilistic Risk Assessment Procedures Guide for NASA Managers and Practitioners, August 2002 (http://www.hq.nasa.gov/office/codeq/doctree/praguide.pdf)

According to NASA requirements, a PRA has to be conducted during project formulation and design concept phases and has to be maintained and updated periodically throughout the system life cycle to support design and operational decisions. Because the PRA models must be synchronized with the system design and operational state-of-knowledge, they are interactive in nature. Furthermore, the focus of PRA models often changes during the lifecycle of the system depending on from where the dominant risk contributors appear to be coming. Because of these properties and in the context of managing risk, a typical NASA PRA can be viewed neither as a static engineering calculation whose results are fixed nor as a single deliverable document.[4]

Evaluation of Uncertainties in PRAs

NASA considers the evaluation of uncertainties as an essential part of evaluating technical risks, in particular the uncertainties associated with the risk scenario probabilities and the risk scenario consequences. To deal with uncertainty as part of the risk function, one must be mindful of the nature of uncertainty and its characterization. According to NASA's PRA Procedures Guide, uncertainty is classified into two broad categories or types: epistemic (state-of-knowledge) uncertainty and aleatory (variability) uncertainty.

- Epistemic uncertainty: that uncertainty associated with incompleteness in the risk analyst's (or analysts') state of knowledge. In the context of modeling of system behavior, there are two categories of epistemic uncertainty:
  - Parameter Uncertainty: uncertainty in the value of a parameter of a model, conditional on the mathematical form of that model.
  - Model Uncertainty: uncertainty in whether the model adequately represents the behavior of the system being modeled.
- Aleatory uncertainty: that uncertainty associated with variation or stochastic behavior in physical properties or physical characteristics of the system being addressed. Aleatory uncertainty is manifested, for example, in the variability of the time at which a failure or a random event will occur. Another example is

---

[4]Risk assessments conducted to support the launch of nuclear or radioactive materials would however be prepared as a single document in accordance with requirements established by PD/NSC-25.

the variations in material properties resulting from variability in manufacturing processes. Another example is the variation in weather properties and characteristics. Human performance also exhibits aleatory uncertainty in its variation from day to day and from individual to individual.

The NASA PRA Procedures Guide provides methods on how to mathematically quantify aleatory and epistemic uncertainty using techniques of probability theory and simulation. For example, the standard method for characterizing uncertainty associated with a parameter value of a risk model (*e.g.*, a failure rate) is to represent it with a probability density function. Similarly, the standard method for propagating uncertainties through a risk model is to use simulation techniques. In the context of managing risk of space systems, it is important to separate the epistemic from aleatory uncertainty. The essential difference between these two types of uncertainty is that the former is, in principle, reducible through the collection of more knowledge (*e.g.*, conducting research), whereas the latter is not as it represents a property of the system being analyzed. Consequently, the control for aleatory uncertainty is very different.

Application of Probabilistic Techniques for Assessment of Programmatic Risks

NASA uses probabilistic techniques to assess programmatic risks. Cost-risk analysis results in a cost estimate value associated with a probability of achieving that value. In cost-risk analysis, four sources of uncertainties are modeled: cost estimating relationship (CER) uncertainty; CER parameter input uncertainty; programmatic uncertainty; and project element correlation uncertainty.

- CER uncertainty is due to the imperfect regression line fit to a set of cost data and is captured by including the standard error or prediction interval as a distribution around the regression line in the statistical convolution. Cost estimators provide the data for modeling of CER uncertainty.
- CER parameter input uncertainty is provided by modeling optimistic, most likely and pessimistic values as triangular (for example) distributions when using the CER in the calculations and statistical convolutions. Engineers provide the data for the modeling of parameter input uncertainty.
- Programmatic uncertainty is captured by modeling programmatic influences on the cost. Both engineers and cost estimators provide the data for the modeling of programmatic uncertainty.
- Finally, correlation uncertainty between the proposed system's elements is modeled through rules of thumb and engineering input. These correlations have to be accounted for since costs in subsystems/components tend to move consistently either in the same direction or opposite directions. Failure to do so will lead to underestimation of cost uncertainty.

The resulting distribution for cost can be interpreted as producing a range of cost estimate values each associated with a probability p that if chosen as a budget the probability that the proposed project will cost that value or less is p.[5]

---

[5] For funding decisions, NASA uses 70% level of probability.

Question 2: Please identify any substantial scientific or technical challenges that you may encounter when conducting risk assessments for your agency.

NASA Response:

There are several significant scientific and technical challenges when conducting risk assessments of space missions:

- Space systems operate in harsh environments. In addition to being subjected to the significant forces during launch and landing, space systems function outside the confines of Earth's atmosphere and are subjected to orbital debris and micrometeoroids. The modeling and evaluation of the effects of these environments on space systems and the uncertainties involved must be factored into the analysis when conducting a PRA.

- Most space systems are designed and operated for a specific mission, such as delivering a satellite to earth orbit, conducting advanced micro-gravity research, or exploring neighboring planets. Because of their unique designs, the system's response to adverse environments and identified initiating events isalso unique. Analysis of the response of one space system is not readily transferable among other systems. Advances in space system design and technology (hardware) also require dedicated physical modeling for specific space systems.

- A space mission is comprised of a number of phases; from launch to orbital operations and possible transit to other planets, and for some missions, entry and landing back on earth. During a mission, the configuration and operation of the systems change; propulsion systems needed for liftoff are not needed outside the confines of earth's gravity; components that must operate in a certain way during one phase may need to operate in different way during another phase. The modeling and assessment of the phased mission's nature of space flight pose challenges.

- Representative reliability and failure data presents a challenge to conducting risk assessment of space systems. There is limited experience data with respect to the operation of systems and components in space.[6] In addition, as technology advances, improved space systems and hardware are fielded that increase energy efficiency and reduce weight. While these systems and component are tested in simulated space environments, there is also limited data on many of these advanced components and systems. Because of scarcity of data, Bayesian approaches need to be employed to combine various sources of data (i.e., available evidence). This presents challenges for how to model the relevance and confidence associated with each piece of evidence systematically.

---

[6]The approach used for system acquisition may also impact the availability of data to support risk assessments. If commercial services are used for a portion of the mission, such as use of a commercial expendable launch vehicle, some or all of the data concerning the performance of the vehicle may be proprietary and access to, or use of the data may be restricted.

- "Margin" in design and operational parameters is an important issue for space exploration. "Margin" in a key parameter is the difference between the value of that key parameter in some operational state and the value of that parameter at which failure will occur. Designers incorporate margin to reduce the chance of failure. Unfortunately, the provision of physical margin in space vehicles is very costly (*e.g.*, extra material strength or shielding adds weight which, in turn, reduces payload delivery capacity to orbit). The determination of the adequacy of margin in a given situation must be key to developing realistic PRA models. Transforming design margins into a probabilistic framework to support PRAs poses significant challenges.

Question 3: What is your current definition of risk assessment, and what types of products are covered by that definition?

NASA Response:

NASA NPR 7120.5 C [6] defines risk assessment as an evaluation of a risk item that determines (1) what can go wrong, (2) how likely is it to occur, and (3) what the consequences are. As stated in response to Question 1, since NASA defines the concept of risk broadly, the subjects of its risk assessments are also broad to include one or more of the three basic program execution domains:

- System technical performance
- Program cost
- Program schedule

NASA considers risk assessment as a necessary element of the risk management process [7] which is required by all programs and projects that provide aerospace products or capabilities—i.e., flight and ground systems, technologies, and operations for space and aeronautics.

Question 4: About how long (that is, from initiation of the risk assessment to delivery to the regulatory decision maker) does it take to produce the various types of risk assessments?

NASA Response

NASA uses risk assessment throughout a program's or project's life cycle, from initial stages of formulation where concepts and preliminary design ideas are developed, through fielding and operation to decommissioning. Since a risk assessment evolves and is updated over the life of the project or program, it can be considered as a "living" risk model with no fixed dates for their final delivery. The level of detail associated with a risk assessment model is dependent on the availability of design and operational information and the nature of the application for which the risk model is intended.

For large programs, where the assessments were conducted after the spacecraft were fielded, i.e., Space Shuttle, the risk assessment required several years to complete. For nuclear missions, where probabilistic and risk techniques are used as part of the safety analyses, the risk assessment is conducted as the mission is planned, the spacecraft and launch vehicles are constructed, and reviews and approvals are attained. The completion of nuclear mission safety analyses require about 3-5 years.

Risk assessments of conceptual designs used to perform trades studies and sensitivity analyses to optimize safety, mission profile and operations have been conducted in several months. These types of risk assessments are typically conducted at a high level.

Questions about OMB's definition of risk assessment and applicability

Question 5: Using the definition of risk assessment described in the OMB Bulletin, are there work products that would now be considered risk assessments that were not previously considered risk assessments? If so, what are they?

NASA Response

One significant area of change relates to our internal policies and directives. OMB Circular A-123, Management's Responsibility for Internal Control, requires management to perform risk assessments to identify internal and external risks that may prevent the organization from meeting its objectives. The results of those risk assessments would be used to identify control activities that could be implemented to ensure agency objectives are met. The OMB Bulletin indicates that influential risk assessments are those that the agency reasonably can determine will have a clear impact on private sector decisions. For NASA, where the majority of our budget is applied to contracted activity, most of our internal controls do not impact the decisions of the private sector. If the special standards for Influential Risk Assessments were applied to every risk assessment performed to determine if an internal policy or directive was required, this could dramatically impact the time to develop, implement, and modify the internal controls. It is not clear, given the emphasis that the Bulletin places on regulatory matters and public use of the risk assessments, that risk assessments performed for internal NASA decision-making purposes need to have this level of regulation.

Questions about type of risk assessment (tiered structure)

Question 6: In your agency, is there currently a clear demarcation between risk assessments used for regulatory analysis and those not used for regulatory analysis? Is this clear at the outset of the risk assessment?

NASA Response

NASA is not a regulator, but rather a user with direct stakes in the technical and programmatic risk metrics that support decision making. NASA never uses its risk models for any regulatory application. Unlike regulatory agencies, NASA owns and operates the subjects of risk assessment. This has several implications for NASA's approach to risk assessment and risk management. Because NASA is interested in technical performance (*e.g.*, safety, mission success), as well as programmatic performance (*e.g.*, cost and schedule), its risk assessments need to address both, preferably in an integrated fashion. At regulatory agencies, the need for regulatory stability and transparency creates an incentive to standardize and hold static the technical approaches used in quantitative risk assessment. At NASA, quite the opposite, because of the application of novel technologies in new environments, there is a need to advance the state-of-the-art in quantitative risk assessment to support decision making aimed at optimizing safety and likelihood of mission success (see Response to Question 2). In this connection, NASA is continuously developing new risk assessment techniques and, as such, needs the flexibility to push the envelope on probabilistic methods and applications. For example, methodological enhancements are needed and are being planned for implementation to handle the dynamic nature of space flights in risk assessment of space missions.

In general, the technical and programmatic risk assessments conducted within NASA would meet the five aspiration goals as described in Section III of the proposed Bulletin (Problem Formulation; Completeness; Effort Expended; Resources Expended; and Peer Review and Public Participation). The significant exception in most cases would involve public participation that would normally not be required in the same sense as a regulatory process affecting the livelihood of the private sector would be.

In the case of environmental compliance and remediation, NASA responds to regulating the agency's requirements in the development of risk assessments for site-specific environmental remediation. These risk assessments reflect the direction, requirements, and processes required by the regulating agency.

Question 7: In your agency, is there currently a clear demarcation between "influential risk assessment" used for regulatory purposes and other risk assessments used for regulatory purposes? Is this clear at the outset of the risk assessment?

NASA Response

This question is not applicable to NASA because technical and programmatic risk assessments performed within NASA are not used for any regulatory purposes. If a regulating agency asks NASA to perform a risk assessment, NASA will perform the assessment in compliance with the technical procedures of the regulating agency.

Questions about impact of the Bulletin on agency risk assessment practices

Question 8: If applicable, please specify provisions in the Bulletin that can be expected to have a substantial positive effect on the quality, conduct, and use of risk assessments undertaken by your agency.

NASA Response

By and large, risk assessments to examine technical risk within NASA meet the provisions that are cited within the Bulletin. The largest benefit to NASA with respect to the performance of risk assessment in the technical arena would be the added emphasis that a higher level external (OMB) requirement provides. Implementation of risk assessment, particularly probabilistic risk assessment, to analyze technical risks is a relatively new activity. If the OMB requirements were to apply to NASA, being able to cite an external requirement reinforces the existing risk assessment requirements established within NASA.

Question 9: If applicable, please specify provisions in the Bulletin that can be expected to have a substantial negative effect on the quality, conduct, and use of risk assessments undertaken by your agency.

NASA Response

The largest potentially detrimental aspect of this Bulletin upon NASA relates to the scope of the Bulletin. The Bulletin indicates that the scope of the document covers risk assessments disseminated by Federal agencies (See "The Requirements of This Bulletin", page 8). This wording infers that the requirements of the Bulletin apply to risk assessments that are prepared specifically for or are likely to be provided external to the agency. This wording is consistent with the significant emphasis that the Bulletin places on use of risk assessments to support definition and implementation of regulations. Later in the definitions section of the Bulletin, however, the scope is significantly broadened when the Bulletin indicates that these rules would apply to any risk assessment document that is made available to the public by the agency or that is subject to release under the Freedom of Information Act. If the Bulletin applies to any internal risk assessment performed within NASA that is releasable under the Freedom of Information Act, there could be a substantial burden to meet all of the requirements contained within the Bulletin. Two examples bear notation.

Within NASA technical areas, many of the benefits of performing risk assessments do not lie in the completion and release of a formal risk assessment report but are realized by performing the risk assessment process among the participants in the design process. The Bulletin indicates that one of its goals is to have the risk assessors engage in an iterative dialogue with the decision makers who will use the assessment. The inference in this text is that the decision maker receives a report at the end of the risk assessment process and then makes a decision[7]. In the use of risk assessment within NASA, it is often the "give and take" with the participants in the risk assessment process that causes design and operational changes to be made to control risks, often at engineering levels lower than that of the ultimate decision maker. Emphasis on delivery of a report rather than the beneficial effects through pursuing the discipline of the process can have a negative effect on the ultimate impact of the risk assessment.

---

[7]Risk assessments related to the launch of nuclear or radioactive materials are conducted in this manner; however, other technical risk assessments within NASA are not of this nature.

A second example has to do with internal controls as defined in OMB Circular A-123, Management's Responsibility for Internal Control. This OMB Circular requires management to perform risk assessments to identify internal and external risks that may prevent the organization from meeting its objectives. The results of those risk assessments then are to be used to identify control activities that can be implemented to ensure agency objectives are met. The OMB Bulletin indicates that influential risk assessments are those that the agency reasonably can determine will have a clear impact on private sector decisions. In NASA, where the majority of the budget is applied to contracted activity, most of our internal controls have no direct application to the private sector; however, they do influence private sector activities. If the special standards for Influential Risk Assessments were applied to every risk assessment performed to determine if an internal policy or directive was required, this could impact the time to develop, implement, and modify the internal controls. Given the emphasis that the Bulletin places on regulatory matters and public use of the risk assessments, it is not clear that risk assessments performed for internal purposes need to have this level of requirement placed upon them.

Question 10: If your agency followed the procedures described in the Bulletin, would it affect the time course for production of the risk assessment (that is, the time required from initiation of the risk assessment to delivery to the regulatory decision maker)? If so, please explain why?

NASA Response

NASA does not provide its programmatic or technical risk assessments to regulatory decision makers so there would be no impact in that area; however, it should be noted that even with the internal risk assessments that are performed to assess technical risk the final delivered report may not be the most important aspect of the risk assessment. NASA accrues much of the benefit from performing its technical risk assessment because of the iterative work performed by the risk assessors in conjunction with the engineers, logisticians, and analysts during the design process. Risks identified during the process are often resolved well before a final report is completed.

As stated earlier, in the case of environmental, safety and health risk assessments, NASA's conduct of site-specific risk assessments reflects the direction and requirements of the regulating agency. NASA must comply with the requirements imposed by the regulating agency and would be subject to any schedule changes or other impacts generated by the regulatory agency's conformance with the Bulletin.

Question 11: One of the Bulletins's reporting standards states the need to be scientifically objective by "giving weight to both positive and negative studies in light of each study's technical quality." Please give an example of how this would be implemented by your agency or department.

NASA Response

NASA is adopting a risk-informed decision-making process which is supported by two major activities: (1) risk assessment and (2) deliberation. NASA considers the deliberation activity as a crucial part of the decision-making process since it evaluates risk assessment results and scrutinize the results to ensure that they are meaningful and the risk models used as the basis of the results are technically sound and traceable [8]. The deliberation activity involves all affected stakeholders that may include, as appropriate, program/project manager, astronauts, NASA workforce, engineering organizations, and safety and mission assurance organizations[8]. Typically these deliberations take place in several forms depending on the context and the nature of decision situation. For example, deliberations can take place as part of the risk assessment peer review activities [9, 10] or as part of the design review or flight readiness review activities [11].

Question 12: Does your agency use risk assessments conducted by external groups? Would it be helpful to you if risk assessments submitted to your agency by external groups, such as consultants and private industry, met the requirements proposed in the OMB Bulletin?

NASA Response

Large-scale risk assessment projects within NASA are often conducted jointly by several groups that include both NASA civil service and contractor analysts. The involvement of contractors in the conduct of risk assessments is necessary because NASA contracts out the majority of its mission execution activities to aerospace sector companies. The domain and discipline knowledge of the external groups who are involved in the development and operation of various aspects of NASA's mission is needed in order to develop realistic risk models. Because of the multi-group and multi-discipline nature of risk assessments and to ensure technical quality and consistency, NASA has developed risk assessment requirements and procedures (*e.g.*, the PRA Procedures Guide) that must be met by all parties involved (internal and external) in the conduct of NASA's risk assessments. NASA's internal use of risk assessments is primarily for non-regulatory purposes and often requires significant innovation in application; therefore, the OMB Bulletin would be of limited help in conducting our risk assessments.

REFERENCES

[1] Space Shuttle Probabilistic Risk Assessment, Volume II, Rev. 1: Model Integration Report, Johnson Space Flight Center, January 2005.

[2] Probabilistic Risk Assessment of the International Space Station: Phase II – Stage 7A Configuration, Volume II – Data Package, Futron Corporation, 2000.

[3] NASA's Exploration Systems Architecture Study, NASA-TM-2005-214062, November 2005.

[4] NASA Smart Buyer Study, 2004

[5] Pluto/New Horizons Interagency Nuclear Safety Review Panel Safety Evaluation Report of August 2005.

---

[8]The safety and mission assurance organizations are independent from the program/project management organizations and provide independent perspective on risk-related issues that affect safety and mission success.

[6] NASA NPR 7120.5C "NASA Program and Project Management Processes and Requirements," March 2005

[7] NASA NPR 8000.4, "Risk Management Procedural Requirements," April 2002.

[8] NASA NPR 8715.3: Chapter 2 (system Safety) of NASA General Safety Program Requirements (updated version pending release)

[9] Final Report of the Independent Peer Review Panel on the Probabilistic Risk Assessment of the Space Shuttle, Prepared for NASA Headquarters Office of Safety and Mission Assurance, April 4, 2005.

[10] Report of the Independent Peer Review Panel on the Probabilistic Risk Assessment of the International Space Station Phase II – Stage 7A Configuration, Prepared for NASA Headquarters Office of Safety and Mission Assurance, June 2002.

[11] Space Shuttle Flight Readiness Review.

EXECUTIVE OFFICE OF THE PRESIDENT
OFFICE OF MANAGEMENT AND BUDGET
WASHINGTON, D.C. 20503

AUG - 3 2006

Dr. Ellen Mantus
Project Director
National Research Council
Division on Earth and Life Sciences
Board on Environmental Studies and Toxicology
500 Fifth Street, NW
Washington, DC 20001

Dear Dr. Mantus:

Enclosed with this letter are the Office of Management and Budget's (OMB's) responses to questions that the National Academies of Sciences (NAS) submitted to OMB on June 28, 2006. We hope these responses will be helpful to the National Research Council Committee as it reviews the OMB Proposed Risk Assessment Bulletin (Proposed Bulletin).

Additionally, your request to OMB asked for "copies of all comments that are submitted by federal agencies on the OMB Bulletin, if possible." At this point in time, OMB has not received any official comment letters on the Proposed Bulletin from Federal agencies that conduct risk assessments. However, staff of one agency did send us comments marked "internal deliberative." Additionally, we have received a comment letter from the Small Business Administration's (SBA's) Office of Advocacy, which is available on that office's website at http://www.sba.gov/advo/laws/comments/omb06_0608.html.

If you should need further information from OMB, please contact Dr. Nancy Beck at 202-395-3258.

Sincerely,

Steven D. Aitken
Acting Administrator
Office of Information
and Regulatory Affairs

Enclosure

OMB-1

1. Dr. Graham discussed the recent perchlorate evaluation as an example that would have benefited from this Bulletin. Does the Bulletin support using a "precursor" of an adverse effect or other mechanistic data as the basis of a risk assessment, as was recommended in the National Academies' perchlorate review?

OMB response:

While the Proposed Risk Assessment Bulletin (Proposed Bulletin) does not speak to specific use of a precursor effect, there is no language in the Proposed Bulletin that precludes the use of a "precursor" of an adverse effect or other mechanistic data as the basis of a risk assessment.

Further, Section V, subsection 7 (page 20) of the preamble of the Proposed Bulletin discusses the standard for characterizing human health effects: "[I]t may be necessary for risk assessment reports to distinguish effects which are adverse from those which are non-adverse." Additionally, Section V, subsection 7 (page 25) of the text of the Proposed Bulletin notes the importance of describing the ramifications of the choice of effect: "Where human health effects are a concern, determinations of which effects are adverse shall be specifically identified and justified based on the best available scientific information generally accepted in the relevant clinical and toxicological communities."

2. Is it correct that those submitting data and risk assessments to the government to obtain product registrations, approvals, and licenses are excluded from the requirements of the Bulletin?

OMB response:

The Proposed Bulletin does not apply to risk assessments performed with respect to individual agency adjudication or permit proceedings (including a registration, approval or licensing) unless the agency determines that: (i) compliance is practical and appropriate and (ii) the risk assessment is scientifically or technically novel or likely to have precedent-setting influence on future adjudications and/or permit proceedings. (Proposed Bulletin, Section II, subsection 2(b), page 23). This exemption applies regardless of who generated the data and the risk assessment.

The OMB Information Quality Guidelines (67 FR 8460 Feb 22, 2002) do not cover adjudicative processes. The OMB Final Information Quality Bulletin for Peer Review (70 FR 2677 Jan 14, 2005) (Peer Review Bulletin) also includes an exemption for "individual agency adjudication or permit proceedings (including a registration, approval, licensing, site-specific determination), unless the agency determines that peer review is practical and appropriate and that the influential dissemination is scientifically or technically novel or likely to have precedent-setting influence on future adjudications and/or permit proceedings." The exemption used in the Proposed Bulletin is consistent with the exemption in the Peer Review Bulletin.

3. Will the Bulletin require further review by OMB staff of risk assessments that have been peer reviewed in accordance with established peer review procedures and standards, including publication in a reputable peer reviewed journal?

OMB response:

The Proposed Bulletin does not require OMB review of any risk assessment. However, under existing authorities and procedures, OMB might review a risk assessment. For example, risk assessments that are part of regulatory impact analyses might be reviewed under Executive Order 12866. Additionally, Section III, subsection 5 (page 23) states: "The agency shall follow appropriate procedures for peer review and public participation in the process of preparing the risk assessment." Agencies should rely on the Peer Review Bulletin to determine appropriate peer review procedures.

4. Public participants in the risk assessment and rulemaking processes – industry groups, environmental groups, other governmental entities, individual scientists – often provide risk assessments for agency consideration. Will these outside assessments be held to the same standards as agency-generated assessments, that is, to the requirements in the Bulletin?

OMB response:

The Proposed Bulletin applies to risk assessments that are made publicly available by an agency, regardless of whether the agency conducted the risk assessment. If third-party submissions are to be used and made publicly available by Federal agencies, it is the responsibility of the Federal Government to make sure that such information meets relevant standards.

5. The 1983 NRC report *Risk Assessment in the Federal Government: Managing the Process* treats "risk assessment" as a term of art that covers four distinct analyses (hazard identification, dose-response assessment, exposure analysis, and risk characterization), each typically based on a number of separate studies and analyses. The OMB Bulletin defines "risk assessment" to apply to "any document" that "could be used for risk assessment purposes, such as an exposure or hazard assessment *that might not constitute a complete risk assessment as defined by the National Research Council.*" What is the advantage of defining risk assessment in this way?

OMB response:

The Proposed Bulletin used a risk assessment definition that "applies to documents that could be used for risk assessment purposes, such as an exposure or hazard assessment that might not constitute a complete risk assessment..."(Proposed Bulletin, Section I, page 8). Many of these individual documents are relied upon by Federal agencies and used in important, and often economically significant, regulatory decisions made by Federal agencies as well as other decision makers. The accuracy, quality, clarity, transparency, and utility of these documents could be improved by meeting, as appropriate, the quality standards outlined in the Proposed Bulletin. As we stated in the OMB Press Release accompanying the Proposed Bulletin, "Transparent and accurate risk assessments are necessary for agencies and other decision makers to make wise risk management decisions during the formation of agency rules and policy decisions."

Additionally, if these individual documents are prepared in a manner consistent with the Proposed Bulletin, this may avoid additional work when these activities are combined to create a comprehensive risk assessment document at a later point in time.

6. The Bulletin discusses the importance of risk assessors interacting with decision-makers. What safeguards will be built into the process to protect the scientific process from being framed by the decision-maker instead of the science?

OMB response:

In Section III, subsection 1 (page 10) of the preamble, the Proposed Bulletin sets forth an aspirational goal of an iterative dialogue between risk assessors and agency decision maker(s). This type of dialogue "will help ensure that the risk assessment serves its intended purposes and is developed in a cost-effective manner." (Proposed Bulletin, Section III, subsection 1, page 10). The standards proposed in the Proposed Bulletin are designed to ensure the quality and objectivity of the scientific process and the science.